OCT Angiography

OCT Angiography

Sanja Sefić Kasumović MD PhD
Ophthalmologist and Head
Private Eye Polyclinic "Dr Sefić"
Sarajevo, Bosnia and Herzegovina

Foreword

Zoran Vatavuk PhD FEBO

JAYPEE The Health Sciences Publisher
New Delhi | London | Panama

Jaypee Brothers Medical Publishers (P) Ltd

Headquarters
Jaypee Brothers Medical Publishers (P) Ltd.
4838/24, Ansari Road, Daryaganj
New Delhi 110 002, India
Phone: +91-11-43574357
Fax: +91-11-43574314
E-mail: jaypee@jaypeebrothers.com

Overseas Offices
JP Medical Ltd.
83, Victoria Street, London
SW1H 0HW (UK)
Phone: +44-20 3170 8910
Fax: +44(0)20 3008 6180
E-mail: info@jpmedpub.com

Jaypee-Highlights Medical Publishers Inc.
City of Knowledge, Bld. 235, 2nd Floor, Clayton
Panama City, Panama
Phone: +1 507-301-0496
Fax: +1 507-301-0499
E-mail: cservice@jphmedical.com

Jaypee Brothers Medical Publishers (P) Ltd.
17/1-B, Babar Road, Block-B, Shyamoli
Mohammadpur, Dhaka-1207
Bangladesh
Mobile: +08801912003485
E-mail: jaypeedhaka@gmail.com

Jaypee Brothers Medical Publishers (P) Ltd.
Bhotahity, Kathmandu, Nepal
Phone: +977-9741283608
E-mail: kathmandu@jaypeebrothers.com

Website: www.jaypeebrothers.com
Website: www.jaypeedigital.com

Inquiries for bulk sales may be solicited at: jaypee@jaypeebrothers.com

OCT Angiography

First Edition: **2019**

ISBN: 978-93-5270-331-9

Printed at: Ajanta Offset & Packagings Ltd., Faridabad, Haryana.

Dedicated to

My parents

Džemila and Mustafa

for their continuous guidance, support and unconditional love throughout every step of my life.

Contributors

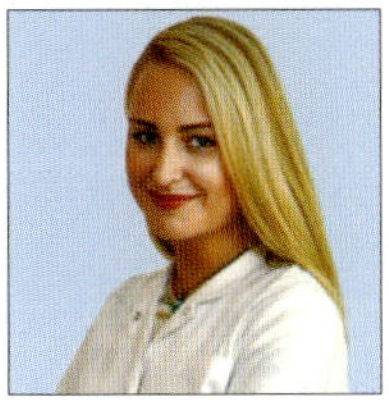

Aida Kasumović MD
Private Eye Polyclinic "Dr Sefić"
Sarajevo, Bosnia and Herzegovina

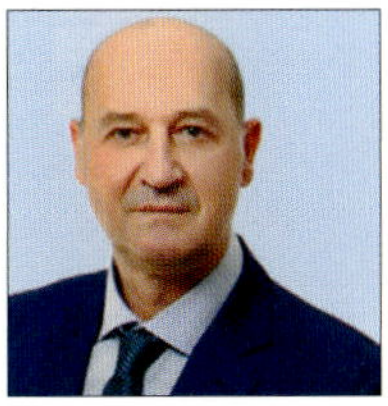

Emir Čabrić MD PhD
Assistant Professor
Medical Faculty
University of Zenica
Director and Head
Department for Ophthalmology
Polyclinic with a Day Care Hospital
Doboj-Jug, Bosnia and Herzegovina

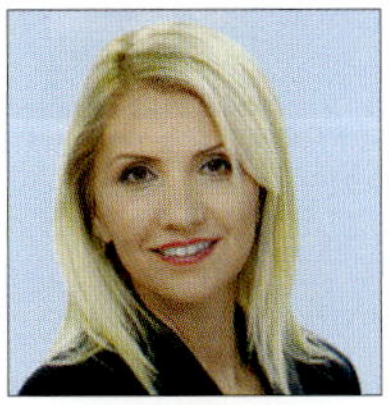

Maja Živković MD PhD
Assistant Professor
Medical Faculty
University of Nis
Eye Clinic, Clinical Center Nis
Nis, Serbia

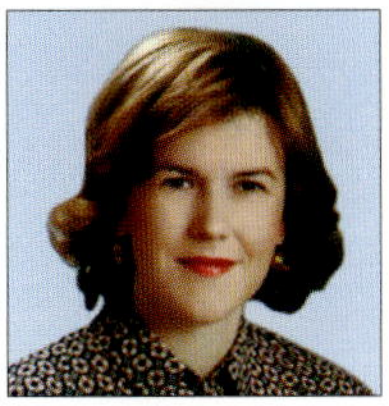

Lejla Muhamedagić MD MSc
The Public Institution Health Center
of Sarajevo Canton
Sarajevo, Bosnia and Herzegovina

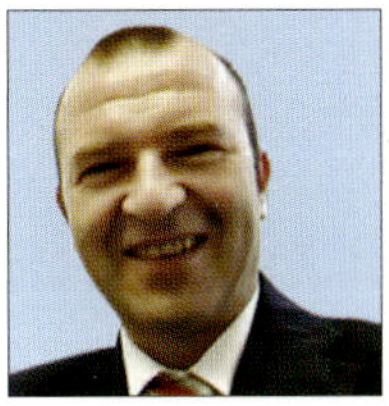

Orhan Lepara MD PhD
Assistant Professor
Faculty of Medicine
University of Sarajevo
Sarajevo, Bosnia and Herzegovina

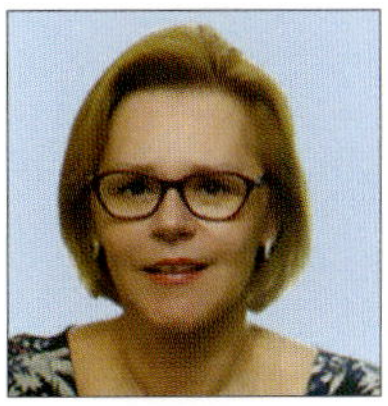

Nesina Avdagić MD PhD
Associate Professor
Faculty of Medicine
University of Sarajevo
Sarajevo, Bosnia and Herzegovina

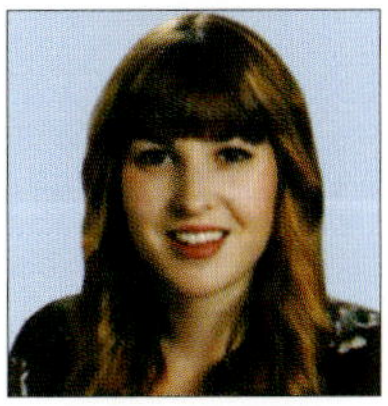

Tatjana Jevtić MD
Emergency Medical Assistance
Center of Sarajevo Canton
Sarajevo, Bosnia and Herzegovina

KLINIČKI BOLNIČK! CENTAR
SESTRE MILOSRDNICE
KLINIKA ZA OČNE BOLESTI
ZAGREB, Vinogradska cesta 29
Predstojnik: Prof.dr.sc. Zoran Vatavuk
Tel: ++ 385 I 37 87 354 Fax.: ++ 385 I 37 68 296

Zagreb, 10.11.2017

Foreword

The book *OCT Angiography* is a handwriting which presents a good example of establishing a correlation with world literature in the field of new, sophisticated ophthalmology diagnostics. It represents a concise and sufficiently detailed monography on the new OCTA diagnostic method in ophthalmology. It is very important to note that the author of the book used their own material with her own descriptions and comments on every single image included, which gives the material a great value and worthiness. Some of pathological cases are presented with ten to fifteen individual images and figures, aiming to help the reader properly read and analyse the patient from beginning to the end. Also, images are organized so the reader can easily compare and understand correlation between them. Documented findings give the physician a possibility of careful comparison with earlier findings of the classic OCT. The author of this work has very skillfully introduced a reader into anatomy, physiology and pathology of the most common diseases of the posterior ocular segment. The book gives also a very good overview of optic nerve pathology and OCTA findings. Monography *OCT Angiography* completes the requirements of educational literature from the domain of diagnostics the posterior eye segment and can serve ophthalmologists, residents of ophthalmology as well as medical students.

Klinički bolnički centar Sestre milosrdnice
Klinika za očne bolesti
ZAGREB
Vinogradska cesta 29
1

Zoran Vatavuk PhD FEBO

Preface

My fascination with the new medical diagnostic technologies started the moment I saw an OCT at Prof. Dr Agarwal's practice 10 years ago and has not passed ever since. That was the moment I entered this new, up to then undiscovered world of retinal analysis which gave me a vast number of possibilities in diagnosing retinal diseases. I was very content with OCT technology for a long period of time, until the analysis of retinal blood vessels became a necessary peace in my retinal story development.

My first encounter with angiography of retinal blood vessels done without a contrast was at a refractive and cataract surgery congress in London in 2014. This, I then realized, opened a door of possibilities such as seeing the changes unrecognizable by previous OCT technology I used. The possibility to look deeper behind the retinal pigment epithelium, finally, with this new technology, become my wish come true.

The vast possibilities such as analysis of blood flow, being able to compare the movement without any form of aggression to retinal layers, offered me the perfection I sought in diagnostics, making me a very happy ophthalmologist. The possibility of constant control, the discovery of changes I never previously thought existed; the continuous, almost daily controls of changes occurring after therapy had all become my everyday reality in my retina cabinet. With OCTA technology, through angioanalytics, I can qualify and quantify the changes occurring which enables me to act accordingly in terms of therapeutic approach.

This book is a story of retinal disease and glaucoma through the lens of OCT angiography. It takes the reader through step-by-step analytics of every single part of retina as well as every single visible flow.

Artefacts, which do hinder the quality of analysis, have been purposefully left visible. The special attention in the book has been given to angioanalytics, analysis of the dynamics of development and drying of new membranes.

Both, the beginners and the experienced ophthalmologists may benefit from the content of this book as it offers many aspects, from the basics to more complicated OCT angiography analytics. I have used my glaucoma knowledge to analyse OCT angiography in glaucoma itself by utilizing the known parameters in OCT analytics of the papilla and the papillary region.

Sanja Sefić Kasumović

Acknowledgments

I owe a very special gratitude to Prof. Dr Asim Kurjak, whose life's work guides me as a true example of professional ideal. He encourages me to have vision where only sky is the limit, who gave me that special piece of strength to persist in publishing the results of my work. His persistence, his vast life and professional experience provided me with the continuous inspiration and guidance in my everyday work. By following his advice, my confidence grew, making me a better, more caring person to my patients, my family, my colleagues and, most importantly, to my children. I hold high hopes to not disappoint this great man in my work and commitment to my patients.

I also owe a very special thanks to Prof. Dr Amar Agarwal and his wonderful spouse. My stay in India has made me, not just a better ophthalmologist but a better person through learning that being humble is the most important human virtue while kindness is the wealth that multiplies through sharing. It is difficult to quantify the gratitude I feel for all that they have taught me, not only about ophthalmology but about the life itself.

Last but not least, I cannot fail to mention my friend and colleague Prof. Vesna Jakšić who has selflessly shared with me her virtues of a good doctor and a good person. I thank her for her letters, the meaningful conversations and the kindness she readily shares with me. I sincerely hope we will get to work and write together, in good faith of our vocation and for the benefit of our patients for at least 100 years to come. Once more, very special thanks.

At the end, my greatest gratitude goes to my best friend, my partner through the journey of life, who has been my support through every single chapter of this book. Without him, not much of this world would make sense.

Contents

CHAPTER 1

Optical Coherence Tomography Angiography

INTRODUCTION

Optical coherence tomography angiography (OCT angiography, OCTA) is a new and noninvasive diagnostic tool in detecting changes in microvascular circulation. It is based on two innovative technologies such as *Split Spectrum Amplitude Decorrelation Angiography—SSADA algorithm* and *Motion Correction Technology—MCT protocol*. OptoVue Company introduced the first OCTA system, AngioVue, at XXXII Congress of European Society of Cataract and Refractive Surgeons (ESCRS) in London, 2014. This novel approach recognizes early retinal and macular disorders differently, and is becoming a part of the standard care in everyday clinical practice in ophthalmology.

OptoVue has developed a completely new and noninvasive approach in microvascular imaging and blood vessels visualization. They can be identified by detecting the movement of the red blood cells, erythrocytes, thus showing the blood flow in specific retinal layers. Microvascular changes can be visualized by using OCTA, a highly sophisticated device that can also visualize the presence of ocular blood flow in the vessels. It is not only modified and improved conventional structural OCT, but a device providing both structural and functional information and the precise location of pathological blood flow. OCTA shows potential efficacy in the evaluation of common disorders involving retinal neovascularization. The system is fundamentally different in comparison to the conventional and well-known fluorescein angiography, since it portrays red blood cells movement, its focus is not on detecting the walls of blood vessels, but on detecting the blood flow. It does not require contrast dye injection, so it is completely noninvasive.

The AngioVue Imaging System acquires different scan sizes with each volume scan acquired in less than 3 seconds. Two imaging volumes are obtained consecutively to perform motion correction later in order to remove the saccadic artifacts.

Segmentation of retinal layers is automatically produced in order to recognize the vascular layers of interest. It is helpful in detecting pathological changes at different depth. In comparison to well-known traditional angiography techniques, AngioVue imaging protocol allows visualization of microvasculature within specific retinal layers without the blurring effects of staining. It provides high-resolution imaging and better penetration. The result is the image that could be segmented and isolated by using the AngioAnalytic software. It provides information that helps to better understand images of inner vascular and outer avascular retinal layers. This imaging system produces images of retinal and choroidal microvasculature and determines early from which layer pathology originates, making it possible to establish retinal changes diagnosis at early stages.

The OCTA shows structural and functional changes in the retinal vascular network in vivo without administration of contrast dye. The result is a precise image of the blood flow in the selected area. It is very important to point out that all pieces of information obtained by OCTA are completely different from those acquired by fluorescein angiography (FA). AngioVue system is capable of detecting blood flow without showing blood vessels walls, by mapping erythrocyte movement. AngioFlow imaging is very fast and does not require pupil dilation. The entire recording process takes only a few minutes. This technique is a noncontact diagnostic procedure. The capillary abnormalities are easily seen. No leakage, staining or pooling is present, and the image may seem 'too sharp' or 'too dry'. OptoVue Avanti high-speed SD-OCT imaging system is a foundation to build the AngioVue imaging system.

The OCTA shows the vascular flow of the retina at three scan sizes: 3 × 3 mm, 6 × 6 mm, and 8 × 8 mm. At 3 × 3 mm and 6 × 6 mm scan sizes, the vessel imaging is clear. For a more detailed analysis, the 3 × 3 mm scans are recommended. The images of OCT angiography with 8 × 8 mm scan are recommended for performing large area scans of the retina giving more of an overview of selected retinal area.

Split Spectrum Amplitude Decorrelation Angiography—SSADA algorithm is developed by David Huang, Center for Ophthalmic Optics and Lasers, Portland, Oregon. The algorithm uses consecutive OCT scans and compares each OCT scan with the subsequent one. The SSADA algorithm uses multiple spectra from single B-scan to improve image quality. Thus, the number of repeated B-scans required for high-quality imaging is reduced. By observing the changes in the pixel intensity at a selected area, a decorrelation value could be generated which means that the marker shows whether there is blood motion or not. It means that the image could present either a highly intensive activity of the blood flow or the regions without any movement and capillary vitality. The SSADA algorithm then generates a flow image, or a functional image of this B-scan. Taking a large number of B-scans make it possible to generate a 3D map of retinal vasculature on the AngioVue system.

Motion Correction Technology *(DualTruc Motion Correction Technology)* is one of many protocols which distinguishes AngioVue system from all the others. MCT was invented by James Fujimoto. MCT provides high-quality imaging through two levels of motion improvement by video tracking (transversal correction) and longitudinal correction after the imaging process. The first level of this powerful MCT algorithm is based on a real-time correction for saccades, blinking or eye drifting; the second level occurs during postprocessing of imaging and corrects smaller levels of motion distortion (<100 μm). Second, two-level approach reduces motion artifact and optimizes the imaging signal.

The SSADA algorithm offers the best quality OCT angiography images. This technology achieves higher signal-to-noise ratio and better and more detailed visualization of the vasculature.

ANATOMIC STRUCTURE OF THE HEALTHY RETINA

Optical coherence tomography image processing of a healthy retina provides the following retinal 'slabs': The inner limiting membrane (ILM), outer boundary of the inner plexiform layer (IPL), the outer boundary of the outer plexiform layer (OPL), and Bruch's membrane (BM) (Fig. 1.1).

The internal limiting membrane presents basal membrane created by *Müller cells (MC)*. The retinal nerve fiber layers (RNFL) are axons of the cells forming the optic nerve. The IPL consists of connections between the axons of bipolar cells and dendrites of ganglion and amacrine cells. The inner nuclear layer (INL) consists of the nuclei of the amacrine cells, bipolar and horizontal cells. The outer nuclear layer (ONL) contains the nuclei of the photoreceptor cells, the synapses between the rod, and cone cells from one side and the bipolar cells from the other side. The ONL consists of the bodies and nuclei of photoreceptor cells. The outer limiting membrane (OLM) separates the inner segments from the photoreceptors nuclei. The photoreceptor layer contains the outer and inner segments of rods and cones. The retinal pigment epithelium (RPE) layer consists of a single layer of cuboid situated under the photoreceptors cells closely interacting with them (Figs. 1.2 and 1.3).

The retina is composed of three vascular networks, one superficial and two deep ones. OCTA system cannot separately visualize two deep layers, so they appear as a uniform layer. Thus, OCTA angiography shows two retinal layers, the superficial and deep retinal networks. The superficial vascular network is located in the ganglion cells layer and the RNFL. The resolution of OCTA SSADA protocol recognizes the superficial vascular network 60 μm below the ILM. The deep vascular network is localized between the INL and the OPL. The protocol recognizes deep vascular layer 30 μm from the internal plexiform layer.

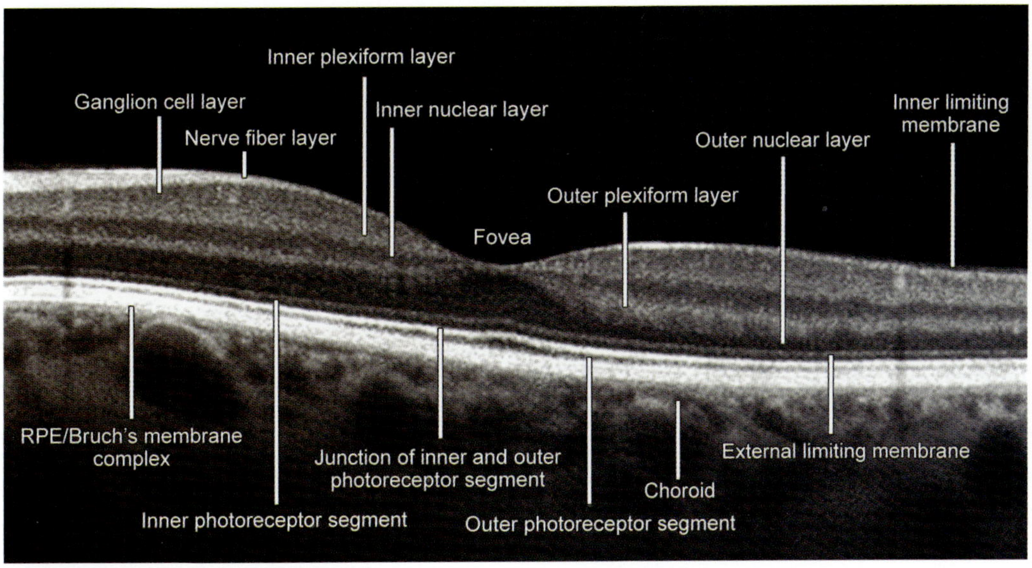

Fig. 1.1: Optical coherence tomography (OCT) B-scan. The image of macula with all anatomic structural layers (slabs) whose understanding and recognition is crucial for proper interpretation of OCT and OCT angiography image. (RPE: retinal pigment epithelium)

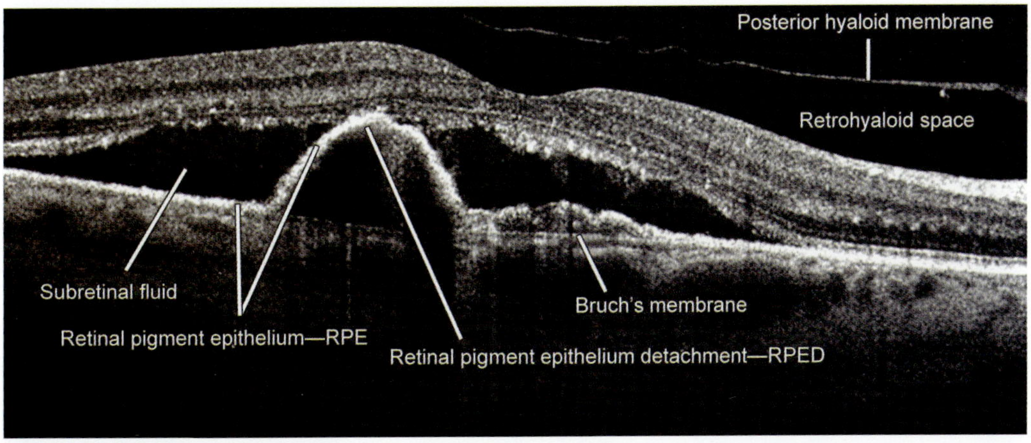

Fig. 1.2: Presentation of pathological changes which could be seen and visualized by the optical coherence tomography. Subretinal fluid, retinal pigment epithelium detachment, and the detachment of the posterior hyaloid membrane can clearly be seen. (RPE: retinal pigment epithelium; RPED: retinal pigment epithelium detachment)

The superficial vascular network is composed of many dense, linearly arranged capillaries radiating towards the fovea, forming the superior and inferior capillary arcades. The capillaries are arranged and interconnected in a way that forms a fine, regular lacy-shaped or spider-web-shaped network around the central oval foveal avascular zone *(FAZ)*. The thickness of the blood vessels is homogenous, without dilated capillaries, capillary loops or meanders. The OCTA image shows blood vessels as white, thread-like structures forming a symmetrical network against a dark background.

Deep vascular network of the inner retina consists of densely distributed, tiny, heavily branched capillaries, connected with superficial layer by anastomotic capillaries. The deep vascular network is denser and rougher than the superficial vascular network. They both form a pattern around the FAZ (Figs. 1.4A and B). The thickness of blood vessels is also the same between the two networks which are connected by small slanted interconnection anastomoses.

These two vascular networks are at the inner vascular retinal level (Figs. 1.5 and 1.6).

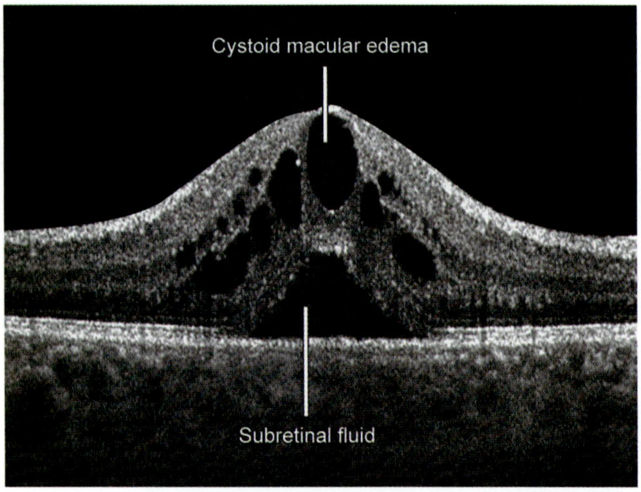

Fig. 1.3: Pathological changes seen by the optical coherence tomography. The image shows the cystoid macular edema and subretinal fluid.

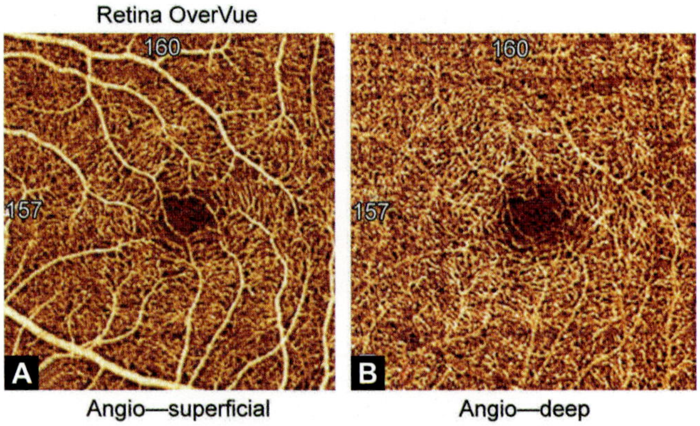

Figs. 1.4A and B: Optical coherence tomography angiography image of the superficial and deep vascular network of a normal and healthy eye (3 × 3 mm). Spider-web-shaped capillaries form a network around the central foveal avascular zone (FAZ).

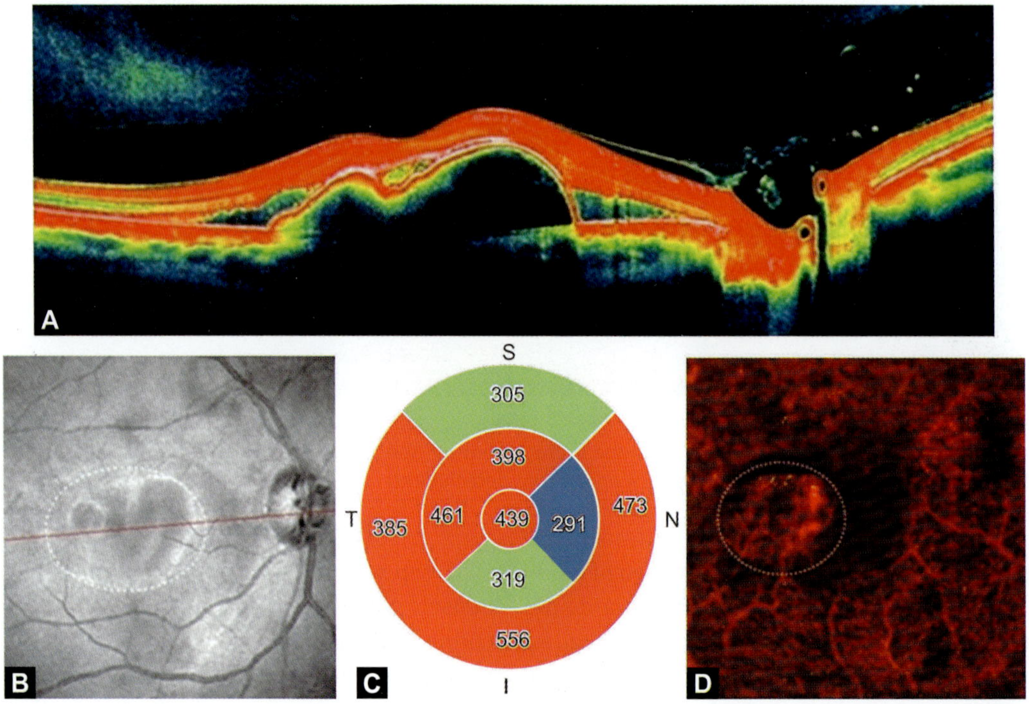

Figs. 1.5A to D: Accurate interpretation of optical coherence tomography (OCT) and OCT angiography (OCTA) images always requires comparison of simultaneous imaging obtained by (A) OCT B-scan, (B) en face OCT, (C) retinal thickness map, and (D) OCTA *split spectrum amplitude decorrelation angiography* algorithm. It is of crucial importance to find out structural and functional information in tandem. (A) A large area of retinal pigment epithelial detachment (*PED*), subretinal fluid, and the detachment of enlarged and thickened posterior hyaloid membrane can be seen in figure. Figure B explains a big hyporeflective zone which corresponds to the PED area. (C) emphasizes the importance of retinal thickness map imaging by showing an increased retinal thickness. Central macular edema (439 µm) and area of paramacular edema are associated with the presence of subretinal fluid. (D) demonstrates the presence of the neovascular membrane in the macular center.

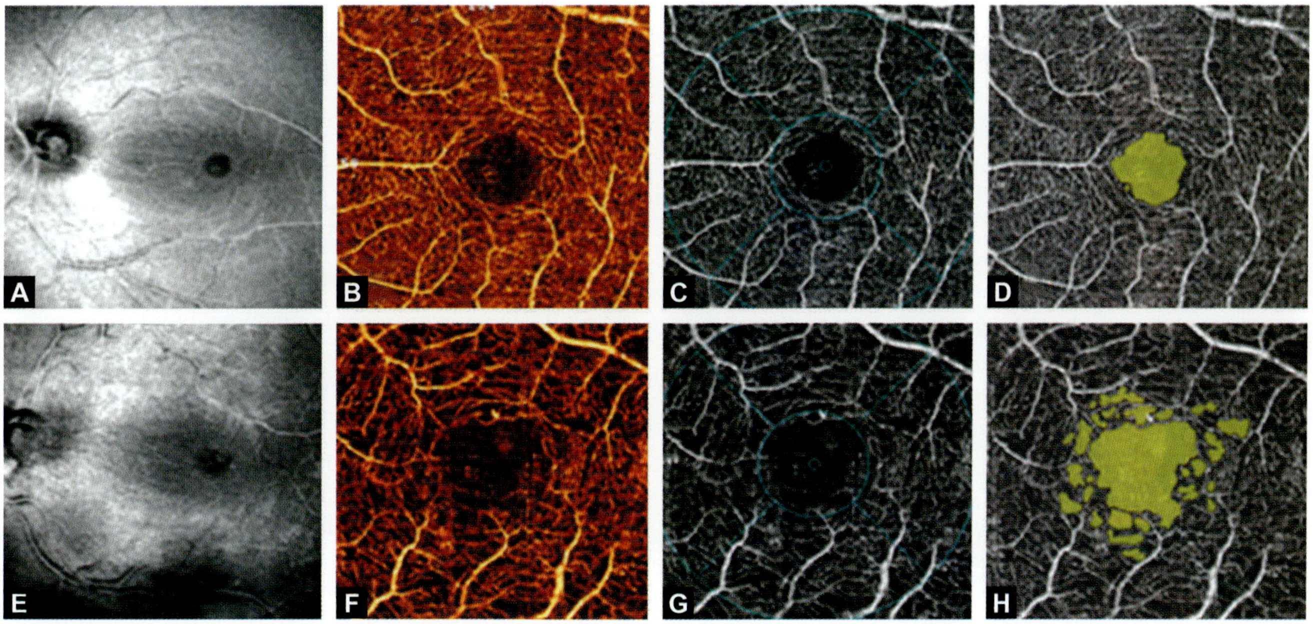

Figs. 1.6A to H: Besides en face optical coherence tomography (OCT) and OCT angiography (OCTA), detailed diagnostic procedure of the eyes requires AngioAnalytics assessment of the FAZ and the detection on nonflow areas in selected region. (A to D) The images of a healthy eye. (A) En face OCT shows a healthy and regular macula and the optic disk with normal flow and normal big blood vessels. (B) The superficial vascular network demonstrates regular structure and appearance on en face angiogram. (C) The en face image of foveal and parafoveal areas. (D) AngioAnalytics shows the FAZ (yellow color) corresponding to the central nonflow region. There are no vascular activities. The foveal avascular zone (FAZ) is regular in size and shape. The parafoveal avascular zones (dropout zones) are not visualized. (E to H). The OCTA images of an eye with nonproliferative diabetic retinopathy. (E) En face OCT shows no evident pathological events. (F) The superficial vascular network displays enlarged and irregular size and shape of the FAZ and enlargement of parafoveal intercapillary areas which are known as 'dropout zones'. (G) En face OCT angiography of foveal and parafoveal area. The FAZ is significantly enlarged in comparison to the healthy eye. (H) AngioAnalytics shows irregular outline of the FAZ, as well as numerous parafoveal areas of capillary dropout. The changes are typical and pathognomonic for nonproliferative diabetic retinopathy.

OPTICAL COHERENCE TOMOGRAPHY ANGIOGRAPHY OF THE HEALTHY RETINA

The superficial inner retinal angiogram of the healthy retina, from the inner retina to the outer retina shows the avascular vitreous and no flow above the ILM, so the en face OCTA image appears black. There are large blood vessels in the superficial vascular plexus, while fine densely arranged capillary network is found in the deep plexus. There is no flow in the FAZ. The outer retina is avascular and OCTA imaging shows it as a dark avascular zone. But, we must be very careful in interpreting this image, since flow projection artifacts from the inner retina can be seen due to shadows cast by the blood flow. These artifacts must be suppressed by *post-processing* software. The choriocapillary layer shows confluent flow, so lobular structure of the choriocapillaris is difficult to recognize because it is densely packed within the macula. The rougher lobules outside the macula would be recognized more easily. The angiogram of deep choroid shows large blood vessels, but this layer is still more difficult to interpret due to flow projection, shadowing, and villous artifacts. Therefore, a part of inner, large choroidal vessels appears as a dark region on both en face OCT angiography and structural OCT. FAZ cannot be visualized in the outer retinal layer nor in choriocapillaris.

In order to detect and analyze standard retinal pathology more efficiently and simply, it is very important to understand the automated segmentation algorithm and layer boundaries within AngioVue imaging system. The automated segmented reference planes could be manually corrected and adjusted depending on imaging requirements. With these options it is possible to clearly define the exact location of pathological processes, their size, and progression within retinal layers. The artifacts and errors could be suppressed and provide clear visualization of vascularization at a specific depth.

AngioVue protocol recognizes:

- *Superficial vascular plexus*: 3 µm below the internal limiting membrane *(inner limiting membrane)* and 15 µm below the internal plexiform layer *(inner plexiform layer)* (Figs. 1.7A and B)
- *Deep vascular plexus*: From 15 µm to 70 µm below the IPL
- *Outer retina*: 70 µm below the IPL to 30 µm below the RPE (Figs. 1.8A and B)
- *Choroidal layer*: It is located from 30 µm to 60 µm below the RPE.

Do not forget to consider the age of the patient. Changes in normal structure and function of the retina are evident during aging. It is very important to compare the right eye to the left eye. The comparison always gives a lot of information to get the final decision on whether the changes are normal and expected or pathological.

OCTA OF A HEALTHY EYE IN A 24-YEAR-OLD PATIENT

Figures 1.9A to D show the OCTA of a healthy eye in a 24-year-old patient.

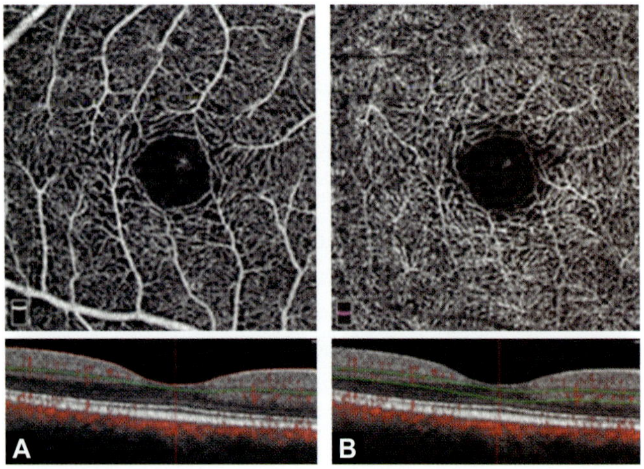

Figs. 1.7A and B: (A) Optical coherence tomography angiography (OCTA) of the superficial vascular plexus (3 × 3 mm). White, thread-like structures against a dark background present the blood flow. Centripetal confluence of the capillaries that form a spider-net symmetric network around the central round avascular zone [foveal avascular zone (FAZ)] can be seen. OCT B-scan marks a layer within the inner retina (between the red and green line), which corresponds to the location of the superficial vascular plexus. B-scan allows depth control of the vascular plexus. (B) OCTA of the deep vascular plexus (3 × 3 mm). A deeper network consists of smaller and less filamentous, tangled capillaries around the FAZ. B-scan shows the point of retinal depth (between two green lines) where deep vascular network spreads.

OCTA OF A HEALTHY EYE IN AN 82-YEAR-OLD PATIENT

Figures 1.10A to D show the OCTA of a healthy eye in an 82-year-old patient.

ANALYSIS OF CAPILLARY LAYERS USING OCTA ANGIOANALYTICS

The OCTA is an irreplaceable diagnostic tool in everyday clinical practice for vascular plexuses visualization and detection of blood vessel flow changes. AngioAnalytics software has recently been developed and approved. It enables additional quantitative evaluation of retinal vascular abnormalities. The data can be saved for comparison and subsequent analysis. AngioAnalytics provides measurements and analysis of the flow areas and the nonflow areas, it generates capillary density map and quantifies the size and appearance of the FAZ.

Flow Area

Flow area measurement is useful in monitoring the development of the neovascular membrane and in patients

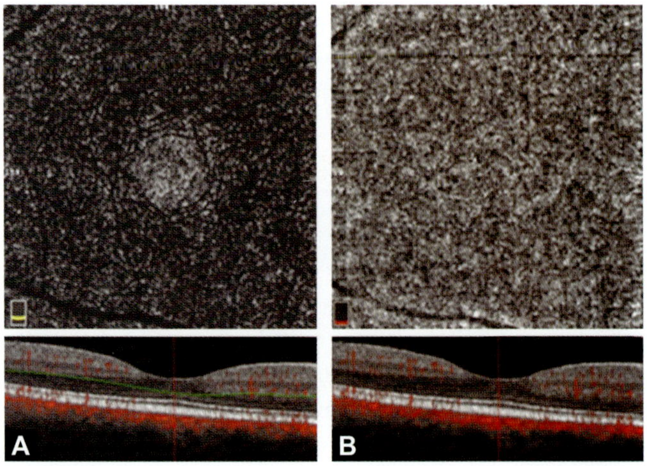

Figs. 1.8A and B: (A) Optical coherence tomography angiography (OCTA) of the outer retina (3 × 3 mm). A dark, avascular zone of the outer retina is shown. The hyperreflective areas present the artifacts caused by flow projection from the inner retinal blood vessels toward the retinal pigment epithelium. The analysis of this layer requires caution since the flow projection artifacts caused by flickering shadows may mimic the presence of capillaries or neovascularizations in the avascular layer. OCT B-scan shows retinal depth that corresponds to outer retina. (B) OCTA of the choriocapillary layer (3 × 3 mm). The flow is presented as a rough lobular structure where capillaries are densely packed.

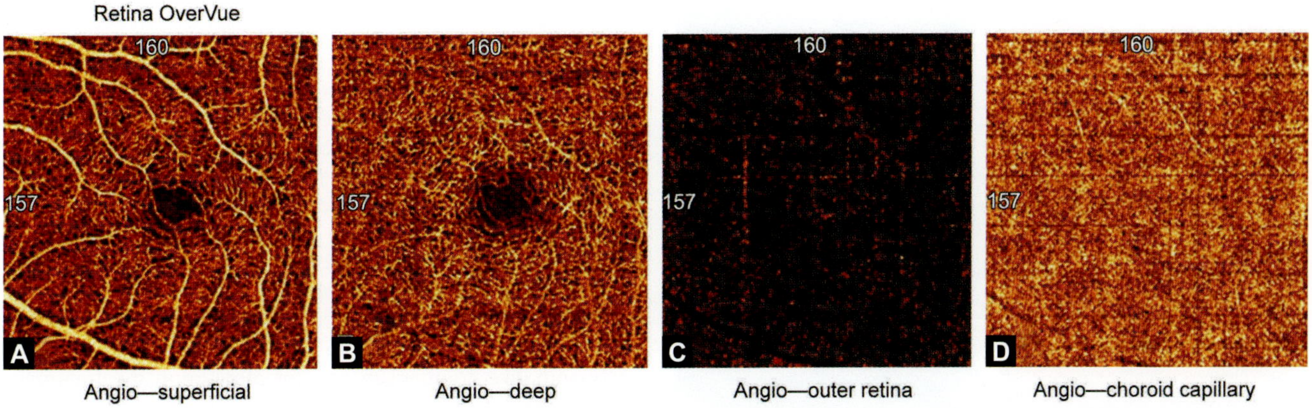

Figs. 1.9A to D: Optical coherence tomography angiography split spectrum amplitude decorrelation angiography protocol of a healthy eye (3 × 3 mm). Illustrations of the (A) superficial capillary plexus, (B) deep capillary plexus, (C) outer retina, and (D) choriocapillary layer. Inner retinal layers show normal vascular texture and normal size of the foveal avascular zone (approximately 0.4 mm in diameter). Avascular zone of the outer retina is dark with minimal visualization of flow projection artifacts. The choriocapillaris vasculature is lobular and dense.

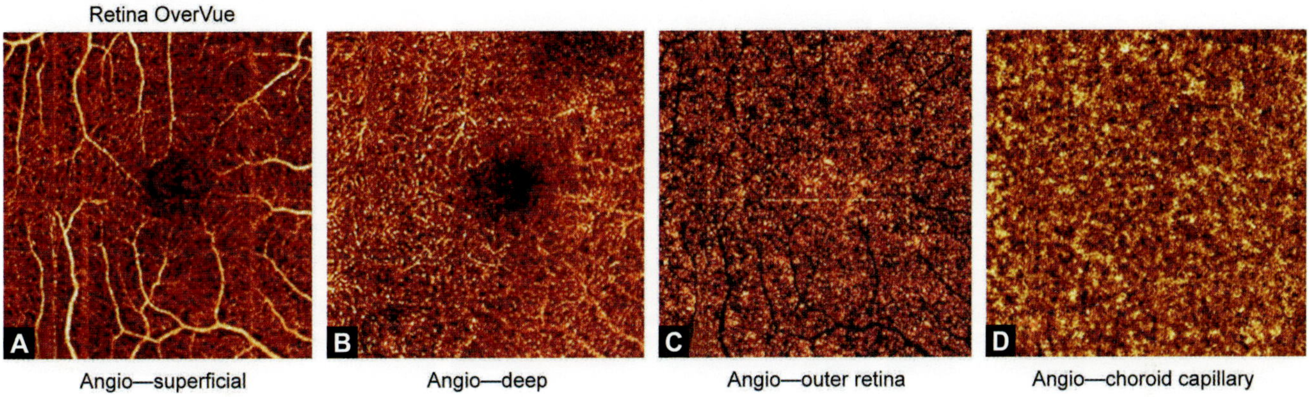

Figs. 1.10A to D: Optical coherence tomography angiography split spectrum amplitude decorrelation angiography protocol of a healthy eye in 82-year-old man (3 × 3 mm). (A) superficial vascular capillary plexus, (B) deep vascular capillary plexus, (C) outer retinal layer, and (D) the choriocapillaris layer are illustrated. Inner retinal layer shows normal vascular network and normal foveal avascular zone considering patient's age. In comparison to Figure 1.9, sclerotic changes of blood vessels and capillaries and their sparse appearance in two vascular plexuses can be visualized. Outer retinal avascular zone shows more intensive flow projection artifacts in comparison to the same zone in a young adult person. The choriocapillaris shows rough and lobular vascularization.

treated with anti-vascular endothelial growth factor (VEGF) therapy and steroids. Unlike the well-known fluorescein where pooling or leakage of the contrast dye masks the capillary network morphology, OCT angiography is dye-free, and allows clear visualization of the flow within retinal vessels in the selected segments. The operator should clearly draw the boundaries of the analyzed segment that is automatically identified by the software and the flow of the selected region is calculated. All the data are stored for comparison and analysis (Figs. 1.11A and B).

Nonflow Area or Vascular Dropout Area

Nonflow areas are regions with vascular damage, ischemia, or vascular dropout. Precise measurements, marking, and region comparison offer new possibilities in monitoring ischemic retinopathies with different etiology. SSADA protocol shows regions with nondetectable separate flow in the superficial and deep vascular plexus. The operator may choose the region of interest and manually color suspicious areas which are automatically colored in yellow by

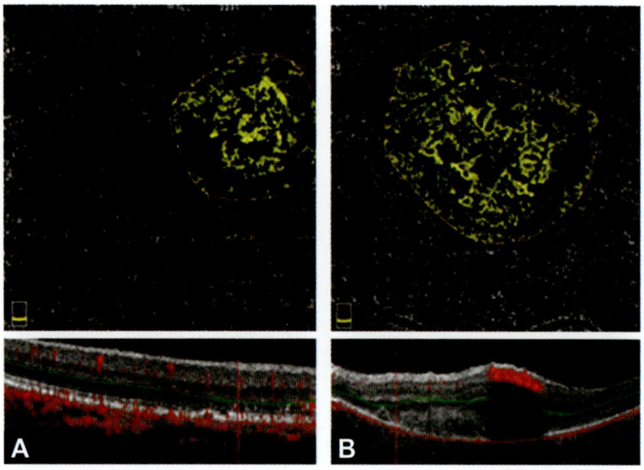

Figs. 1.11A and B: Optical coherence tomography (OCT) angiography AngioAnalytics of the flow in the outer retina in two examples with choroidal neovascularization (CNV). By choosing the specific area of interest, the software analyses of blood vessels shows regions with flow using the yellow color, while avascular regions remain dark. (A) Type 2 CNV in a ball-of-wool-shaped pattern and a surrounding halo. (B) Type 2 CNV, but with larger neovascularization which is coral-shaped. A dark halo can be observed around some parts of the neovascularization. The software displays numerical data about the flow in the selected region, important for quantitative comparison and for monitoring the treatment response. In the lower part of image, OCT B-scans are presented showing the depth of analyzed layers.

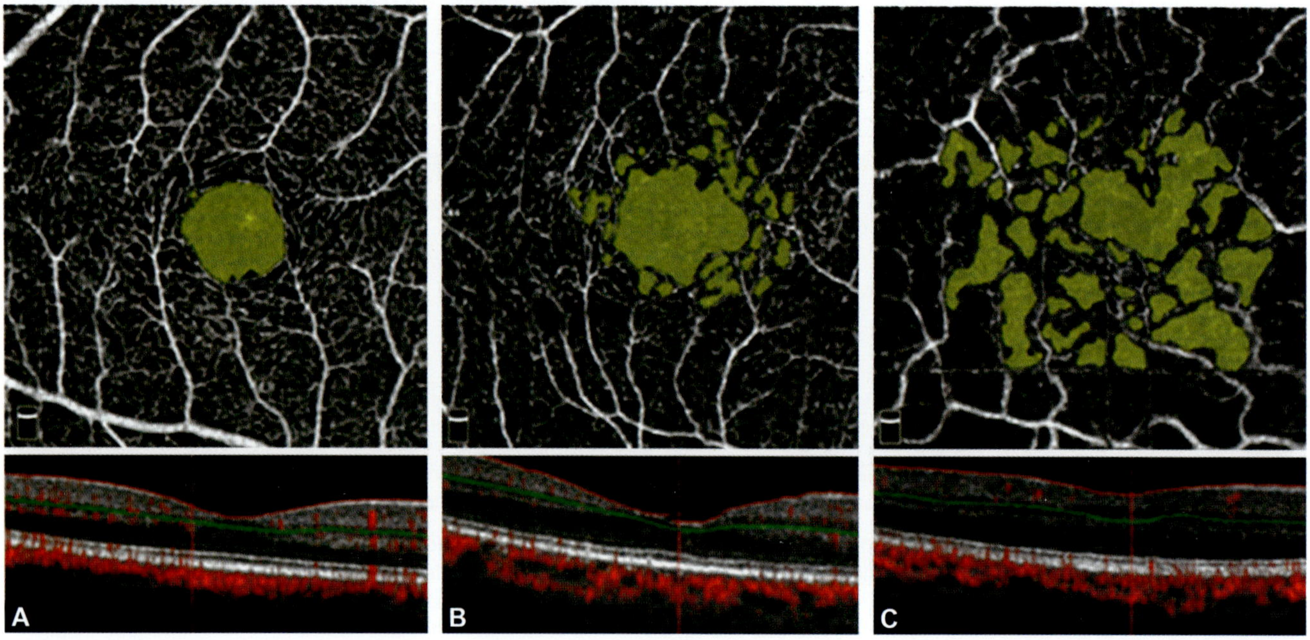

Figs. 1.12A to C: AngioAnalytics of nonflow regions in the superficial retinal layer of a healthy eye, nonproliferative diabetic retinopathy eye, and ischemic diabetic retinopathy eye. By analyzing nonflow area, the software shows all the regions of vascular dropout in yellow by mouse click selection. (A) Central region of the foveal avascular zone (FAZ) demarcated in yellow is visualized in the healthy eye. The software automatically shows numeric data of the FAZ and nonflow area size. In this example, FAZ measures 0.352 mm^2 representing a physiological value. Enlarged perifoveal intercapillary areas and vascular defects are not visualized. A regular, symmetric, and dense superficial vascular network is seen. (B) In the eye with nonproliferative diabetic retinopathy, the FAZ and perifoveal intercapillary area (vascular dropout) appear enlarged and slightly irregular with numerous microaneurysms (not relevant for this analysis). Nonflow area in this example measures 0.797 mm^2, a value higher than the physiological one. (C) The eye with ischemic diabetic retinopathy shows yellow zones of different size that present the regions of vascular dropout. The regular oval FAZ is not seen, so the surface of the selected nonflow regions is 1.620 mm^2.

software if they are ischemic. Software can also calculate the size of ischemic nonflow regions. These data are automatically saved for further monitoring and comparison (Figs. 1.12A to C).

Flow Density Map

This type of AngioAnalytics has recently been available and designed for separating flow and nonflow regions on one map. It automatically calculates numerically the

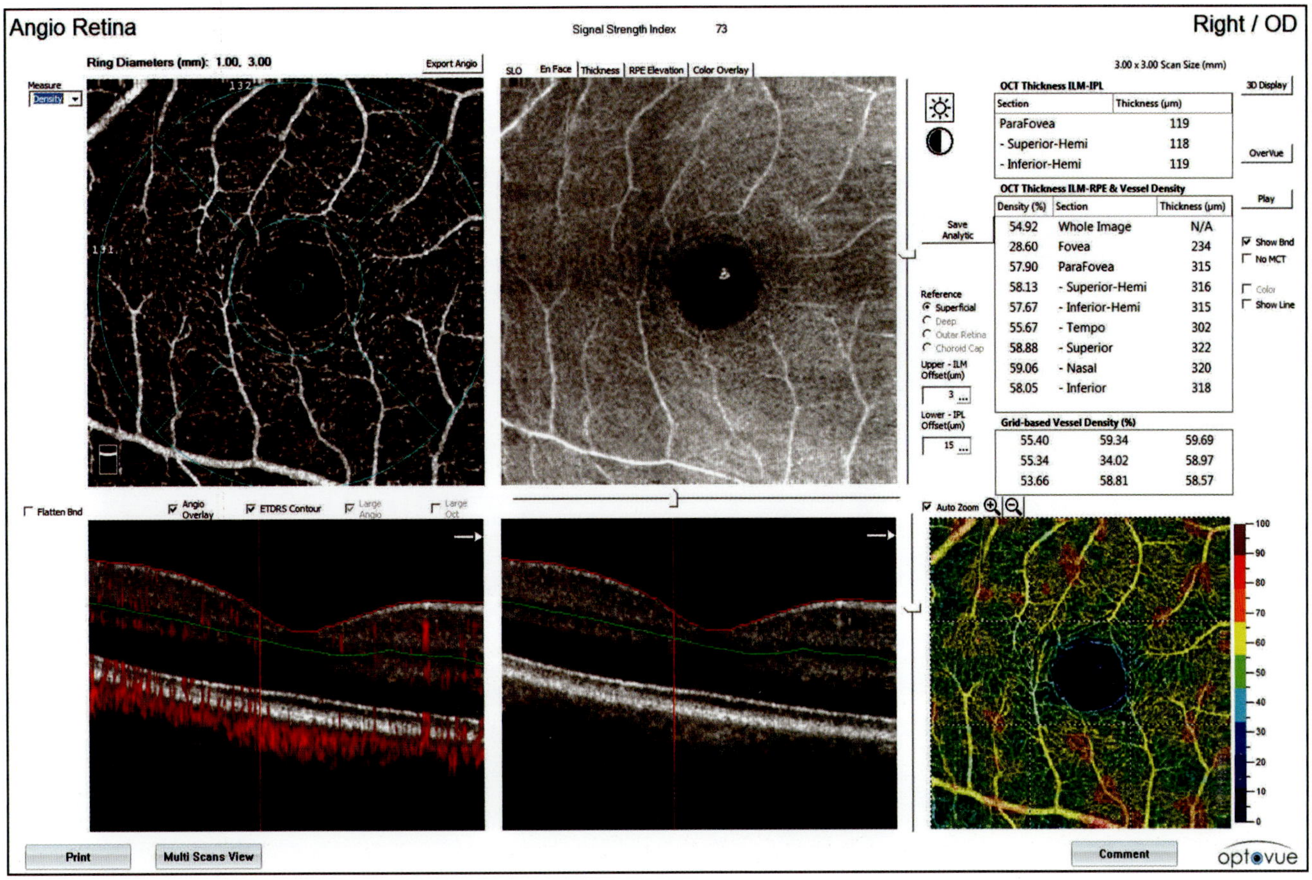

Fig. 1.13: Flow density map of the superficial vascular layer in a healthy eye. Central angiography shows normal superficial vascular network, corresponding en face optical coherence tomography angiography (OCT) image, and OCT-B scan in the lower part showing the localization of the analyzed superficial layer of the inner retina. In the lower right corner of the Figure, flow density map illustrates prevailing yellow-orange areas that indicate regions with vascular flow. A normal, blue avascular foveal avascular zone is in the central zone. The chart in the upper-right part of the Figure shows numeric values of flow density in segments, expressed as percentage.

percentage of flow and nonflow region, or a color-coded scale can be used. The scale shows the results in cool and warm colors with cool blue areas corresponding to the areas of weak and reduced flow, while warm yellow-orange areas indicate areas of medium-high flow density. Flow density map also estimates segmented vascularization density, expressed as the percentage on en face angiogram. This analysis provides information on mean capillary network density in each macular and paramacular sector. The calculation of capillary network density may be applied for both the superficial and deep vascular plexus. This application of AngioAnalytics is used in all vascular occlusive disorders, in monitoring diabetic retinopathy, and in estimating regression changes after laser photocoagulation and/or anti-VEGF treatment (Figs. 1.13 and 1.14).

OCTA COMPARISON TO FLUORESCEIN AND INDOCYANINE GREEN ANGIOGRAPHY

Fluorescein angiography and indocyanine green angiography (FAG and ICG) have been the gold standards of retinal vascular imaging until recently. Compared to these two methods, a newly developed method, OCTA has many advantages and differences. SSADA protocol is a noninvasive method, does not require patient's preparation nor intravenous contrast dye, it is fast, and images can be acquired in a few minutes. FAG and ICG are methods requiring intravenous injections that can result in many side effects such as nausea, vomiting, and rarely anaphylaxis. The noninvasive nature of OCTA allows

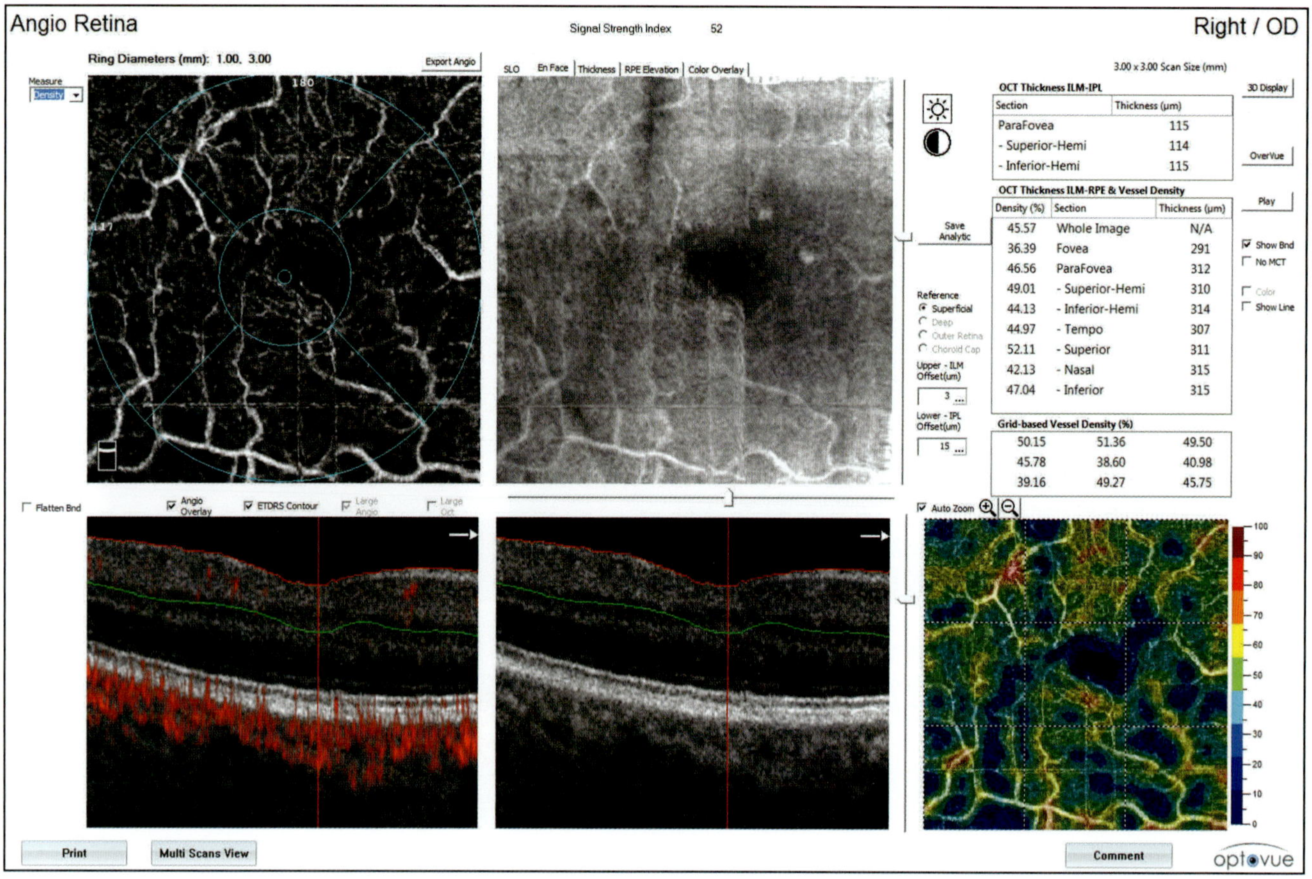

Fig. 1.14: Flow density map of the superficial vascular layer of an eye with ischemic diabetic retinopathy. The center of angiography illustrates superficial vascular network with the foveal avascular zone without margins, enlarged intercapillary nonflow spaces, and thin irregular blood capillaries. A corresponding en face optical coherence tomography angiography (OCT) is also illustrated; OCT B-scan in the lower part shows the localization of the analyzed superficial layer of the inner retina. Flow density map (lower right) illustrates cool blue regions indicating the areas with low or completely reduced flow. Few regions are in warm colors, they are mostly pale and indicate progressive attenuation of vascularization in this layer. The chart (upper-right) shows numeric values of flow density in segments, expressed as percentage.

more frequent and better follow-up and monitoring of the therapeutic response. Dye leakage in FAG is a vital sign in recognizing vascular pathologies such as neovascularization or microaneurysms. It is important to note that OCTA cannot show leakage because it does not employ a dye; vascular pathologies are detected by the other methods based on depths and vascular abnormality pattern. Choroidal neovascularizations (CNVs) are illustrated as clear vascular models present above the RPE (type 2 CNV), or between the Bruch's membrane and the RPE (type 1 CNV). OCTA measures and analyzes the regions of capillary dropout and neovascularizations as well as the regions with high flow with more precision because there is no dye leakage and image staining as in FAG.

SUGGESTED READING

1. Campbell JP, Zhang M, Hwang TS, et al. Detailed vascular anatomy of the human retina by projection-resolved optical coherence tomography angiography. Sci Rep. 2017;7:42201.
2. Chalam KV, Sambhav K. Optical coherence tomography angiography in retinal diseases. J Ophthalmic Vis Res. 2016;11(1):84-92.
3. Chen CL, Wang RK. Optical coherence tomography based angiography [invited]. Biomed Opt Express. 2017;8(2):1056-82.
4. Coscas G, Lupidi M, Coscas F. Heidelberg spectralis optical coherence tomography angiography: technical aspects. Dev Ophthalmol. 2016;56:1-5.
5. Coscas G, Lupidi M, Coscas F. Image analysis of optical coherence tomography angiography. Dev Ophthalmol. 2016;56:30-6.

6. de Carlo TE, Romano A, Waheed NK, et al. A review of optical coherence tomography angiography (OCTA). Int J Retina and Vitreous. 2015;1:5.
7. Fang PP, Lindner M, Steinberg JS, et al. Clinical applications of OCT angiography. Ophthalmologe. 2016;113(1):14-22.
8. Gao SS, Jia Y, Zhang M, et al. Optical coherence tomography angiography. Invest Ophthalmol Vis Sci. 2016;57(9):27-36.
9. Hoon M, Okawa H, Della Santina L, et al. Functional architecture of the retina: development and disease. Prog Retin Eye Res. 2014;42:44-84.
10. Jayadev C, Jain N, Sachdev S, et al. Utility of noninvasive imaging modalities in a retina practice. Indian J Ophthalmol. 2016;64(12):940-43.
11. Jia Y, Bailey ST, Hwang TS, et al. Quantitative optical coherence tomography angiography of vascular abnormalities in the living human eye. Proc Natl Acad Sci U S A. 2015;112(18):E2395-402.
12. Lumbroso B, Huang D, Chen JC, et al. Clinical OCT angiography atlas, 1st edition. New Delhi: Jaypee Brothers Medical Publishers; 2015. pp. 1-20.
13. Lumbroso B, Huang D, Souied E, et al. Practical handbook of OCT angiography, 1st edition. New Delhi: Jaypee Brothers Medical Publishers; 2016. pp. 1-21.
14. Shoughy SS, Kozak I. Selective and complementary use of optical coherence tomography and fluorescein angiography in retinal practice. Eye Vis (Lond). 2016;3:26.
15. Son T, Wang B, Thapa D, et al. Optical coherence tomography angiography of stimulus evoked hemodynamic responses in individual retinal layers. Biomed Opt Express. 2016;7(8):3151-162.
16. Spaide RF, Curcio CA. Evaluation of segmentation of the superficial and deep vascular layers of the retina by optical coherence tomography angiography instruments in normal eyes. JAMA Ophthalmol. 2017;135(3):259-62.
17. Wylęgała A, Teper S, Dobrowolski D, et al. Optical coherence angiography: a review. Medicine (Baltimore). 2016;95(41):e4907.
18. Zhang A, Zhang Q, Chen CL, et al. Methods and algorithms for optical coherence tomography-based angiography: a review and comparison. J Biomed Opt. 2015;20(10):100901.

CHAPTER 2

Choroidal Neovascularization

INTRODUCTION

Choroidal neovascular membrane (CNVM) or choroidal neovascularization (CNV) is the formation of new blood vessels that grow beneath the retina and threaten the central vision.

Choroidal blood vessels are classified on the basis of their morphology, the type of their branching, the presence of vascular loops, localizations of loops, and according to their capillary density, thickness and appearance.

Morphologically, newly formed blood vessels may have various appearances. They can be filamentous, medusa-shaped, coral-shaped, or have a bicycle-wheel pattern, pruned tree pattern or a 'ball of wool' pattern. Sometimes, they can also appear as a glomerulus-shaped lesion.

Capillaries inside the neovascularization, according to their density may be more or less tight, and they usually vary in thickness. Some of capillaries may appear gentle and thin, while some of them may be thicker, straighter, more rigid, and robust.

Vascular loops are generally localized in the very periphery of the CNV where they merge and develop the neovascular formation that may have the appearance of a wheel, fan or coral.

ETIOLOGY AND EPIDEMIOLOGY

Choroidal neovascularization is the most frequently seen in the age-related macular degeneration (ARMD), in its exudative form, where abnormal blood vessels grow from the choriocapillaris. They break through Bruch's membrane, extend and merge under the retinal pigment epithelial space, presenting subepithelial neovascularization type I (occult type, CNV I). If the pathologic blood vessels develop and grow in pre-epithelial subretinal space, they are referred to as neovascularized blood vessels type II (classic membrane, CNV II). The presence of exudates and hemorrhage may be present in both types. The development of CNVM may also be associated with presumed ocular histoplamosis syndrome, myopic macular degeneration, and traumas, although it may occur as an idiopathic entity. ARMD is the most common cause of vision loss in the population over 50 years of age in the developed countries. Up to 90% of the visual acuity loss in ARMD is caused by the development of CNV. Myopia is the second most frequent cause of CNV in the United States and Europe, meaning that CNV occurs in 5–10% of myopic patients.

The mechanism of CNV development is not yet fully understood. It is believed that any pathological process involving the retinal pigment epithelium (RPE) and Bruch's membrane can lead to the secondary complications such as the development of CNV. RPE cells produce *pigment epithelium derived factor* (PEDF) that has an inhibitory effect on CNV development (inhibitor of angiogenesis). On the other hand, *vascular endothelial growth factor* (VEGF) starts to produce due to the hypoxia, hyperglycemia, activation of protein kinase C, increased production of free radicals, and activation of oncogenes and cytokines. The VEGF is a factor in ocular angiogenesis that stimulates the development of CNV. The balance between concentrations of inhibitors (PEDF) and stimulators of angiogenesis (VEGF) directly influences the growth of CNV.

SYMPTOMS AND SIGNS

Patients often complain on painless vision loss, metamorphopsia, central or paracentral scotoma, color disturbances, and apparent change in image size. Clinical manifestations in patients with CNV include a subretinal hemorrhage, accumulation of subretinal fluid, lipid exudates, RPE detachment, and subretinal fibrosis (disciform scar).

TYPES OF CHOROIDAL NEOVASCULARIZATION

Type 1 CNV is known as an occult neovascularization, located beneath the RPE causing its shallow elevation. Thus, type 1 CNV is most commonly localized between elevated RPE and Bruch's membrane. In the case of fibrovascular tissue proliferation, the elevated RPE may look stratified. Subretinal fluid is also frequently present and the risk of pigment epithelium perforation is high. Morphology of type 1 CNV varies. It can be coral, fan or medusa-shaped, or have a bicycle-wheel pattern, pruned tree pattern or a 'ball of wool' pattern. If left untreated, Type 1 CNV will evolve and form a fibrovascular plaque. Hemorrhages and outer retinal layer lesions in later phases of CNV evolution are frequently seen. Irreversible fibrosis occurs at a later stage.

Type 2 CNV is known as a classic neovascularization, develops in the subretinal space above the RPE. Type 2 new blood vessels may penetrate into the outer retinal layer which is avascular in healthy eyes. Type 2 CNV is generally smaller than type 1 CNV. This type of neovascularization is almost always accompanied by the intraretinal fluid (diffuse edema or cystoid edema) and fluid pooling under the retina that may result in a shallow retinal detachment. Morphologically, these neovascularizations are similar in shape as the type 1 CNV. Pigment epithelial detachments are not usually present, but hemorrhages are frequent. If left untreated, these new blood vessels may grow surprisingly fast according to some studies even about 9 mm per day.

Type 4 CNV or mixed neovascularization type consists of type 1 and type 2 CNV components in the same eye, along with the shallow pigment epithelial detachment, subretinal fluid, cystoid edemas, hemorrhages, and alterations in outer retinal layers. This type of CNV involves two or more parallel, flat vascular formations localized at several retinal levels. Type 2 CNV vessels are placed above the RPE having a rounded or fan-like shape with numerous dense vascular loops at the periphery. Deeper down under the RPE and above Bruch's membrane, one or more irregular and significantly larger type 1 neovascularizations are present. If left untreated, this type of neovascularization slowly progresses to a fibrovascular plaque. Hemorrhages occur very frequently as well as edemas and hard exudates. Disruption of outer retinal layer and severe damage of photoreceptors can also take place. Irreversible fibrosis occurs in later stages.

Type 3 CNV is a distinct type of neovascularization that may occur in neovascular ARMD. This type of CNV has predilection for the neurosensory retina and is usually accompanied by a telangiectatic formations. Terms that were previously used for this type of CNV include *retinal angiomatous proliferation (RAP)* and *chorioretinal anastomosis* [*retinal choroidal anastomosis (RCA)*]. Type 3 CNV involves a focal neovascular proliferation from the deep retinal layer (essentially RAP), an intraretinal neovascular extension from underlying occult type 1 CNV (essentially RCA), and *de novo* breaks in the Bruch's membrane with neovascular infiltration into the retina.

DIAGNOSTICS

The first step in the diagnostic procedure is a clinical examination of the fundus when an experienced ophthalmologist may detect greyish or altered regions that may be suspicious of CNV. Detailed anamnesis is a very important segment of examination helping to yield information on risk factors relevant for the development of CNV (age, previous myopias, the presence of diabetes or some other conditions relevant for the development of CNV). By the fundus examination a clinician can also sometimes observe subretinal hemorrhages, subretinal fluid pooling, and lipid exudates. An optical coherence tomography (OCT) has always significantly contributed the diagnostics. For a long period of time, fluorescein angiography (FAG) and indocyanine green angiography (ICG) have been necessary for a diagnosis in conditions suspicious of CNV.

The introduction of optical coherence tomography angiography (OCTA) made the CNV diagnosis much easier both for patients and doctors. It can clearly visualize, measure, and monitor neovascular membranes. Patients may undergo OCTA imaging many times and still avoid the risk of side effects even without standard pupillary dilation. OCTA enables deep and segmented analysis of retinal microcirculation. The advantages of OCTA in comparison to FAG are numerous including noninvasive high-resolution imaging, 3D images with the possibility of segmentation during the analysis, avoidance of the injection of a contrast dye, and acquisition imaging time is less than 5 minutes. FAG provides better visualization of a wide peripheral field, but it is an invasive method that requires administration of a contrast dye, the presence of reanimation team (since the incidence of anaphylactic shock is 1:25,000); the image resolution is poor and the procedure costs is more. Also, it cannot separately visualize the retinal layers, but only superficial retina; the image is 2D and the whole procedure is time-consuming, since the dynamics of the blood flow analysis takes about 5–30 minutes.

The OCTA is a fast, effective, and safe method at diagnosing a disease. Recognition of neovascular membrane (CNV) in its early stages is of extreme importance since they achieve better prognosis and can start their treatment on time. Anti-VEGF therapy as a monotherapy or in combination with laser photocoagulation is a preferred therapy in a daily practice in cases when the patient's status, changes, and therapeutic effects can be monitored daily by the angiography imaging technique. The OCTA can clearly show a CNV regression signs and the disease withdrawal. The software is also irreplaceable in differentiating the type of microvascular change since it can clearly visualize the affected layer. OCTA clearly separates the four retinal layers—the superficial and deep layer of inner retina, the outer retina and choriocapillaris. Neovascularizations can be visualized in separate layers as well as those that spread and perforate the RPE. OCTA also has a possibility of quantitative monitoring of the activity and growth of neovascular changes by using AngioAnalytics quantification software. The software allows a quantification of the flow in the area with neovascularization.

Detection of Choroidal Neovascularizations by the OCTA

Type 1 CNV always appears beneath the RPE and the blood flow cannot be observed in avascular outer retinal layer. This type of neovascularization may eventually spread into the outer retina and break through the RPE. Type 1 CNV most commonly forms an extensive capillary network and is characterized by a high flow index. Type 1 CNV is generally larger and wider than type 2 CNV. Different morphology types of these neovascularizations have previously been mentioned in this chapter. Morphology of the CNV is always clearly presented so there is no room for suspicion about the diagnosis. Capillaries can be densely or sparsely arranged. They can also appear thin and have curved course, or be thicker and straighter. Vascular loops can be seen in the periphery of the CNV taking part in the formation of neovascularization shapes that resemble a 'ball of wool', bicycle-wheel, or a fan. Loops can be sparsed, or frequent and dense with a complex arborization and branching. Neovascularization usually has one feeder trunk, or a bundle of feeder blood vessels that deliver blood. Type 1 CNV can be seen in en face angiogram of choroidal layer. CNV capillary network may also be visualized on the en face OCT presenting itself as a hyperreflective neovascular membrane in choroidal part.

Type 2 CNV presents itself as a new vascular structure above the RPE and the flow can be visualized in the outer retina which is normally avascular. Newly-formed blood vessels subsequently spread more widely into the outer avascular retinal zone. Type 2 CNV is always smaller than the type 1 CNV. The blood flow index in this type of neovascularization is also high and the morphology is similar to type 1. Neovascularizations are more often observed in the form of a fan and in a 'bicycle-wheel' shape with the loops at the periphery. The margin between pathologically altered blood vessels and normal retina can be clearly observed. Capillaries in the affected area are usually densely packed, thin, and numerous. After the repeated treatment, capillaries become wider and thicker with a rough appearance (arterialization), while the thinner capillaries disappear. CNV always presents one larger feeder trunk or a bundle of feeder capillaries with centrifugal branches that form a bicycle-wheel or fan-shape on one side. Fluid is also often present especially if the new vessels penetrate into the neuroepithelium. Subretinal fluid accumulation can also be seen as well as small spaces of cystoid edema. Hemorrhages and alterations in the outer retina, fibrosis, and severe damage of the photoreceptor layer may occasionally be seen. Both in CNV 1 and CNV 2, a dark halo surrounding the neovascularization is usually present.

Type 4 CNV includes the presence of two or more newly formed vascular networks in two parallel retinal layers (simultaneous presence of type 1 CNV and type 2 CNV in one eye). Neovascularization may initially be located under the RPE, progress in time and penetrate through the RPE and eventually reach the outer retina. Neovascular networks are extensive and have a high flow index. Morphologically, they have the forms as CNV 1 and CNV 2 in corresponding layers. The density of the network may vary and densely packed capillary network may be seen as well as a sparse network with thin capillaries. As a consequence of arterialization and relapse, the vessel network may appear thicker, straighter, and more rigid. Vascular loops may be seen in the periphery of the neovascularization and they can be frequent and dense or sparse and thin. OCTA angiogram reveals a classical neovascularization type 2 in the outer retinal layer, most commonly in the shape of a fan or bicycle-wheel with a thin and dark halo around the vessels. Under the RPE and above Bruch's membrane in the same eye one or more type 1 neovascularizations can be seen. Type 1 CNVs are much larger, wider, and more irregular. They have numerous, thicker vascular loops. The fluid is present in almost all cases and is associated with a shallow detachment of RPE, neuroepithelial detachment, and with the formation of a diffuse or cystoid edema.

Type 3 CNV is a special type of neovascularization that occurs usually in neovascular form of ARMD and can be now better analyzed by the OCTA. OCTA shows characteristic retinal-retinal anastomosis that occurs in a deep vascular plexus and form a tuft-shaped, high-flow structure that ends in the outer retina, finally adjoining in the sub-RPE level. The tuft-shaped lesion corresponds to a small glomerular-shaped lesion which is seen in the choriocapillary layer on the OCTA. OCTA confirms the hypothesis that the most cases of type 3 neovascularization are characterized by the intraretinal vascular complex formation in the deep capillary network of the inner retina.

MORPHOLOGICAL FORMS OF NEOVASCULARIZATIONS

Figures 2.1 to 2.4 show the morphological forms of neovascularizations.

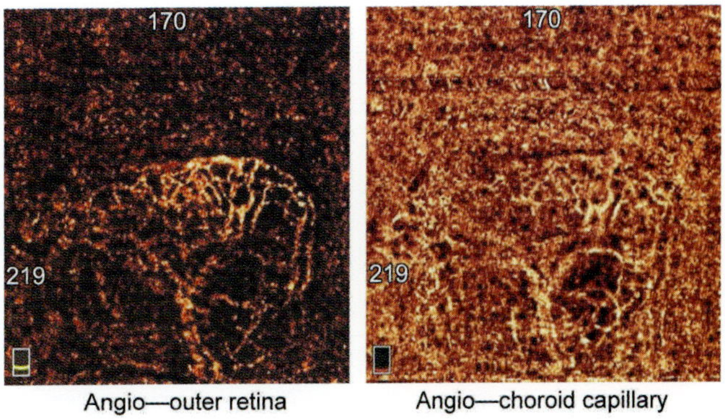

Fig. 2.1: An optical coherence tomography angiography of the outer retinal layer and choriocapillaris (3 × 3 mm). A type 2 choroidal neovascularization (CNV), which is fan-shaped is presented. Capillary loops at the periphery of the neovascularization are illustrated. Capillaries are rough, thick, and sparse. A dark halo around the neovascularization cannot be seen suggesting that it is an active form of CNV which intensively spreads into the surrounding tissue.

EXAMPLES OF EYES WITH NEOVASCULARIZATION SHOWN BY THE OCTA

Figures 2.5 to 2.21 show some examples of eyes with neovascularization shown by the OCTA.

THERAPY

The fundamental principle in CNVMs is anti-VEGF therapy.

Vascular Endothelial Growth Factor

Vascular endothelial growth factor is a glycoprotein substance important in inducing angiogenesis (development of tiny blood vessels) in physiological and pathological conditions. Besides stimulating neovascularization, VEGF has an effect on increased permeability of blood vessels. Neovascularization plays an important pathophysiological role in tumorogenesis and in vision loss caused by ischemic retinal disorders or wet ARMD. Hypoxia is a major inducer of increased VEGF production, but it also causes increased expression of VEGF receptors on endothelial cells. The VEGF family includes five glycoprotein growth factors—VEGF-A, VEGF-B, VEGF-C, VEGF-D, and placental growth factor (PIGF). VEGF-A is the most common cause of ocular pathologies causing angiogenesis and increased permeability of blood vessels acting through the receptors VEGFR1 (also known as FLT-1) and

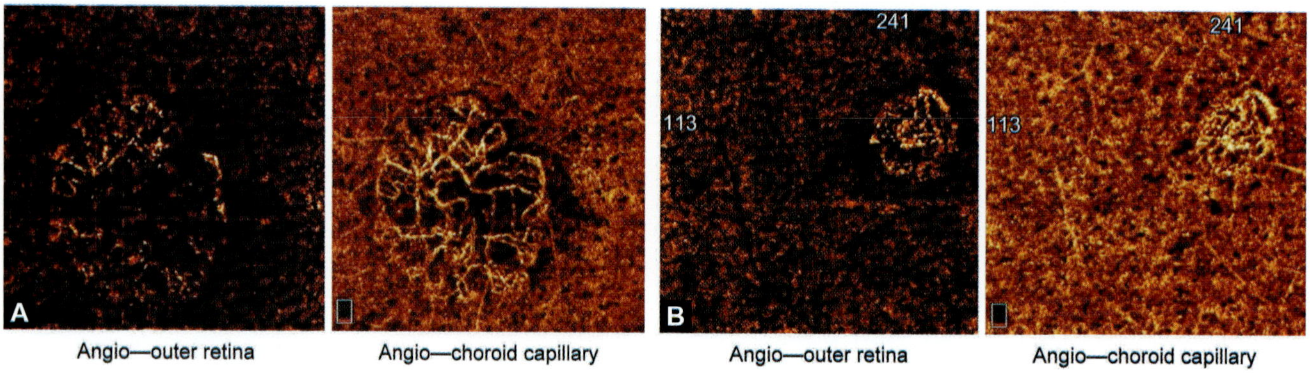

Figs. 2.2A and B: An optical coherence tomography angiography of the outer retina and choriocapillaris in two different examples that present type 2 neovascularization (3 × 3 mm). Both examples in both retinal layers illustrate the type 2 neovascularization with a 'bicycle-wheel' shape. Numerous vascular loops can be seen in the very periphery of the circular neovascularization. In both cases, in the outer retina, a dark halo clearly differentiates the neovascularization from the surrounding tissue. A sparse and larger neovascularization is illustrated in Figure A, while the Figure B illustrates neovascularization with densely packed capillaries which is smaller in size.

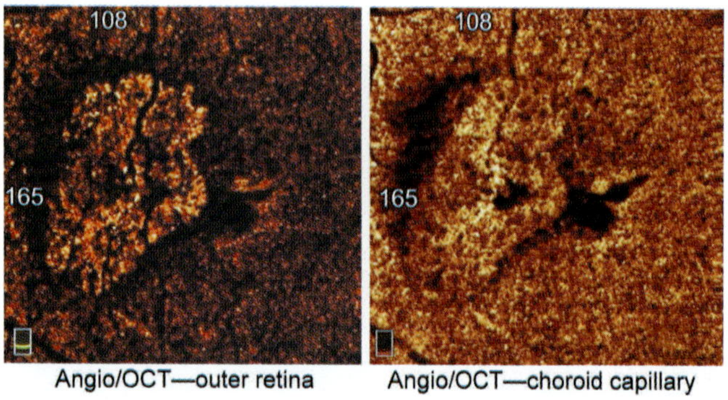

Fig. 2.3: An optical coherence tomography angiography (OCTA) of the outer retina and choriocapillaris (3 × 3 mm). A coral-shaped type 2 choroidal neovascularization (CNV) is illustrated. Neovascularization consists of numerous small, densely intertwined and packed capillaries that mutually form numerous loops. A dark thin halo can be seen around the CNV in both layers but especially in outer one.

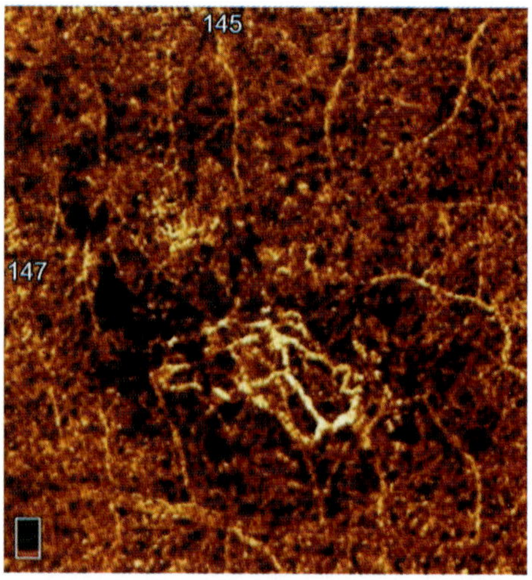

Fig. 2.4: An optical coherence tomography angiography of the choroidal layer (3 × 3 mm) shows in this example a type 1 choroidal neovascularization (CNV) with a filamentous vascular structure and tangled new blood vessels. This type of neovascularization can often be seen in the cases of age-related macular degeneration and epitheliopathy. Vascular loops are sparse and only a few can be visualized. Also a dark halo can be observed only little at one part of CNV. This is an active change which widely spreads into the surrounding tissue and can perforate the retinal pigment epithelium.

VEGFR2 (also known as KDR). Since VEGF-A is the main cause in ocular disease pathology, it is preferentially targeted by the drugs from VEGF inhibitors group.

Inhibitors of VEGF

Angiogenesis is a process of vital importance in the eye development, but also in pathogenesis of different ocular diseases such as diabetic retinopathy, ARMD, corneal vascularization, rubeosis iridis, retinopathy of prematurity, retinal vein occlusion, neovascular glaucoma, and many others. Since there is a wide range of ocular diseases caused by angiogenesis and VEGF, a new therapeutic approach has been developed by using vascular endothelial growth factor inhibitors. VEGF inhibitors or anti-VEGF drugs are substances that block the growth and the development of neovascularization by the mechanism of competitive inhibition. They can be used in the treatment of numerous ocular diseases in whom new pathological blood vessels or macular edema develop. Out of all vascular endothelial

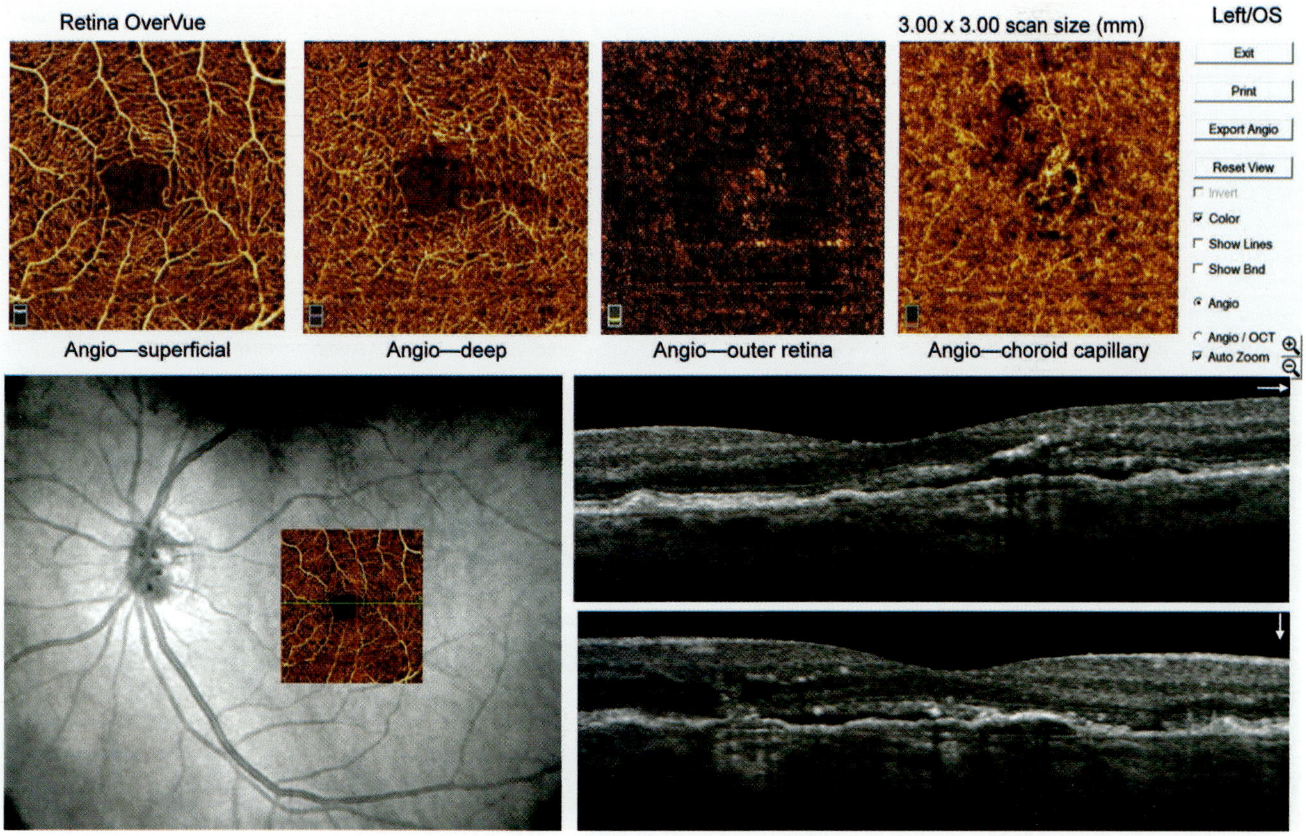

Fig. 2.5: An optical coherence tomography angiography finding in an eye with a wet form of age-related macular degeneration. The finding shows illustrations of OCTA split spectrum amplitude decorrelation angiography protocols of all retinal layers (3 × 3 mm), fundus photography, and an OCT B-scan of the macular region. Superficial and deep vascular plexus show no pathological changes. Foveal avascular zone is regular in size and shape. Outer retina is avascular and shows a minimal flow projection artifact. A filamentous type 1 neovascularization can be seen in the choriocapillaris. It is a small roundish hyperreflective vascular structure, with densely packed new blood vessels and a discrete black surrounding halo zone. The OCT B-scan shows irregular, wavy, hyperreflective, and thickened retinal pigment epithelium with a sporadic discontinuation, a shallow sensory retinal detachment, and accumulation of intraretinal fluid.

growth factors, VEGF-A is the most dominant in ocular pathology, and is a mediator both in retinal and choroidal angiogenesis. Nine isoforms of this growth factors have been identified in humans so far, including—VEGF121, VEGF145, VEGF148, VEGF162, VEGF165, VEGF165b, VEGF183, VEGF189, and VEGF206. It has been confirmed that its level in the vitreous is proportional to the severity of diabetic retinopathy, being highest in patients with proliferative diabetic retinopathy and diabetic macular edema. Its inhibition by the use of anti-VEGF treatment is currently the cornerstone for the therapy for age-related macular degradation and diabetic retinopathy as well. The aim of anti-VEGF treatment is to suppress pathological neovascularizations and disease progression, and to arrest visual acuity impairments progression.

Anti-VEGF drugs may be divided into three main pharmacological classes:

1. Drugs targeting all VEGF isoforms
2. Drugs inhibiting VEGF receptors
3. Drugs inhibiting VEGF downstream signaling.

The first anti-VEGF drug was introduced in clinical practice in 1997 by Gordon et al. in the treatment of advanced malignancy. Anti-VEGF agent they used was bevacizumab (Avastin), a humanized anti-VEGF antibody that blocks all VEGF isoforms. In the first phase, bevacizumab was investigated for the treatment of advanced malignancy and its minimal toxicity was observed. In the second phase of investigation, the efficacy of bevacizumab combined with fluorouracil and leucovorin as chemotherapeutic drugs in terms of longer survival rate in patients

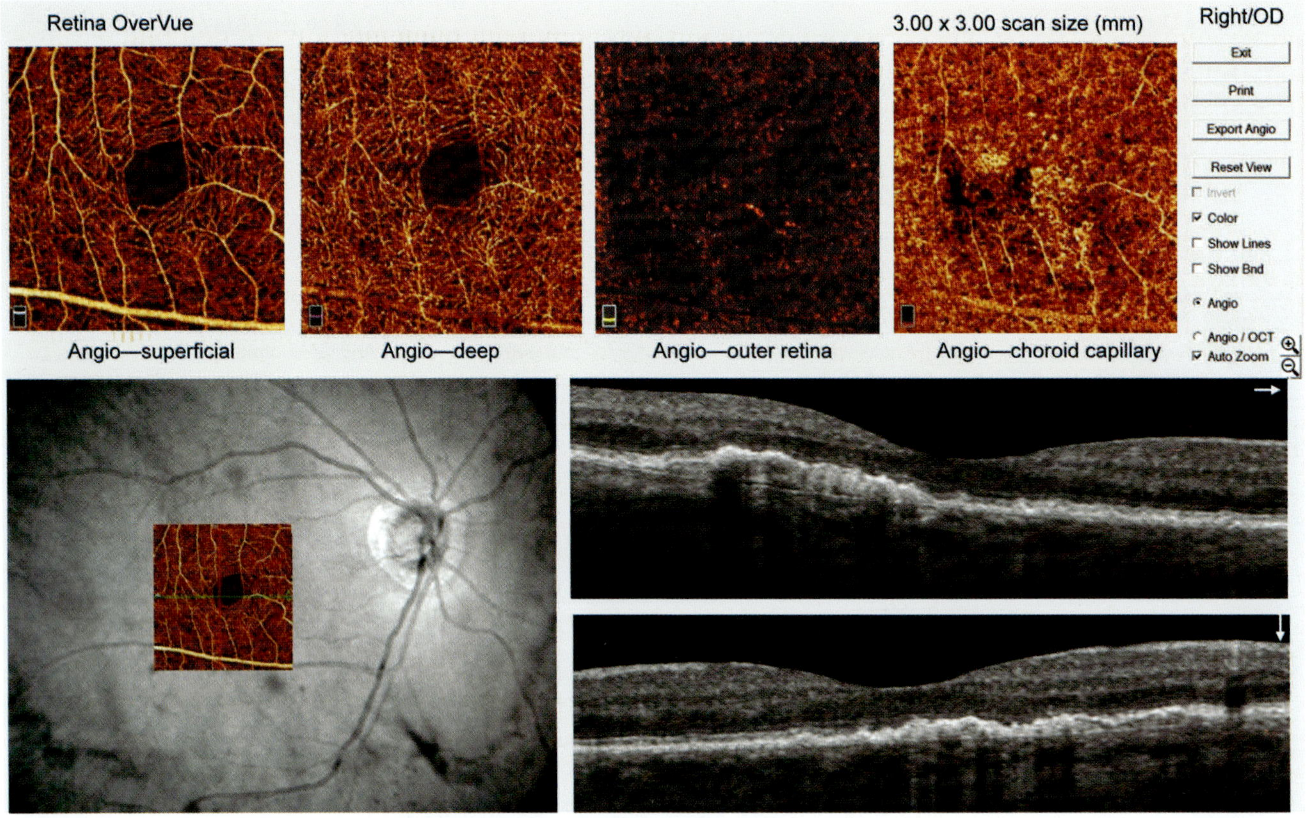

Fig. 2.6: An optical coherence tomography angiography finding of an eye with the wet form of age-related macular degeneration shows OCTA split spectrum amplitude decorrelation angiography scanning protocols of all retinal layers (3 × 3 mm), fundus photography, and OCT B-scan of the macular area. The en face angiogram of the choroidal area shows a few bud-like, hyperreflective, and densely packed neovascularizations without surrounding dark halo. The outer retina is avascular without the retinal pigment epithelium (RPE) perforation. The superficial and deep vascular network is regular, dense, and symmetric. An OCT B-scan shows an irregular and thickened RPE with subretinal hyperreflective thickening and focal RPE elevation.

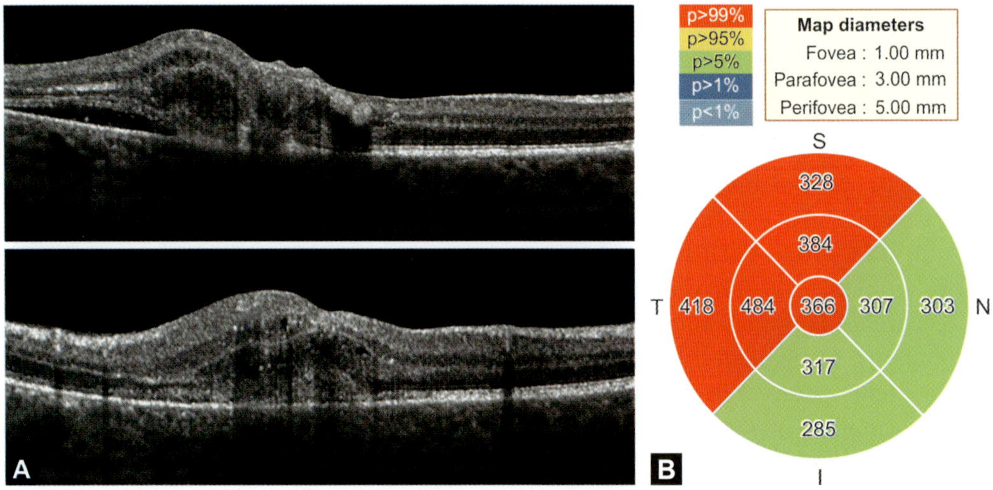

Figs. 2.7A and B: (A) An optical coherence tomography B-scan of the macular region in the patient with wet form of age-related macular degeneration. Small cystoid changes with intraretinal fluid can be seen in the inner retina, as well as the subretinal edema with sensory retinal detachment. Retinal pigment epithelium is thinned and disrupted in the center. In the outer retina, in its central part, a blurred hyperreflective zone that is suspected on choroidal neovascularization can be visualized. (B) Retinal thickness map shows segments of macular thickening in the central, superior, and temporal regions.

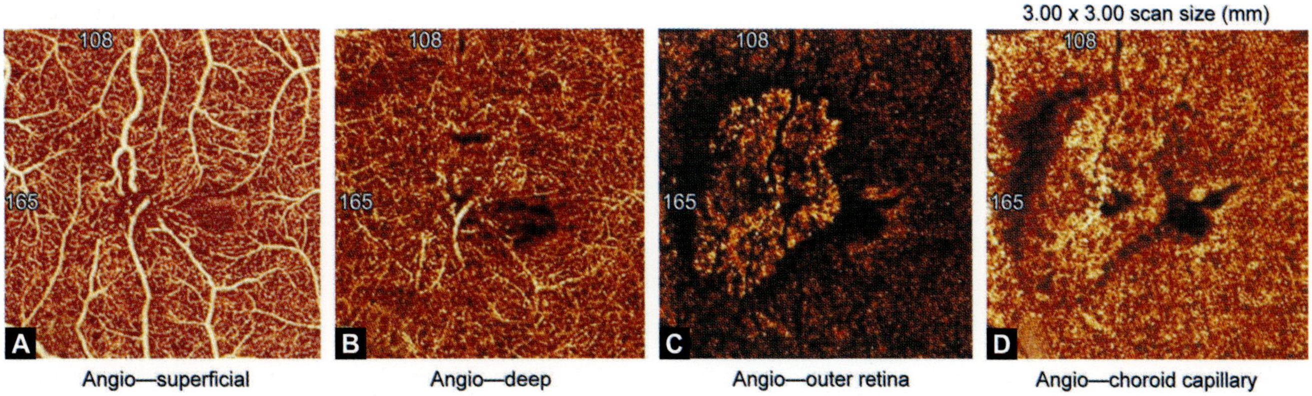

Figs. 2.8A to D: The optical coherence tomography angiography split spectrum amplitude decorrelation angiography protocol of the same eye as in the previous image with presented vascularization of retinal layers (3 × 3 mm). Superficial vascular plexus and deep vascular plexus show altered appearance, foveal avascular zone is not clearly visualized, and numerous anastomoses can be seen between two layers. In the outer retina, as well as in choriocapillaris, central neovascularization is visualized in the coral-shaped form which is composed of a great number of densely packed capillaries. This is the type 2 choroidal neovascularization, since the vascular structure perforated through the retinal pigment epithelium and can be visualized in the outer retinal avascular layer. A dark halo is visualized around the neovascularization in both layers, but is especially pinpointed in the outer retina.

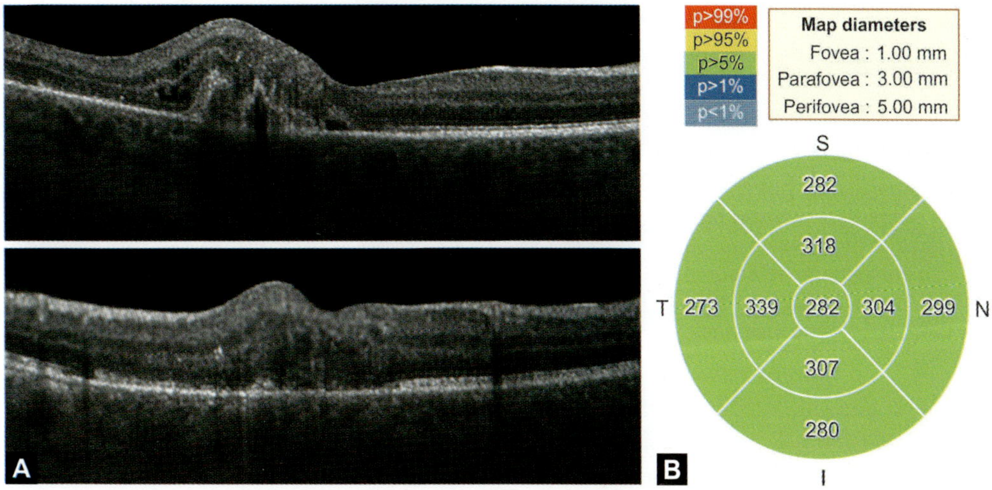

Figs. 2.9A and B: An optical coherence tomography (OCT) B-scan and retinal thickness map of the same eye as in Figures 2.7 and 2.8, after three intravitreal ranibizumab injections. Both OCT B-scan images confirm an obvious reduction of subretinal edema and hyperreflective tissue in outer retina. Retinal pigment epithelium is still irregular and perforated in places. The retinal thickness map shows a significantly decreased values of macular area thickness. Each segment has physiological thickness according to the OCT software.

with colorectal carcinoma was significantly better in comparison to patients treated only with chemotherapeutic drugs. Similar results were obtained in the third phase of investigation in the terms of bevacizumab efficacy in combination with chemotherapy in patients with metastatic colorectal cancer. By analyzing these results, Food and Drug Administration (FDA) approved bevacizumab in combination with chemotherapy for the treatment of metastatic colorectal carcinoma in 2004, but not for the treatment of ophthalmic diseases.

Parallel to the development of anti-VEGF therapy in carcinomatous diseases, a new therapeutic strategy in the treatment of ophthalmic diseases in which VEGF and angiogenesis play an important part was initiated. The first disease treated with anti-VEGF drugs was neovascular ARMD, and the first anti-VEGF therapy is used to treat this

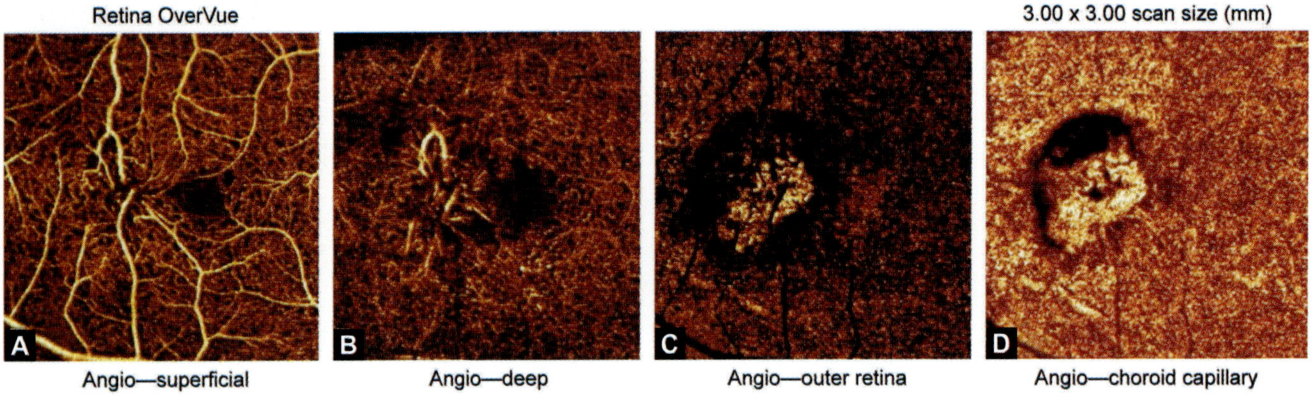

Figs. 2.10A to D: The optical coherence tomography angiography split spectrum amplitude decorrelation angiography imaging protocol of the same eye as in Figures 2.7 and 2.8 with en face angiograms of retinal layers after three injections of ranibizumab (3 × 3 mm). In the outer retinal layer and in choriocapillaris, almost a twice smaller neovascularization can be seen, as well as a smaller ramification and significantly greater dark halo around the choroidal neovascularization (CNV). Also, a loss of small gentle capillaries in the very center of neovascularization can be observed. All of those changes implicate the inactivity of dried CNV. A few irregular, rigid, and shrunk blood vessels in the deep vascular plexus are observed. The foveal avascular zone can be clearly visualized, but its shape is still slightly irregular.

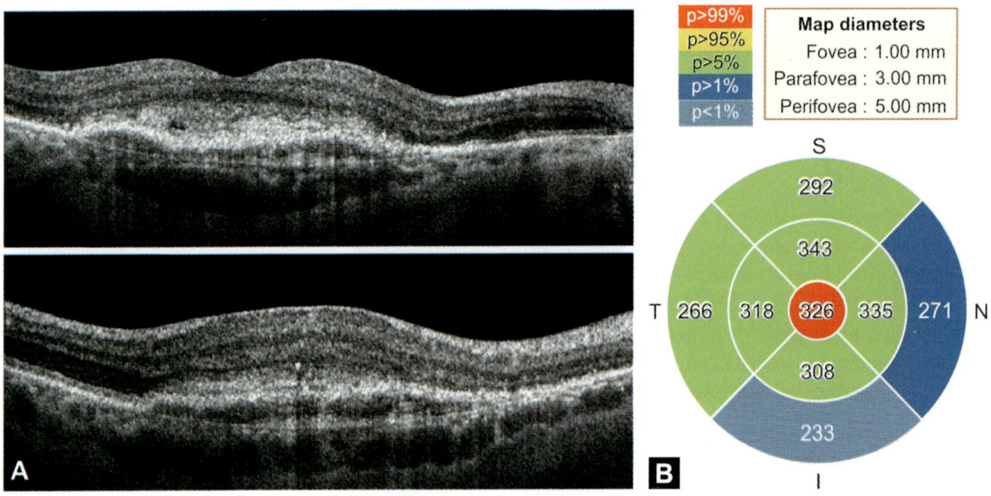

Figs. 2.11A and B: (A) An optical coherence tomography B-scan of an eye with wet form of age-related macular degeneration shows a subretinal hyperreflective tissue thickening, irregular and thickened retinal pigment epithelium, along with its flat elevation, and accumulation of intraretinal and subretinal fluid. (B) Retinal thickness map shows an increased values in the very center.

ocular disease was pegaptanib (Macugen). It is an RNA aptamer that binds and neutralizes VEGF165 isoform (and probably also VEGF188, although this has not been evidence based yet). Considering the fact that this drug targets only one isoform of the VEGF, its use has declined and has largely been substituted by bevacizumab and ranibizumab which block all VEGF isoforms. However, it is necessary to mention the efficacy of this drug in the treatment of certain types of macular edema, as evidenced by some recent studies.

Bevacizumab (Avastin®)

After approving bevacizumab for cancer therapy, and given the role of VEGF in the pathogenesis of neovascular ARMD, bevacizumab began to be used in the treatment of this disease as an '*off-label*' use.

Bevacizumab is a recombinant humanized monoclonal immunoglobulin G1 antibody targeting all forms of VEGF-A. This drug is produced in genetically engineered Chinese hamster ovary cells and binds to VEGFR1 (FLT-1)

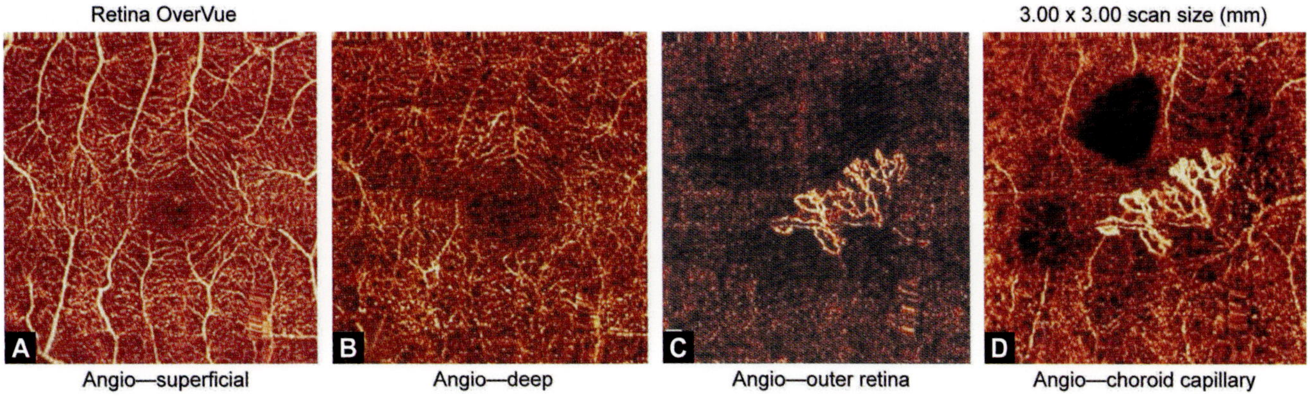

Figs. 2.12A to D: An optical coherence tomography angiography split spectrum amplitude decorrelation angiography imaging protocol of the same eye as in Figure 2.11 (3 × 3 mm). Superficial and deep vascular network do not show significant vascular alterations. A couple of mild capillary dropouts, along with a slight change in foveal avascular zone shape, can be observed. A filamentous, thread-like choroidal neovascularization (CNV) is observed in the outer retina and in choriocapillaris. A dark halo around the CNV cannot be seen, but a few surrounding regions with a capillary flow dropout are observed in the choriocapillaris. The angiogram illustrates a developed, active form of neovascularization type 2.

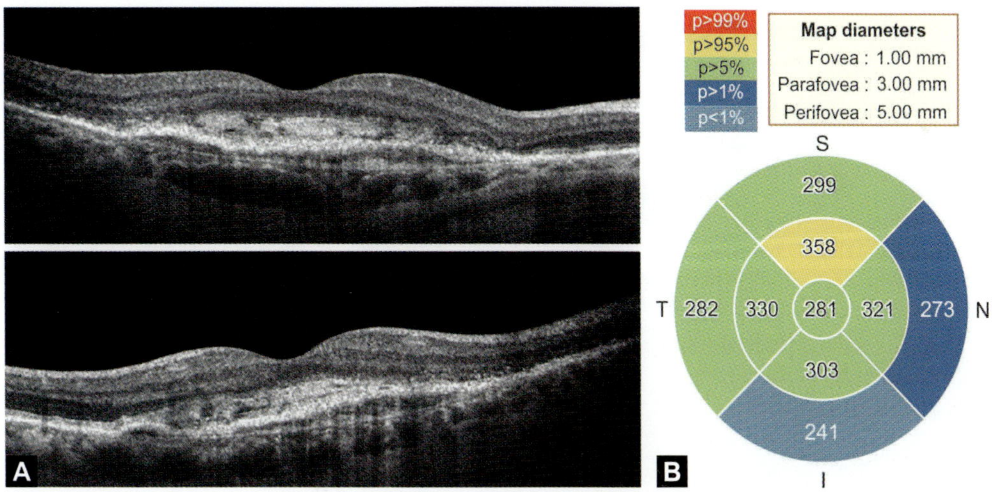

Figs. 2.13A and B: The optical coherence tomography B-scan and retinal thickness map of the same eye which is presented in Figs. 2.12A and B, only a day after the application of first intravitreal ranibizumab injection. It seems like the hyperreflective tissue is thinner, compared to the previous scans, and there is no subretinal fluid. Retinal pigment epithelium is slightly less elevated, but it shows irregularities and segmental perforations. The retinal thickness map illustrates decreased numeric values of central macular thickness.

and VEGFR2 (KDR) endothelial receptors, thus inhibiting the biological activity of human VEGF, both in vitro and in vivo conditions. Bevacizumab has a molecular weight of 149-kD. In ophthalmic diseases, bevacizumab was first used in the treatment of wet ARMD, then in other ophthalmic diseases such as proliferative diabetic retinopathy, retinopathy of prematurity, corneal neovascularization, retinal vein occlusion, neovascular glaucoma, and others. It has been registered in vitro that bevacizumab decreases VEGF-induced permeability and proliferation of cultured porcine choroidal cells, inhibits VEGF-stimulated proliferation of monkey choroidal cells, and inhibits VEGF-stimulated migration human umbilical vein endothelial cells.

One of the first studies on bevacizumab efficacy in patients with neovascular ARMD was conducted by Michels et al. who observed improved visual acuity, as well as improvements in OCT and angiographic parameters after the systemic application of this drug. The same authors also pointed out a promising evidence on the safety of this drug application due to favorable results

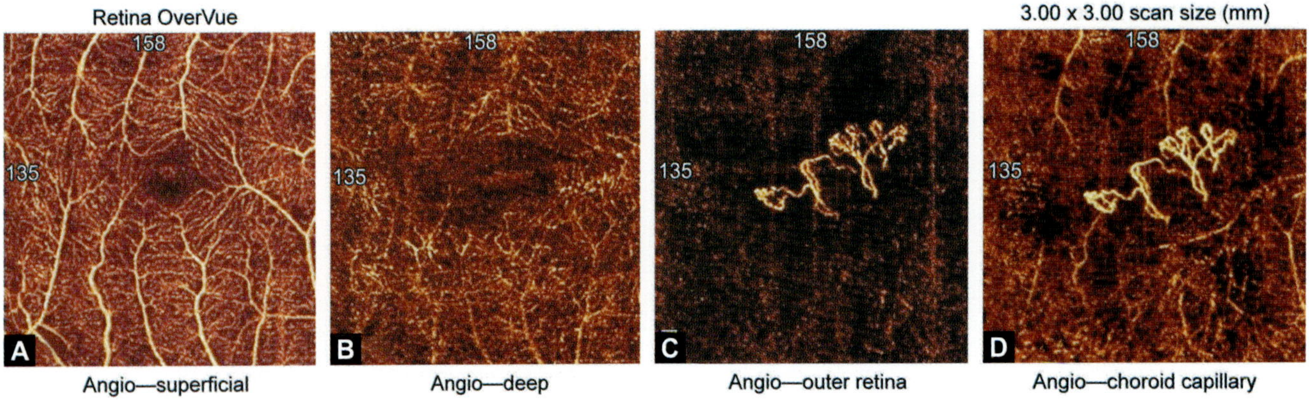

Figs. 2.14A to D: The optical coherence tomography angiography split spectrum amplitude decorrelation angiography imaging protocol of the same eye as in Figures 2.11 and 2.12 with en face angiograms of retinal layers (3 × 3 mm), a day after the application of first intravitreal ranibizumab injection. Significantly less active membrane is shown due to the fact a dark surrounding halo started to form. Choroidal neovascularization is also less branchy and dense, and compared to the state before the therapy is definitely more sparse. Deep vascular plexus exhibits altered shape and size of the foveal avascular zone, and also numerous tiny microaneurysms. Superficial inner retinal layer appears regular.

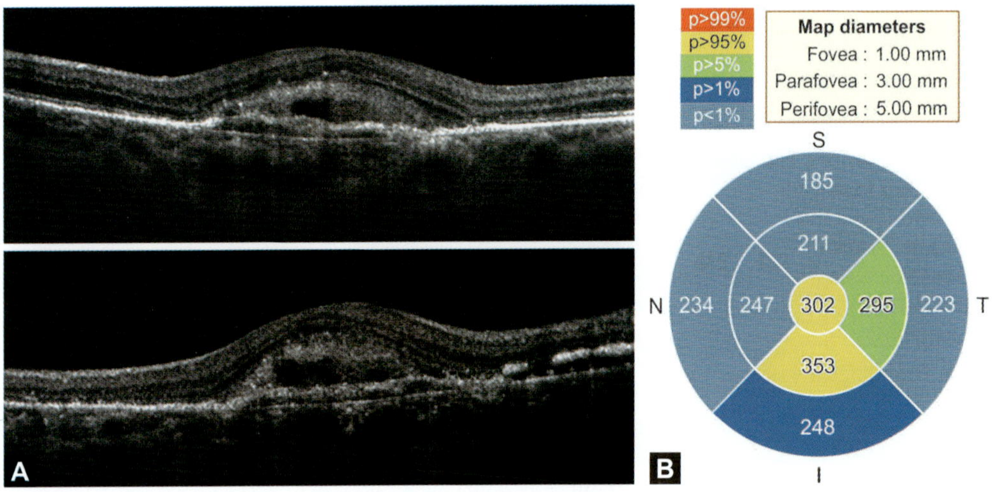

Figs. 2.15A and B: (A) An optical coherence tomography B-scan of the macular area in an eye with neovascularization. A macular thickening with the central subretinal hyporreflective edema, blurred hyperreflective subretinal tissue, and focal elevation of rough, wavy, and thickened retinal pigment epithelium is shown. Hyperreflective spots which are indicative of cholesterolosis, and hyperreflective posterior hyaloid membrane are seen in the vitreous. (B) Retinal thickness map shows a most of segments colored in blue representing the thinner retina, but the center is colored in yellow indicating the central macular thickening.

of their study. Shortly after that, many researchers started intravitreal administration of this drug. One more reason for intravitreal administration of this drug was the evidence on bevacizumab systemic side effects with high-dose administration in cancer patients who experienced complications such as gastrointestinal perforations, neutropenia, and an increased risk of fatal hemorrhage. In accordance with this evidence, the researchers recommend intravitreal administration in the treatment of ophthalmic diseases, although the applied doses are significantly lower. The studies investigated that the incidence of severe side effects of bevacizumab intravitreal administration showed low rates of adverse side effects and no significant systemic risk of this drug administration. The beneficial effects of bevacizumab have been reported in a wide range of ophthalmic diseases. A study has recently

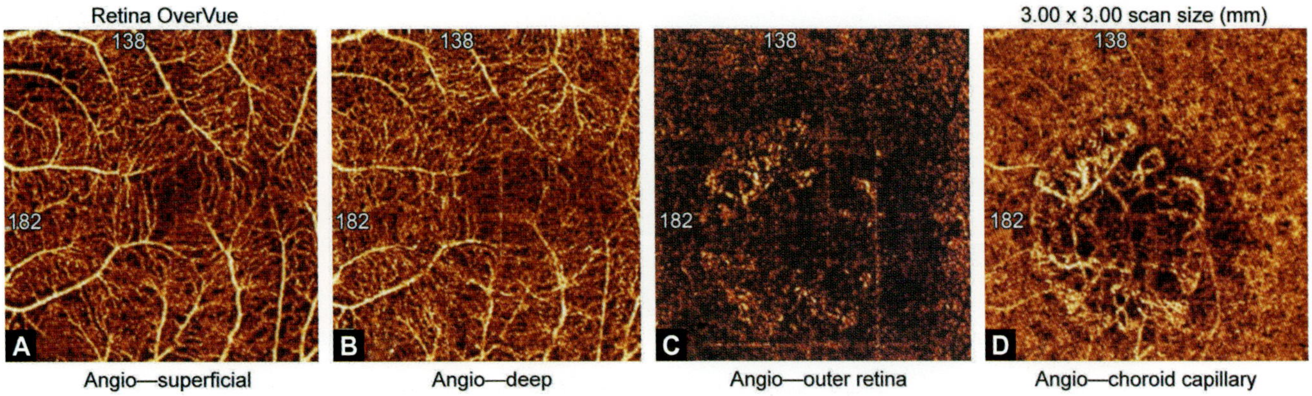

Figs. 2.16A to D: The optical coherence tomography angiography split spectrum amplitude decorrelation angiography imaging protocol of the same eye as in Figure 2.15 (3 × 3 mm). Superficial and deep vascular networks do not show significant vascular changes. A wide, branched and blossomed choroidal neovascularization (CNV) is in the form of a bicycle-wheel pattern can be visualized in the outer retina and even more clearly in the choroidal layer. Numerous vascular loops can be seen at the very periphery of the neovascularization as well as a dark halo in some parts around the CNV. AngioAnalytics software is recommended to verify the exact depth of the CNV.

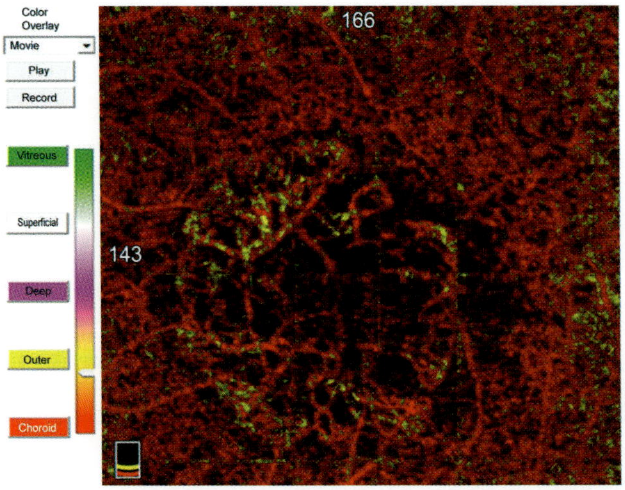

Fig. 2.17: AngioAnalytics software shows the exact depth using a red and yellow colors as markers. If the capillary vessels appear in the outer retina, software automatically marks those with yellow color. A reddish-yellow 'bicycle-wheel' shaped neovascular formation indicating a perforation through the retinal pigment epithelium and proliferation into the outer retina is illustrated. AngioAnalytics clearly demonstrate that it is a type 2 choroidal neovascularization.

been conducted and confirmed that an early intravitreal application of bevacizumab inhibits corneal neovascularization. By examining the effects of intravitreal bevacizumab in patients with diabetic macular edema, an improvement in vision in the treated eye has been confirmed in 55% of patients. The administration of this drug statistically significantly decreases the central macular thickness in an edema caused by branch retinal vein occlusion. A significantly better outcome in patients with proliferative diabetic retinopathy has also been proved in the cases when an intravitreal injection of bevacizumab is applied prior to panretinal laser photocoagulation. A recent study conducted in Serbia showed that intravitreal administration of this drug effectively blocks pathophysiological process of neovascularization in patients with ARMD. After the patients with ARMD were stratified into classical, minimally classical, and occult type, the authors demonstrated that after intravitreal bevacizumab injection in patients with classical and minimally classical type, a statistically significant improvement of corrected visual acuity was observed after 4–6 weeks.

The results of a great number of studies published so far have shown on experimental and electrophysiological tests on humans and animals that intravitreal administration of bevacizumab manifests positive effects in many ophthalmic diseases, no retinal toxicity, and no serious systemic or ocular adverse events were encountered. Another advantage for this drug is its cost-effectiveness.

Ranibizumab (Lucentis®)

Ranibizumab is fragmented humanized recombinant monoclonal antibody produced in *Escherichia coli* cells by recombinant DNA technology. This drug has the same mechanism of action as bevacizumab meaning that it binds with high affinity to the VEGF-A isoforms. Thus,

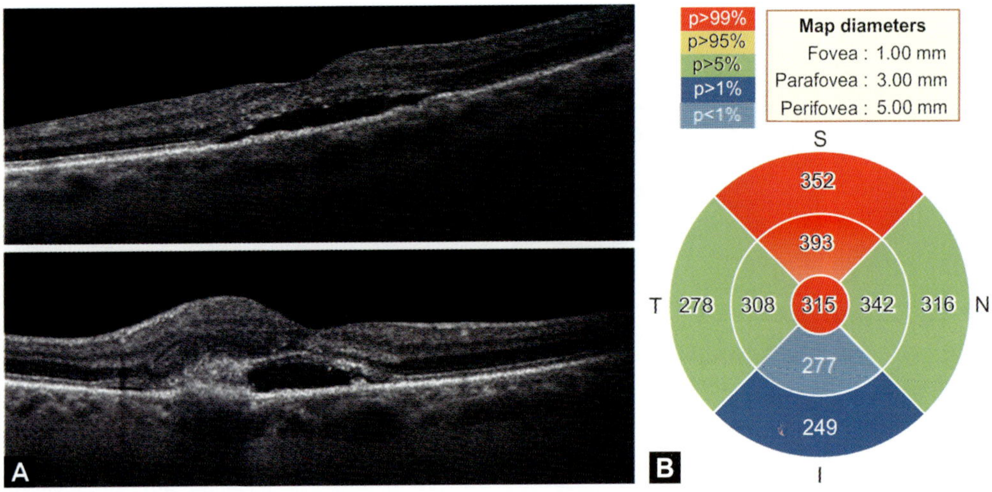

Figs. 2.18A and B: (A) An optical coherence tomography B-scan of the macular area in a patient with wet form of age-related macular degeneration. Scan shows a sensory retinal detachment and hyperreflective subretinal tissue on the very edge of sensory detachment. Retinal pigment epithelium is irregular, thickened in places, as well as perforated on the same place where the hyperreflective tissue is. (B) Retinal thickness map shows the thickening centrally and in the superior area, while the thinning in inferior area. Nasal and temporal parts correspond to the physiological finding.

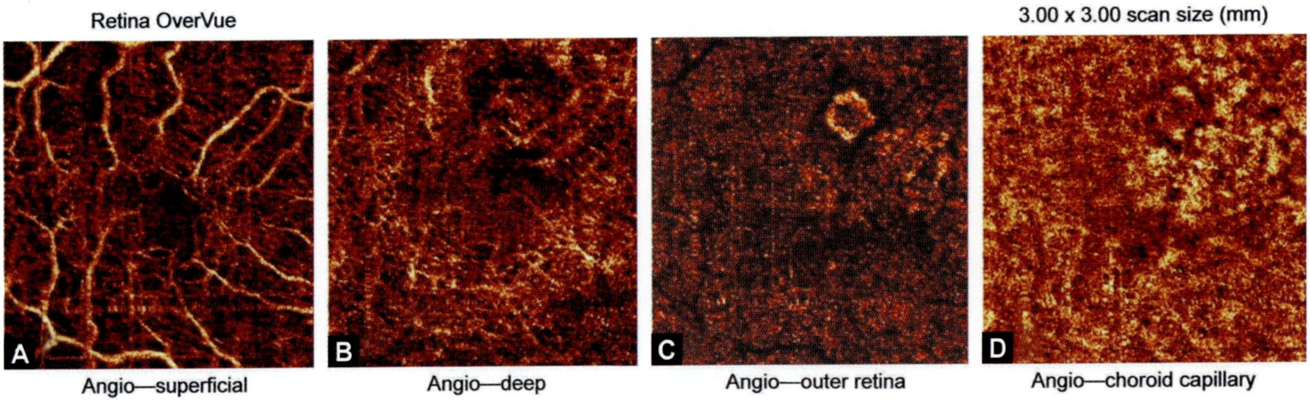

Figs. 2.19A to D: The optical coherence tomography angiography split spectrum amplitude decorrelation angiography (SSADA) imaging protocol of the same eye as in the Figs. 2.18A and B (3 × 3 mm). A superficial and deep vascular plexuses show a sclerotic changes in capillaries, along with the slightly changed foveal avascular zone (FAZ). Vascular dropouts can be seen around the FAZ. A small, rounded neovascularization with sharp margins, which perforated the retinal pigment epithelium, can be seen in the outer retinal layer [type 2 choroidal neovascularization (CNV)], while a significantly larger, densely branched, blossomed vascular structure is present in the choroidal layer (type 1 CNV). Findings indicate the presence of the mixed neovascularization (type 4 CNV).

binding of VEGF-A to its receptors VEGFR1 and VEGFR2 is prevented. The application of this drug was approved in 2005 for the treatment of subretinal neovascularization in ARMD. Unlike bevacizumab, its molecular weight is significantly lower (49 kDa) and it has a shorter half-life. As an antibody fragment characterized by low molecular mass, this drug can penetrate all retinal layers and reach the target tissue. On molar basis, ranibizumab is 5–20-fold a more potent drug than bevacizumab. Since it competitively inhibits VEGF-A in the extracellular space in all retinal layers, its application is indicated for the treatment of many diseases such as ARMD, diabetic retinopathy, retinal vein occlusion, diabetic macular edema, choroidal neovascularization in pathologic myopia, and many others. The studies that investigated the incidence of serious harmful effects after its intravitreal application showed

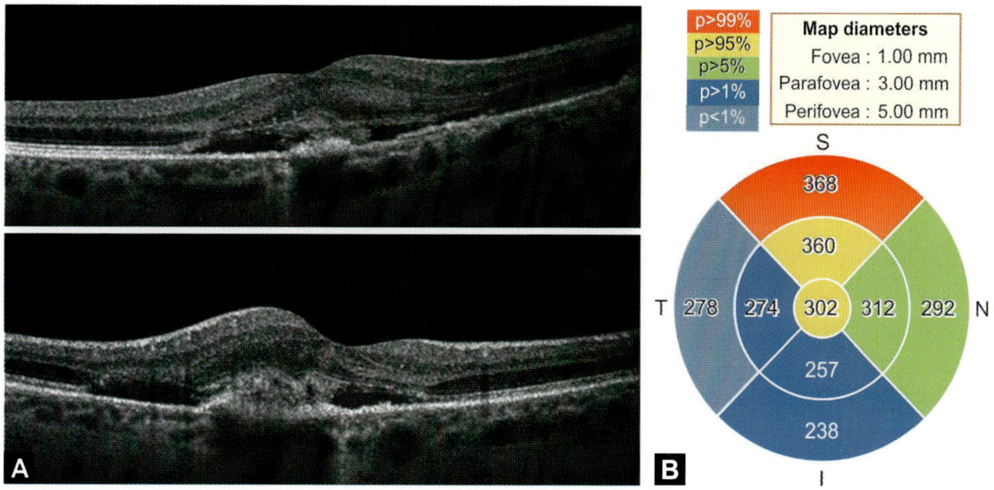

Figs. 2.20A and B: An optical coherence tomography B-scan and retinal thickness map of the same eye as in Figures. 2.19A and B, scanned a day after the second intravitreal aflibercept injection. A shallower subretinal edema can be observed along with the clearly limited hyperreflective subretinal tissue and perforated retinal pigment epithelium. Retinal thickness map reveals decreased thickness values in the central and superior parts comparing to the ones before therapy.

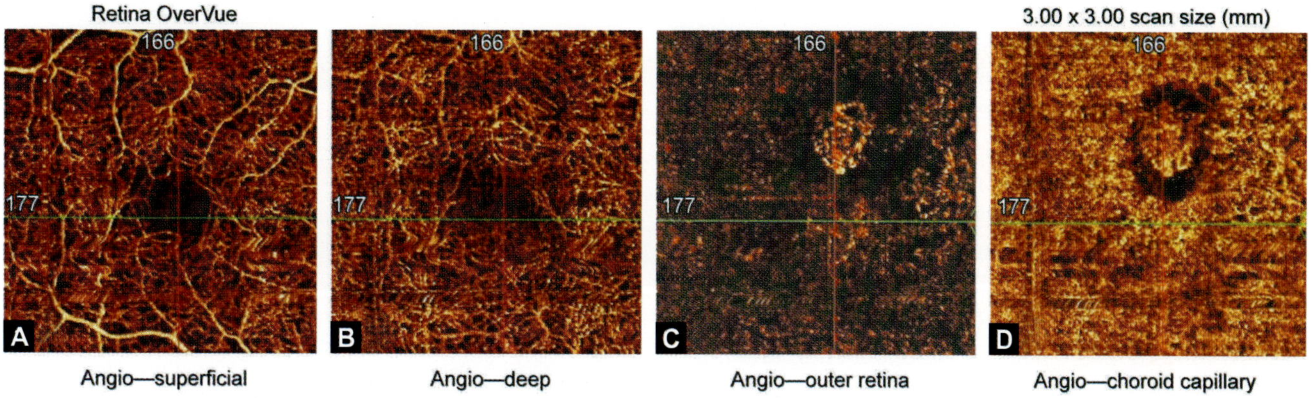

Figs. 2.21A to D: The optical coherence tomography angiography split spectrum amplitude decorrelation angiography imaging protocol of the same eye as in Figs 2.20A and B, scanned a day after the second intravitreal aflibercept injection. Superficial and deep vascular plexuses show no significant changes, but in the outer retina clearly bounded choroidal neovascularization (CNV) is shown. The same vascular structure is seen in the deep choroid. In both angiograms, a black halo which surrounds the neovascularization, is observed. Blossoming type 1 CNV cannot be visualized anymore, so now it is a clear type 2 neovascularization. Neovascularization becomes inactive due to the formation of a dark halo zone around it, and loss of tiny little capillaries inside itself. Of course, this patient is recommended for the third intravitreal anti-vascular endothelial growth factor injection.

that they occur rarely, and there is no significant systemic risk associated with this drug application. On the other hand, its benefits are numerous.

A great number of studies published so far showed that the intravitreal application of ranibizumab statistically significantly improves visual acuity, or results in its stabilization in a huge percentage in patients with ARMD. It has also been proved that intravitreal administration of ranibizumab, in the follow-up period of 2 years prevents vision loss and leads to visual acuity improvement in patients with minimally classical or occult choroidal neovascularization in ARMD. During 1-year follow-up it has also been proved that intravitreal application of ranibizumab with a rapid or delayed laser application was significantly a more efficient treatment modality in comparison to laser monotherapy without ranibizumab injection in the treatment of diabetic macular edema. Application of ranibizumab in combination with verteporfin photodynamic therapy in the period of 6 months achieves complete regression of polyps in patients with polypoidal choroidal vasculopathy. Intraocular ranibizumab injection is effective in the treatment of macular edema following branch retinal vein occlusion.

Although proved to be a very effective drug for lots of ophthalmic diseases, a disadvantage of ranibizumab is that it is significantly more costly than bevacizumab.

Aflibercept (Eylea®)

Aflibercept is a relatively new drug for neovascular ARMD approved by the FDA in 2011 known in the scientific literature as *VEGF-trap*. It is a fusion protein with a molecular weight of 115 kDa. Unlike ranibizumab and bevacizumab, aflibercept binds VEGF-A, VEGF-B, and placenta growth factor that is believed to play an important role in the neovascular ARMD progression. Aflibercept neutralizes biological activities mediated by VEGF including retinal and choroidal neovascularization, thus potentially decreasing retinal edema, subretinal fluid, and hemorrhages. Considering the fact that aflibercept has a significantly higher binding affinity for VEGF, prolonged therapeutic effects of a drug in the eye, and prolonged intervals between two treatments are potentially possible. The advantage of fewer treatments is beneficial because patients are less likely to experience side effects associated with intravitreal injection application. It is essential to mention that aflibercept has low immunogenic potential due to its human amino acid sequences content.

Significant results of the application of this drug were first evidenced in ARMD therapy, then in other ophthalmic diseases accompanied by the retinal vascular changes. By monitoring the effects of aflibercept intravitreal injection in exudative ARMD, it has been shown that visual acuity is significantly better and stabilized in majority of patients, and that there is not a statistically significant difference between aflibercept and ranibizumab effects. A study that monitored the efficacy of neovascular age-related degeneration by using aflibercept in patients who had previously been treated with bevacizumab and/or ranibizumab concluded that aflibercept is an alternative drug for patients previously treated with aforementioned drugs. Aflibercept therapy managed to solve the problem of persistent exudative fluid accumulation that could not be removed with the application of bevacizumab and/or ranibizumab. The results obtained in this group of patients showed statistically significant improvement of the best corrected visual acuity and visual acuity stability, significant decrease in central foveal thickness as well as a decrease in macular volume as seen on the OCT scan. Similar results were obtained after the application of aflibercept therapy in patients with diabetic macular edema.

SUGGESTED READING

1. Amadio M, Govoni S, Pascale A. Targeting VEGF in eye neovascularization: What's new?: A comprehensive review on current therapies and oligonucleotide-based interventions under development. Pharmacol Res. 2016;103:253-69.
2. Boyer DS, Hopkins JJ, Sorof J, et al. Anti-vascular endothelial growth factor therapy for diabetic macular edema. Ther Adv Endocrinol Metab. 2013;4(6):151-69.
3. Brown DM, Campochiaro PA, Bhisitkul RB, et al. Sustained benefits from ranibizumab for macular edema following branch retinal vein occlusion: 12-month outcomes of a phase III study. Ophthalmology. 2011;118(8):1594-602.
4. Castillo MM, Mowatt G, Elders A, et al. Optical coherence tomography for the monitoring of neovascular age-related macular degeneration: a Systematic Review. Ophthalmology. 2015;122(2):399-406.
5. Chan CK, Jain A, Sadda S, et al. Optical coherence tomographic and visual results at six months after transitioning to aflibercept for patients on prior ranibizumab or bevacizumab treatment for exudative age-related macular degeneration (an American Ophthalmological Society thesis). Trans Am Ophthalmol Soc. 2014;112:160-98.
6. Chawla R, Mittal K, Vohra R. Optical coherence tomography angiography study of choroidal neovascularization associated with focal choroidal excavation. Ophthalmic Surg Lasers Imaging Retina. 2016;47(10):969-71.
7. Chen WL, Chen YM, Chu HS, et al. Mechanisms controlling the effects of bevacizumab (avastin) on the inhibition of early but not late formed corneal neovascularization. PLoS One. 2014;9(4):e94205.
8. Costanzo E, Miere A, Querques G, et al. Type-1choroidal neovascularization lesion size: indocyanine green angiography versus optical coherence tomography angiography. Invest Ophthalmol Vis Sci. 2016;57(9):OCT307-13.
9. Fong AH, Lai TY. Long-term effectiveness of ranibizumab for age-related macular degeneration and diabetic macular edema. Clin Interv Aging. 2013;8:467-83.
10. Gerding H, Monés J, Tadayoni R, et al. Ranibizumab in retinal vein occlusion: treatment recommendations by an expert panel. Br J Ophthalmol. 2015;99(3):297-304.
11. Heier JS, Campochiaro PA, Yau L, et al. Ranibizumab for macular edema due to retinal vein occlusions: long-term follow-up in the HORIZON trial. Ophthalmology. 2012;119(4):802-9.

12. Ho VY, Yeh S, Olsen TW, et al. Short-term outcomes of aflibercept for neovascular age-related macular degeneration in eyes previously treated with other vascular endothelial growth factor inhibitors. Am J Ophthalmol. 2013;156(1):23-28.
13. Homayouni M. Vascular endothelial growth factors and their inhibitors in ocular neovascular disorders. J Ophthalmic Vis Res. 2009;4(2):105-14.
14. Karadžić J, Kovačević I, Ljikar J, et al. Pharmacological intravitreal treatment for macular edema in branch retinal vein occlusion - three-month results. Med Pregl. 2015;68(9-10):295-300.
15. Kim LA, D'Amore PA. A brief history of anti-VEGF for the treatment of ocular angiogenesis. Am J Pathol. 2012;181(2):376-9.
16. Koh A, Lee WK, Chen LJ, et al. EVEREST study: efficacy and safety of verteporfin photodynamic therapy in combination with ranibizumab or alone versus ranibizumab monotherapy in patients with symptomatic macular polypoidal choroidal vasculopathy. Retina. 2012;32(8):1453-64.
17. Kuehlewein L, Bansal M, Lenis TL, et al. Optical coherence tomography angiography of type 1 neovascularization in age-related macular degeneration. Am J Ophthalmol. 2015;160(4):739-48.
18. Lee J, Rosen R. Optical coherence tomography angiography in diabetes. Curr Diab Rep. 2016;16(12):123.
19. Major JC Jr, Wykoff CC, Mariani AF, et al. Comparison of spectral-domain and time-domain optical coherence tomography in the detection of neovascular age-related macular degeneration activity. Retina. 2014;34(1):48-54.
20. Malihi M, Jia Y, Gao SS, et al. Optical coherence tomographic angiography of choroidal neovascularization ill-defined with fluorescein angiography. Br J Ophthalmol. 2017;101(1):45-50.
21. Mastropasqua R, Di Antonio L, Di Staso S, et al. Optical coherence tomography angiography in retinal vascular diseases and choroidal neovascularization. J Ophthalmol. 2015;2015:343515.
22. Mavija M. Šta je novo u liječenju senilne makularne degeneracije. Acta Ophthalmologica. 2014;40(2):29-40.
23. Michels S, Rosenfeld PJ, Puliafito CA, et al. Systemic bevacizumab (Avastin) therapy for neovascular age-related macular degeneration twelve-week results of an uncontrolled open-label clinical study. Ophthalmology. 2005;112:1035-47.
24. Nakao S, Kaizu Y, Oshima Y, et al. Optical coherence tomography angiography for detecting choroidal neovascularization secondary to punctate inner choroidopathy. Ophthalmic Surg Lasers Imaging Retina. 2016;47(12):1157-161.
25. Novais EA, Adhi M, Moult EM, et al. Choroidal neovascularization analyzed on ultrahigh-speed swept-source optical coherence tomography angiography compared to spectral-domain optical coherence tomography angiography. Am J Ophthalmol. 2016;164:80-8.
26. Regatieri CV, Branchini L, Duker JS. The role of spectral-domain OCT in the diagnosis and management of neovascular age-related macular degeneration. Ophthalmic Surg Lasers Imaging. 2011;42(Suppl):S56-66.
27. Risimić DS. Primena VEGF inhibitora u oftalmologiji. Zbornik radova i sažetaka, II Kongres oftalmologa Bosne i Hercegovine, Banja Luka, Maj 2012. Str: 132-135.
28. Risimić DS. Uticaj intravitrealne terapije inhibitorima angiogeneze na funkcionalni nalaz kod različitih tipova subretinalne neovaskularne membrane. Zbornik radova i sažetaka, I Kongres oftalmologa Republike Srpske, Bijeljina, Maj 2015. Str: 95-100.
29. Sarwar S, Clearfield E, Soliman MK, et al. Aflibercept for neovascular age-related macular degeneration. Cochrane Database Syst Rev. 2016;2:CD011346.
30. Schachat AP, Thompson JT. Optical coherence tomography, fluorescein angiography, and the management of neovascular age-related macular degeneration. Ophthalmology. 2015;122(2):222-3.
31. Shahzad R, Siddiqui MA. Choroidal neovascularization secondary to best vitelliform macular dystrophy detected by optical coherence tomography angiography. J AAPOS. 2017;21(1):68-70.
32. Sulzbacher F, Kiss C, Munk M, et al. Diagnostic evaluation of type 2 (classic) choroidal neovascularization: optical coherence tomography, indocyanine green angiography, and fluorescein angiography. Am J Ophthalmol. 2011;152(5):799-806.
33. Sulzbacher F, Pollreisz A, Kaider A, et al. Identification and clinical role of choroidal neovascularization characteristics based on optical coherence tomography angiography. Acta Ophthalmol. 2017;95(4):414-20.
34. Takahashi H, Shibuya M. The vascular endothelial growth factor (VEGF)/VEGF receptor system and its role under physiological and pathological conditions. Clin Sci (Lond). 2005;109(3):227-41.
35. Tan AC, Dansingani KK, Yannuzzi LA, et al. Type 3 neovascularization imaged with cross-sectional and en face optical coherence tomography angiography. Retina. 2017;37(2):234-46.
36. Torrecillas-Picazo R, Cerdà-Ibáñez M, Almor Palacios I, et al. Analysis and follow-up of type 1 choroidal neovascularisation with optical coherence tomography-angiography after antiangiogenic treatment. Arch Soc Esp Oftalmol. 2017; 92(6):265-72.
37. Varma P, Walia S. Bevacizumab (Avastin) for ocular disorders. IJPR. 2013;3(4):59-68.

CHAPTER 3

Dry Age-related Macular Degeneration

INTRODUCTION

Age-related macular degeneration (ARMD) is a bilateral, but asymmetric degenerative disease of the macula causing loss of central vision. There are two basic types of macular degeneration--nonexudative (dry form) and exudative (wet form). Vision loss in the dry form of ARMD happens slowly, occurring over several years or decades, while in the exudative form of ARMD, vision loss occurs considerably faster over the course of a few months. In the last stage of the disease, there is an absolute central scotoma, while the peripheral vision is preserved. Recently, great progress has been made in gene discovery and mechanistic studies which clearly indicate that ARMD involves the interaction of multiple genetic and environmental factors.

Dry ARMD is associated with drusen and/or retinal pigment epithelium (RPE) abnormalities, possible pigment epithelial detachment (PED), and often progresses to geographic macular atrophy.

EPIDEMIOLOGY AND ETIOLOGY

Age-related macular degeneration is the leading cause of visual impairment in the elderly patients across developed countries and the third leading cause of global blindness. The prevalence of ARMD has been reported across a range of populations and measures as high as 25% for the over 75-year age group.

The etiology and pathogenesis of ARMD are incompletely defined. The identification of genes that have a substantial impact on the risk for ARMD is not only facilitating the diagnosis and screening of populations at risk but is also elucidating key molecular pathways of pathogenesis. At the beginning of the disease, lipids are deposited below the Bruch's membrane and visible drusen start to form. At the same time, Bruch's membrane thickens, the elastin and collagen within it degenerate and calcify, while the accumulation of exogenous proteins and lipids takes place. Consequently, photoreceptors start to damage and loss of vision acuity happens.

SYMPTOMS AND SIGNS

The disease is characterized by a gradual, moderate decrease of vision acuity over several months or years. Signs and symptoms of dry ARMD include difficulty with night and color vision and with changing light conditions (specifically changes in Amsler grid self-evaluation), difficulty with reading and making out faces and metamorphopsia. In the case of geographic atrophy, slow but certain loss of vision may be more pronounced (absolute central scotoma) than with the exudative form of ARMD.

Drusen are usually the earliest clinical sign which can be most often seen on the posterior pole, although they can be found on all parts of the retina. They are clinically seen as yellowish-white deposits located deep in the retina between Bruch's membrane and the RPE. By size, drusen are divided into small (<63 μm), intermediate (63–125 μm) and large (>125 μm) drusen.

Hard drusen are small and round with very sharp borders often seen in perfectly healthy eyes and they do not increase the risk for neovascular ARMD. These well-defined deposits are light yellow and thought to be less harmful. They become more common with age and may or may not indicate the early development of ARMD.

Soft drusen are intermediate and large. Their edges are not as clearly defined as hard drusen. Soft drusen have a tendency to cluster and merge with one another demonstrating confluence. This soft type of drusen increases the risk for the occurrence and progression of the neovascular ARMD. Patients who have soft drusen will often have more serious changes in vision than those who have only hard drusen. Drusen, by themselves, do not cause damage to central vision. However, patients may have slightly impaired contrast sensitivity, metamorphosis and difficulty in adapting to light and darkness. One of the main complaints is difficulty in reading. A smudge or blurry spot may appear in the center of their vision field.

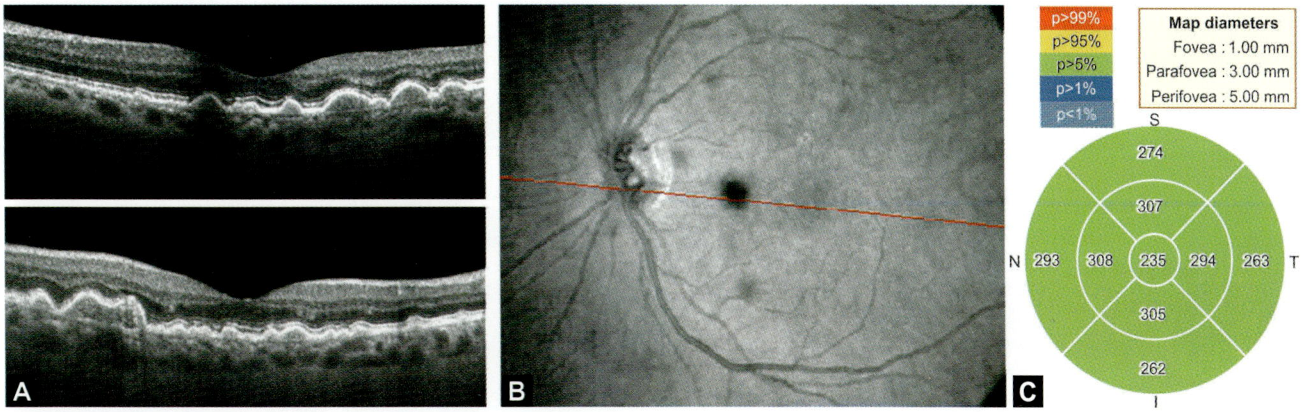

Figs. 3.1A to C: (A) An optical coherence tomography (OCT) B-scan of the macula in a 70-year-old male patient with ARMD. The image demonstrates confluent drusen between the RPE and Bruch's membrane which cause small protrusions and give a characteristic wavy appearance of RPE at OCT B-scan. Irregular and wavy RPE is visible in the whole central part of retina; (B) Shows a fundus photography with an optic disc and large retinal blood vessels, a small dark area of the macula and between these two areas––a dark dot which corresponds to vitreous opacities; and (C) Presents a retinal thickness map which shows the numerical values in the physiological range (green color in all segments of the map). (RPE: retinal pigment epithelium; ARMD: age-related macular degeneration)

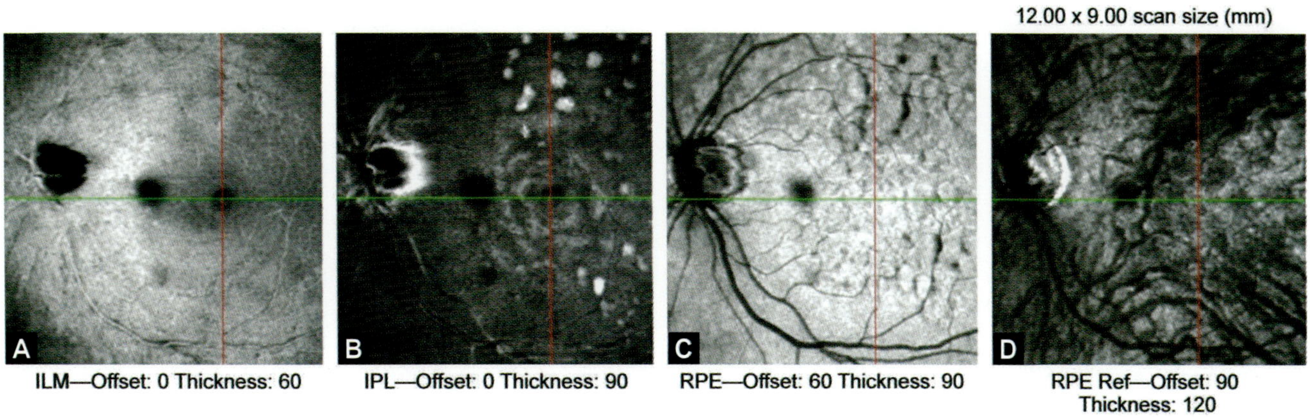

Figs. 3.2A to D: En face OCT of the corresponding retinal layers of the same eye as depicted in the Figure 3.1 (12 × 9 mm). (A) Superficial part of the inner retina which corresponds to the fundus photography in Figure 3.1B; (B) Deep part of the inner retina with sharply bounded hyperreflective areas, irregularly scattered on the retina, and circular changes of paramacular area corresponding to changes in the outer part of the retina and the choroidal part; and (C) Shows the outer part of the retina and choroid (D) with granulated and lobular changes of the whole posterior pole. The dark dot between the macula and the optic disc in all retinal layers corresponds to vitreous opacities.

Geographical atrophy is clinically manifested as areas of hypopigmentation or depigmentation of the RPE and indicates the regions of the outer retina loss. Firstly, small and discrete areas occur, and they merge with each other over the time. Visual acuity can be significantly damaged if changes include the foveal area. Atrophy is most commonly found in the areas of the first drusen appearances.

DIFFERENTIAL DIAGNOSIS

- Neovascular ARMD
- Pattern dystrophy
- Vitelliform macular dystrophy
- Stargardt disease
- Toxic maculopathy or drug-induced maculopathy (Chloroquine derivatives, phenothiazine, canthaxanthin)
- Multifocal choroiditis
- Macular telangiectasia type 2.

DIAGNOSTICS

Age-related macular degeneration is diagnosed by a clinical examination of the macula, fundus photography, fundus autofluorescence (FAF), optical coherence tomography (OCT), fluorescein angiography (FA) and optical coherence tomography angiography (OCTA).

Funduscopic examination in patients with suspected ARMD includes drusen or geographic atrophy. The color fundus photography also shows the drusen, changes in RPE and geographic atrophy. OCT is the current gold standard for the diagnosis of ARMD. The drusen are seen as small deposits below the Bruch's membrane. OCT shows geographic atrophy as the absence and change of outer retinal layers. The absence of subretinal and/or intraretinal fluids is the leading sign demonstrating that dry macular degeneration does not turn into a very serious wet form of the ARMD. Fluorescein angiography (FAG) can be used to confirm the diagnosis, or determine and

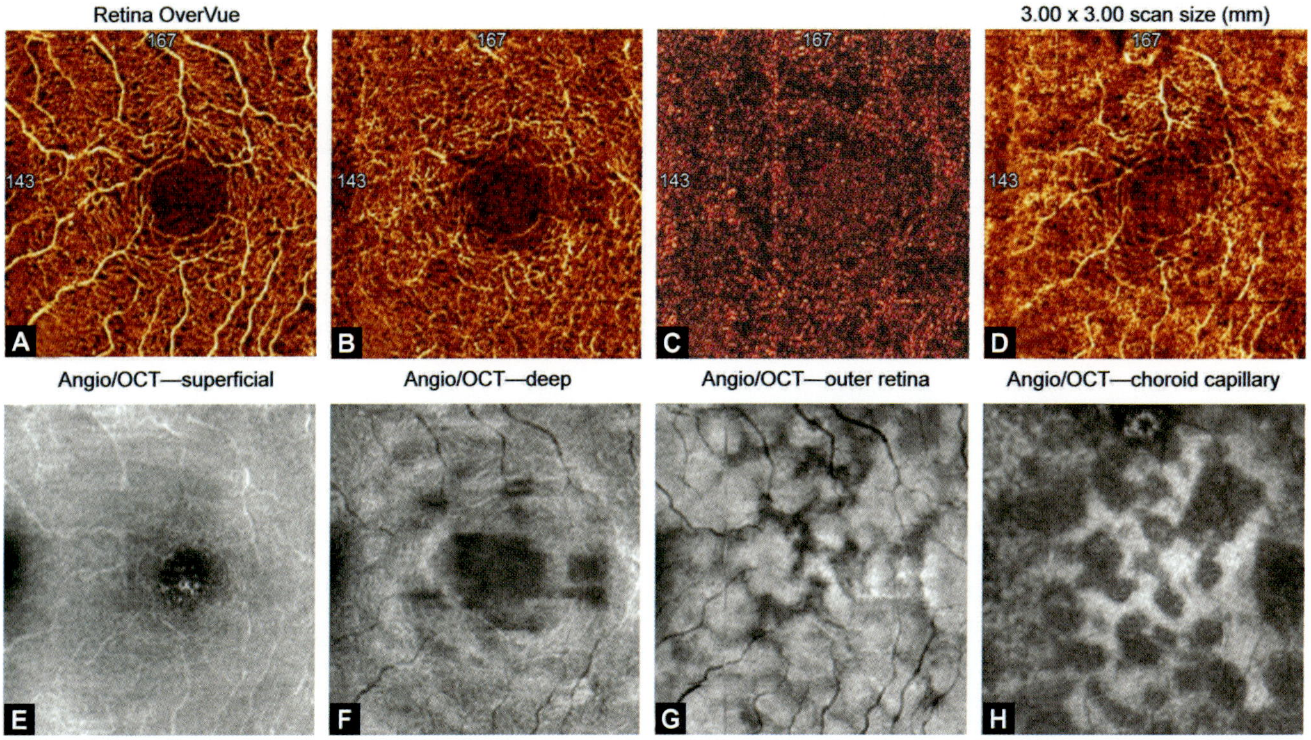

Figs. 3.3A to H: An OCTA SSADA protocol of retinal layers (3 × 3 mm) along with en face OCTs, the same eye as depicted in Figures 3.1 and 3.2. (A and B) Showing en face angiograms of superficial and deep vascular plexus which are regular and correspond to the age of the patient. The FAZ is regular in size and shape; (C) The outer retina is dark without neovascularization; (D) The choroidal part shows a network that looks a lot like superficial one. Granulated and lobular shape of the choroid is lost. The CNV is not visible, and that indicates the dry form of ARMD; and (E to H) Showing en face OCT of the corresponding retinal layers of the same eye. The outer retina and choriocapillaris show typical changes which correspond to the dry ARMD. Visible hyporeflective areas that look like a leopard pattern are dense and confluent in the choroidea. (FAZ: foveal avascular zone; ARMD: age-related macular degeneration; OCT: optical coherence tomography; OCTA: optical coherence tomography angiography; CNV: choroidal neovascularization)

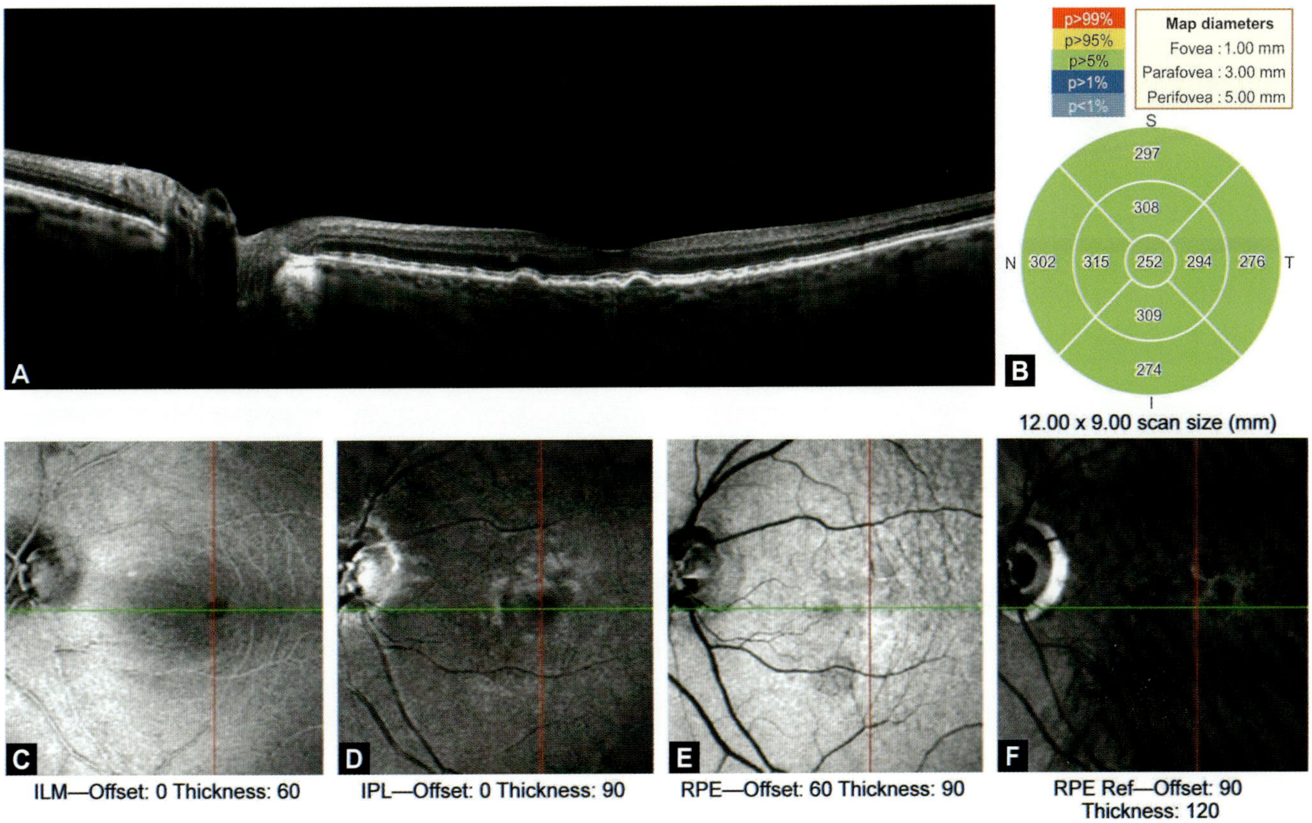

Figs. 3.4A to F: (A) An optical coherence tomography (OCT) B scan of the macula and optic disc in a 68-year-old female patient with the dry form of age-related macular degeneration. The image demonstrates the drusen between RPE and the Bruch's membrane of the macula. The separation of hyperreflective posterior hyaloid membrane is also visible; (B) The retinal thickness map shows the numerical values in the physiological range; and (C to F) Showing en face OCT images of the same eye (12 × 9 mm). The macula and optic disc are visible in all retinal layers. The superficial part of the inner retina seems regular, while paramacular changes can be seen in the deep part of the inner retina as well as in the outer retina and choroid.

prove the existence of choroidal neovascularization. In dry form of ARMD, there is no visible leak in the late phase.

Optical coherence tomography angiography is a new, noninvasive method for easier and faster diagnosing of the absence of neovascularization, but is also irreplaceable in monitoring the disease and in treatment follow-up (*see* Figs. 3.1 to 3.5).

THERAPY

There is no clearly defined treatment for dry ARMD. Recommendations for patients include avoiding or quitting the smoking, using glasses with ultraviolet protection, regular physical activity, maintaining an ideal body weight, natural hygiene diet with antioxidant vitamin and mineral supplements (lutein, zinc, copper and omega-3 fatty acids). Controlling diabetes, hypertension and lipid profile are very important. Ophthalmic studies [Age-related Eye Disease Study (AREDS) and Age-related Eye Disease Study 2 (AREDS2)] show that supplements--vitamin C (500 mg), vitamin E (400 IJ), zinc oxide (80 mg), copper oxide (2 mg), lutein (10 mg) and zeaxanthin (2 mg)--reduce the risk of the progression of the advanced form of dry ARMD and/or occurrence of the neovascularization in 25% of patients with ARMD within 5 years. Depending on the development and complications of the disease, ophthalmological examination is recommended every 3–12 months. There is a long tradition of recommending self-testing by means of the plain Amsler metamorphopsia grids. The decrease in vision acuity and metamorphopsia are often one of the clinical signs of a transition taking place from the dry form to the neovascular, wet form of ARMD.

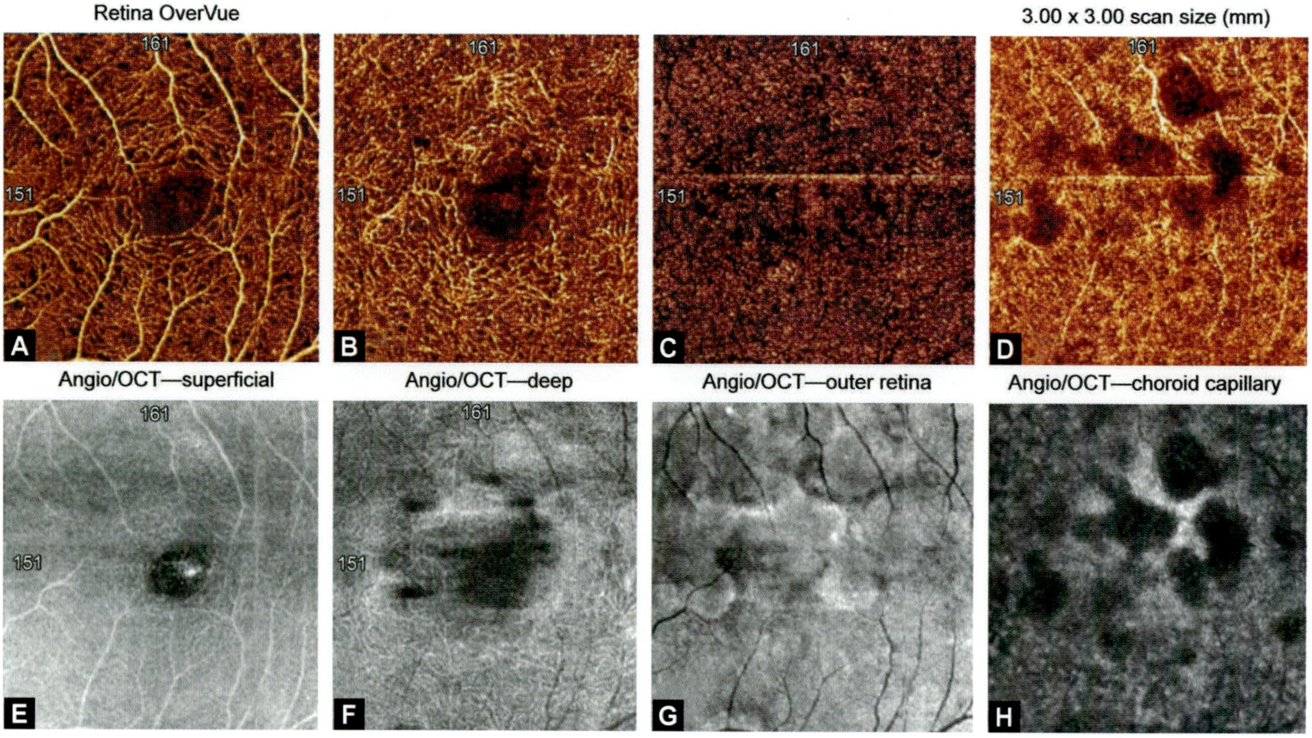

Figs. 3.5A to H: An OCTA SSADA protocol (3 × 3 mm) and en face OCT of the corresponding retinal layers of the same eye as depicted in Figure 3.4. (A and B) Showing en face angiograms of superficial and deep vascular plexus with no pathological changes; (C and D) In the outer retina and especially in the choroidal part (D), dark 'drop out' areas varying from small to big in size which correspond to an atrophy are visible. The neovascularization is not visible; and (E to H) Showing en face OCT of the corresponding retinal layers. In the deep part of the inner retina, hyporeflective central areas which correspond to FAZ are visible as small, surrounding, suspected cystic forms. Typical dark areas which form a leopard pattern are visible in the choroidal part. (FAZ: foveal avascular zone; OCT: optical coherence tomography; OCTA: optical coherence tomography angiography)

BIBLIOGRAPHY

1. Age-Related Eye Disease Study 2 Research Group. Lutein + zeaxanthin and omega-3 fatty acids for age-related macular degeneration; the Age-Related Eye Disease Study 2 (AREDS) randomised clinical trial. JAMA. 2013;309(19):2005-15.
2. Bird AC. Therapeutic targets in age-related macular disease. J Clin Invest. 2010;120(9):3033-41.
3. Ferris FL III, Wilkinson CP, Bird A, et al. Clinical classification of age-related macular degeneration. Ophthalmology. 2013;120(4):844-51.
4. Ferris FL, Davis MD, Clemons TE, et al. A simplified severity scale for age-related macular degenerations: AREDS Report No.18. Arch Ophthalmol. 2005;123(11):1570-74.
5. Klein R, Cruickshanks KJ, Nash SD. The prevalence of age-related macular degeneration and associated risk factors. Arch Ophthalmol. 2010;128(6):750-8.
6. Kuno N, Fujii S. Dry age-related macular degeneration: recent progress of therapeutic approaches. Curr Mol Pharmacol. 2011;4(3):196-232.
7. Nagiel A, Sadda SR, Sarraf D. A promising future for optical coherence tomography angiography. JAMA Ophthalmol. 2015;133(6):629-30.
8. Puliafito CA. OCT angiography: the next era of OCT technology emerges. Ophthalmic Surg Lasers Imaging Retina. 2014;45(5):360.
9. Yanoff M, Duker JS. Ophthalmology. 3rd edition. London: Mosby Elsevier Publishers; 2009.

CHAPTER 4

Neovascular/Exudative/Wet Age-related Macular Degeneration

INTRODUCTION

Age-related macular degeneration (ARMD) is a condition characterized by the appearance of pathological neovascular membrane arising from choriocapillaris. ARMD is the leading cause of blindness in the elderly population, aged 65 years and above.

EPIDEMIOLOGY AND ETIOLOGY

The growth of choroidal neovascular membrane (CNV) is the leading cause of vision loss in the elderly population in developed countries. Although appearance of the wet form of ARMD is quite rare (10% of the total number of patients), this form of disease causes blindness in 90% of the affected population. The pathophysiological mechanism of disease is still quite unclear. The mechanism by which dry and slow progressive macular degeneration turns into a wet neovascular form is not yet fully explored. Clinical signs such as confluent drusen, large soft drusen and focal hyperpigmentation of retinal pigment epithelium (RPE) may be risk factors which cause slowly progressive dry macular degeneration to turn into a very serious form of disease with very poor prognosis. The disease is usually bilateral, although both eyes are not always equally affected. In developed countries in 2011, a total of 200,000 patients with severe visual impairment due to the wet form of ARMD were registered. It is estimated that the number of patients with severe and permanent vision impairment due to the wet form of ARMD will reach up to 500,000 by 2030.

SYMPTOMS AND SIGNS

The patient has decreased visual acuity in one or both eyes, distorted vision (metamorphopsia) and sometimes photopsy, central scotoma or difficulties in adaptation to darkness. Fundus examination can reveal subretinal and intraretinal accumulation of fluid; retinal, subretinal or sub-RPE bleedings; lipid exudates or greyish-green membranous formation in the foveal area. RPE detachment can also be present.

DIFFERENTIAL DIAGNOSIS

- Central serous chorioretinopathy (CSCR)
- Idiopathic choroidal neovascular membrane
- Myopic choroidal neovascularization
- Best's disease (Vitelliform macular dystrophy)
- Ocular histoplasmosis syndrome (OHS)
- Angioid streaks
- Choroidal rupture
- Other macular dystrophies—North Carolina, Doyne's, Sorsby.

DIAGNOSTICS

Clinical examination can usually detect changes in the fundus in both eyes, although they may be asymmetric. Visual acuity is decreased. The Amsler test helps to diagnose and reveal the appearance of relative central scotoma and distortion of vision. Wet ARMD is always marked by the presence of CNV associated with other clinical manifestations, such as subretinal fluid, subretinal hemorrhage and lipid exudates. Fundus photography is not required for the diagnosis of ARMD, but it is helpful in visualizing the presence of drusen, retinal pigmentary changes, intraretinal and subretinal hemorrhage, as well as CNV. Optical coherence tomography (OCT) and optical coherence tomography angiography (OCTA) are the main diagnostic tools for ARMD. These diagnostic procedures precisely pinpoint the location of the neovascularization. However, OCTA is also irreplaceable in monitoring and in treatment follow up. Fluorescein angiography (FAG) can be used to confirm the diagnosis and determine the type of neovascularization, wherein the late leakage of fluorescein indicates the region with an active CNV (Figs. 4.1 to 4.36).

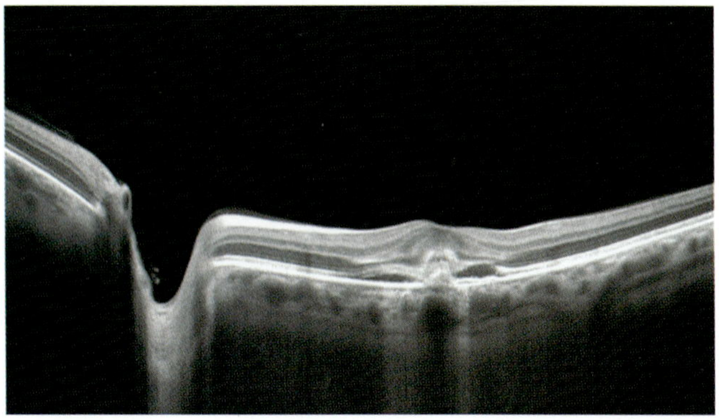

Fig. 4.1: An OCT B-scan of the retina and optic papilla in a 67-year-old male patient. The image demonstrates changes that lift off the macula; subretinal fluid accumulation and hyperreflective tissue cluster in the macular area are highly indicative of the presence of CNV. Posterior vitreous detachment can also be seen above the retina. (CNV: choroidal neovascular membrane; OCT: optical coherence tomography)

THERAPY

Patients with neovascular membrane are treated with intravitreal anti-vascular endothelial growth factor (VEGF) injections. The initiation of ranibizumab treatment in the ANCHOR (Anti-VEGF antibody ranibizumab for the treatment of predominantly classic choroidal neovascularization in age-related macular degeneration) and MARINA (Minimally classic/occult trial of the Anti-VEGF Antibody Ranibizumab in the treatment of Neovascular Age-related macular degeneration) trials resulted in Food and Drug Administration (FDA) approval of ranibizumab in 2006, with clear instructions and protocols for use. The MARINA study was a two-year-long randomized, double-blind study of monthly ranibizumab application in classical or occult CNV caused by the wet form of ARMD. In the group of eyes treated with ranibizumab, visual acuity

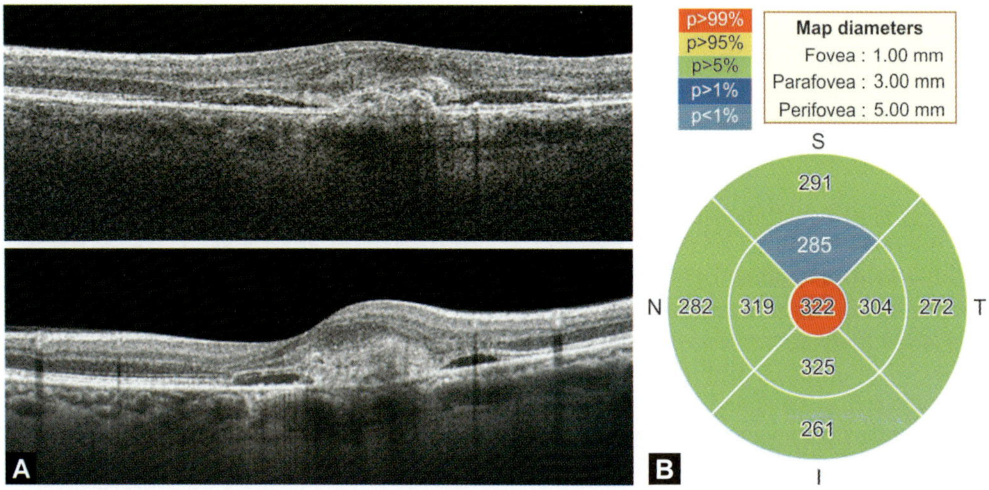

Figs. 4.2A and B: (A) An OCT B-scan of the same eye as in Figure 4.1. Subretinal fluid and hyperreflectivity of the tissue accumulated in macula can be observed more accurately. RPE is accumulated, wavy and interrupted on certain sites. The posterior hyaloid membrane can also be seen; and (B) Retinal map thickness with increased central macular thickness of 322 μm. (RPE: retinal pigment epithelium; OCT: optical coherence tomography)

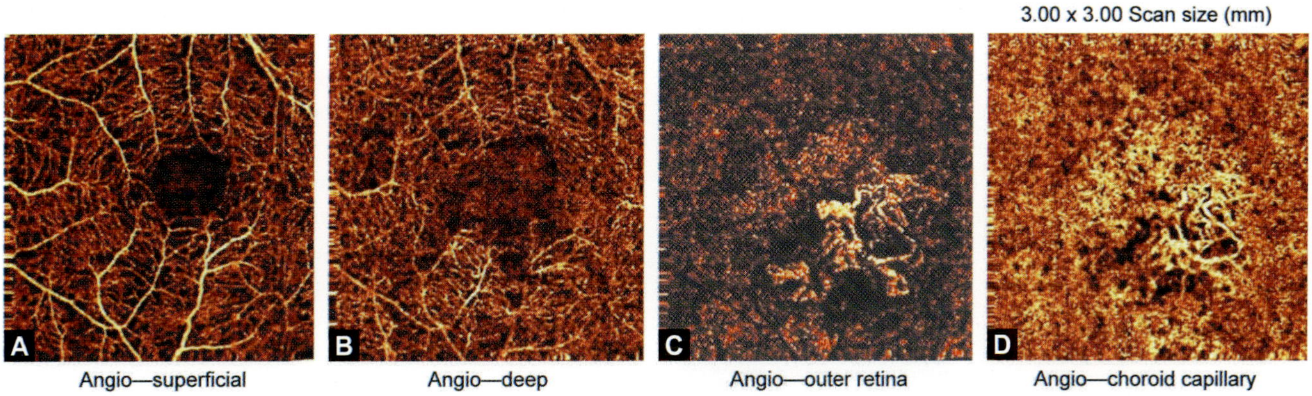

Figs. 4.3A to D: The OCTA SSADA protocol of the same eye as seen in the Figures 4.1 and 4.2 (3 × 3 mm). (A and B) The en face angiogram shows superficial and deep vascular plexus in which a symmetrical, regular and dense network of capillaries can be observed. The FAZ is regular in shape and physiological size in the superficial vascular plexus, while it is slightly increased and irregular in the deep vascular layer; (C) Outer retina reveals an irregular, filamentous, thread-like formation in the macular area, actively expanding into the surrounding tissue. The same neovascular change, although larger, can be observed at the same location in the choriocapillaris; and (D) The described change is CNV type 2, which perforated RPE and is actively spreading into the surrounding retina. (FAZ: foveal avascular zone; OCTA: optical coherence tomography angiography; CNV: choroidal neovascular membrane; RPE: retinal pigment epithelium)

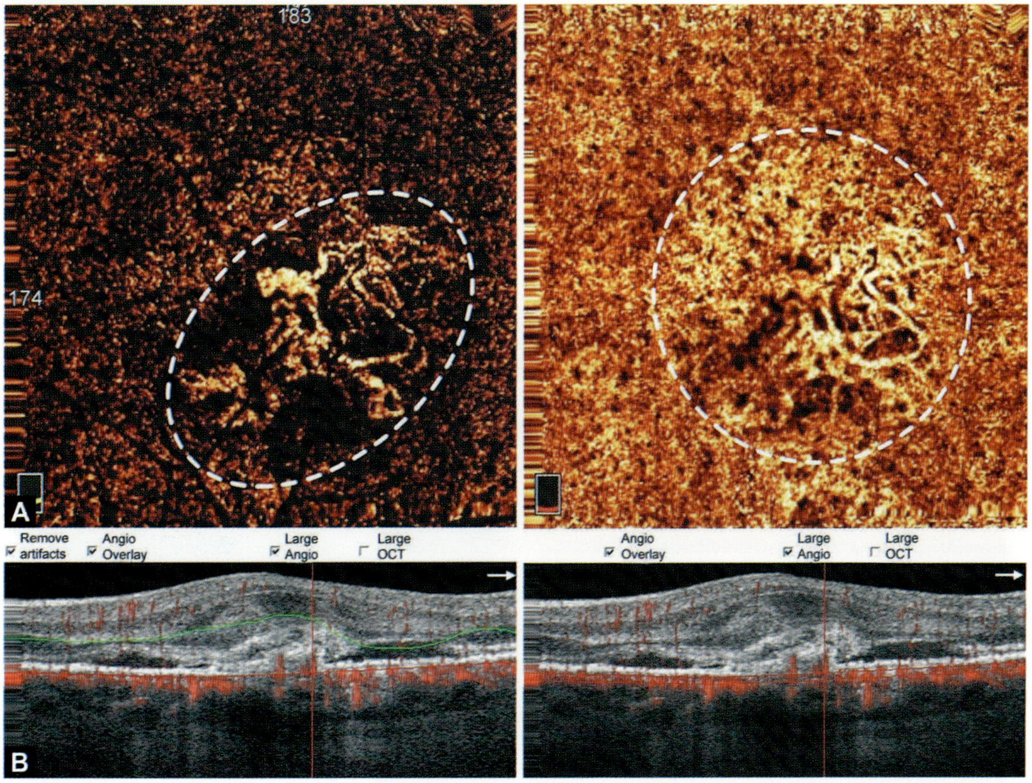

Figs. 4.4A and B: The en face angiogram of (A) the outer retina; and (B) choriocapillary layer with the corresponding OCT B-scans of the macular area. On both angiograms, the filamentous, irregular and branchy neovascular membrane is highlighted. The OCT B-scan shows the perforation of RPE and precisely localizes hyperreflective tissue within horizontal borders of the outer retina. (RPE: retinal pigment epithelium; OCT: optical coherence tomography)

was recovered for 7 letters, while in the untreated group of eyes there was a loss of visual acuity of about 10 letters. The ANCHOR study is a multicenter, randomized, double-blind study that compares the monthly administration of ranibizumab and verteporfin photodynamic therapy in patients with predominant classical CNV in ARMD. The study was performed over a period of 2 years and the results suggest that 90% of the patients treated with ranibizumab did not experience dramatic vision loss of about 15 letters, while such vision loss was present in 66% of patients in the control group that were treated with verteporfin photodynamic therapy.

VEGF is a vascular endothelial growth factor. Today, anti-VEGF drugs are widely used in the treatment of retinal diseases. There are three anti-VEGF drugs in use. "Off-label" remedy Avastin (bevacizumab) continues to be used in daily practice. Lucentis (ranibizumab) and Eylea (aflibercept) are drugs whose active molecules block the release of VEGF, stop CNV growth and the formation of macular edema. Conventional laser photocoagulation is not to be disregarded as a treatment method for central macular pathology nor Iridex, a yellow laser. Supplements of vitamins, diet, and smoking cessation are recommended during treatment of ARMD, particularly if

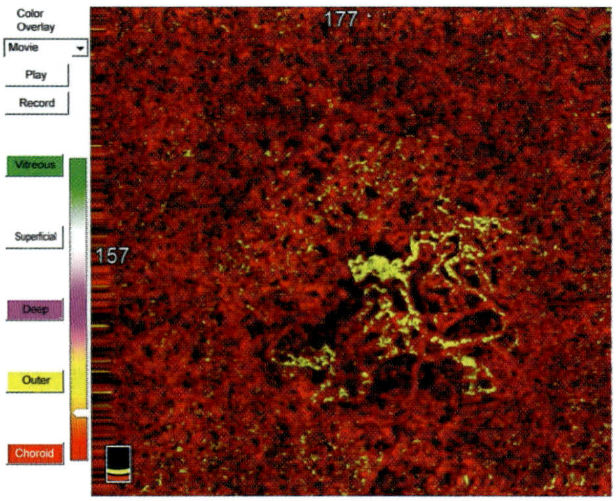

Fig. 4.5: The optical coherence tomography angiography software allows the visualization of four angiography layers marked in different colors, so neovascular localization can be even more certain and reliable. The image shows neovascularization colored in red and yellow indicating that it is situated in the choroidal layer and outer retina.

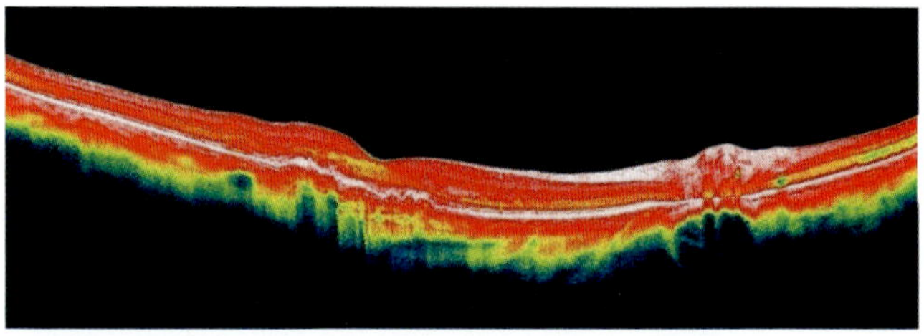

Fig. 4.6: An OCT B-scan of the retina and optic papilla in a 74-year-old female patient. Irregular and wavy RPE is visible in the macula. (RPE: retinal pigment epithelium; OCT: optical coherence tomography)

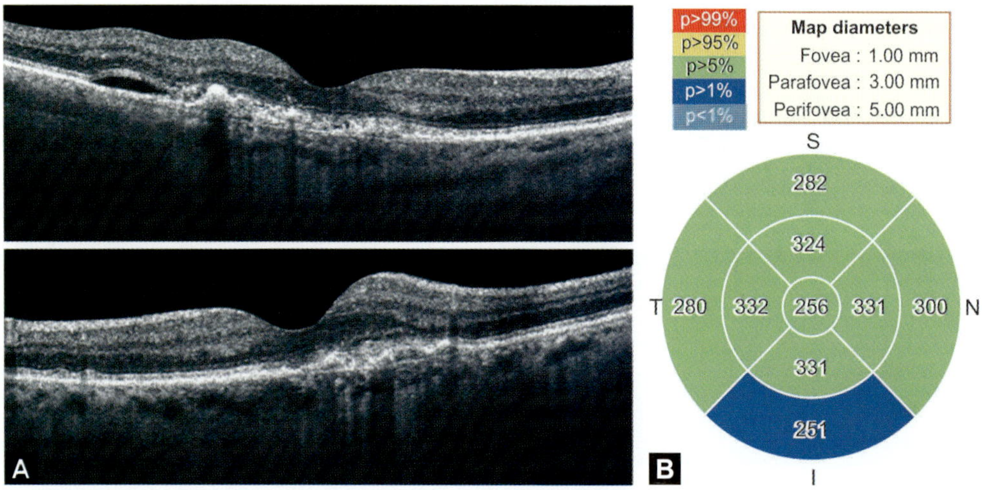

Figs. 4.7A and B: The OCT B-scan of the same eye as presented in Figure 4.6. This scan clearly shows: (A) Irregular, thickened RPE, but on this section shallow subretinal fluid accumulation can also be seen; (B) Retinal map thickness shows the numerical values in the physiological range, slightly decreased in the perifoveolar inferior part. (RPE: retinal pigment epithelium; OCT: optical coherence tomography)

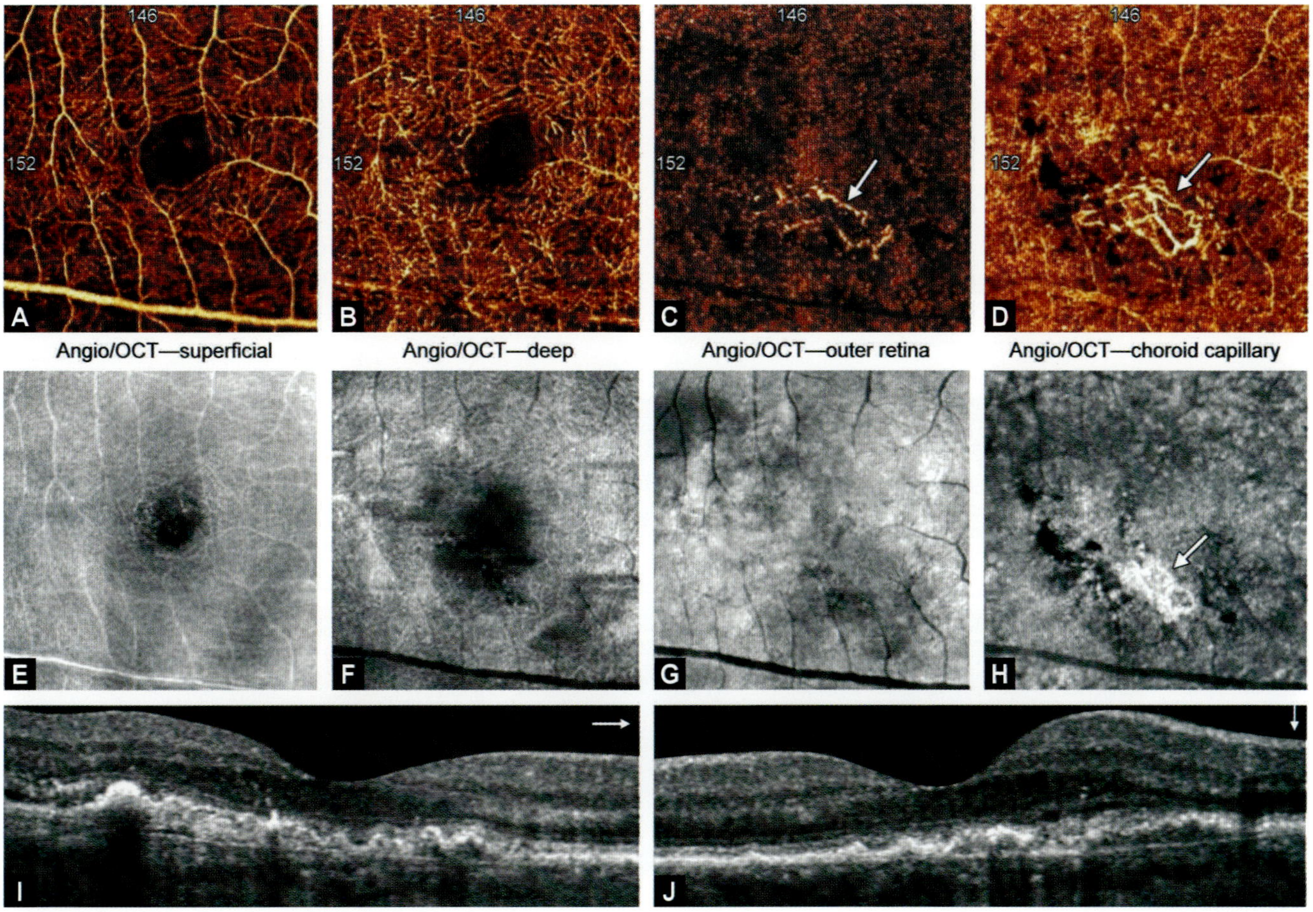

Figs. 4.8A to J: The OCTA SSADA protocol (3 × 3 mm), en face OCT and OCT B-scan of the corresponding retinal layers of the same eye as depicted in Figure 4.7. (A to D) Shows en face angiograms of the retinal layers. The superficial vascular plexus is composed of densely and symmetrically arranged capillaries. (A) The FAZ is regular in size and shape. The deep vascular plexus corresponds to the age of the patient; (B) Capillaries are slightly sclerotically aberrated. The shape of FAZ is slightly changed; (C) Showing the outer retina with both the RPE and Bruch's membrane perforated, and discrete filamentous capillaries (arrow) visible in the center. This is indicative of the patient having the wet form of ARMD and CNV type 2; (D) In the choroid capillary layer (arrow), a neovascular nest of capillaries with a surrounding dark halo is shown; (E to H) Demonstrating en face OCT of corresponding retinal layers, with the inner parts of the retina being regular in appearance, whilst the outer part of the retina, namely the choroidal part shows fibrosing, hyperreflective changes of structure that correspond to CNV. Hyporeflective areas that match areas of subretinal fluid on the OCT B-scan can also be seen; and (I and J) Showing OCT B-scans of the corresponding macular area. The irregular, wavy and partially accumulated RPE is seen, as well as a small site of PED at the margin of the subretinal edema. The comparison of OCT B-scans and en face, frontal OCT angiography images are vital and compulsive for the correct localization, measurement and pathology monitoring. (CNV: choroidal neovascular membrane; OCT: optical coherence tomography; RPE: retinal pigment epithelium; FAZ: foveal avascular zone; OCTA: optical coherence tomography angiography; PED: pigment epithelial detachment; ARMD, age-related macular degeneration)

the other eye shows signs of dry macular degeneration. The recommended formula follows the guidelines of the AREDS (Age-Related Eye Disease Study) and includes taking vitamin C (500 mg), vitamin E (400 IU), zinc oxide (80 mg), copper oxide (2 mg), lutein (10 mg) and zeaxanthin (2 mg). Patients who are in the process of treating CNV should be frequently followed-up, even every month. Follow-up is recommended until the signs of disease stabilization are obtained. 80% of patients treated with anti-VEGF therapy show improvement and recovery of visual acuity. Despite the aggressiveness of anti-VEGF therapy, 20% of patients develop signs of CNV progression and macular edema.

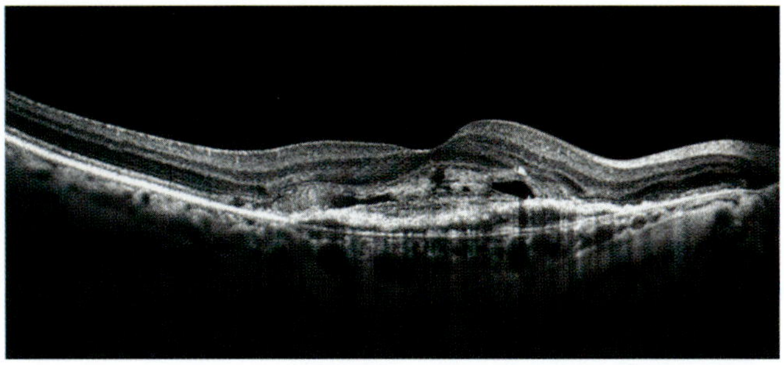

Fig. 4.9: An OCT B-scan of the retina in a 62-year-old female patient. The macula is elevated due to hyperreflective tissue change in the outer part of the retina. In this section, subretinal fluid accumulation is also visible. Macular changes are highly suspected in CNV. Also, RPE is irregularly grouped and lost in places. (CNV: choroidal neovascular membrane; OCT: optical coherence tomography; RPE: retinal pigment epithelium)

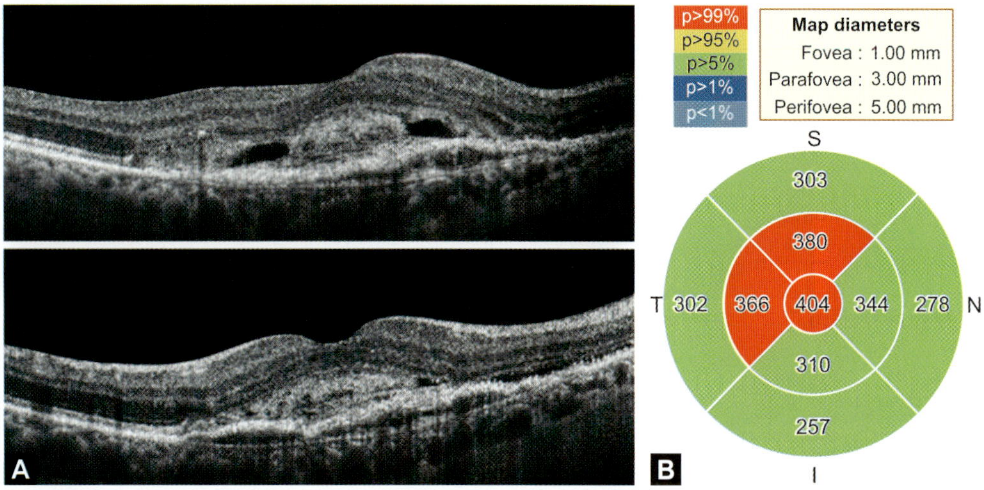

Figs. 4.10A and B: (A) The OCT B-scan of the macular area of the same eye depicted in Figure 4.9. Hyperreflective subretinal tissue is more accurately observed in this image. The edges also present with an accumulation of subretinal fluid. RPE is irregular and thickened; (B) Retina map shows increased macular thickness, with a central value of 404 μm. (OCT: optical coherence tomography; RPE: retinal pigment epithelium)

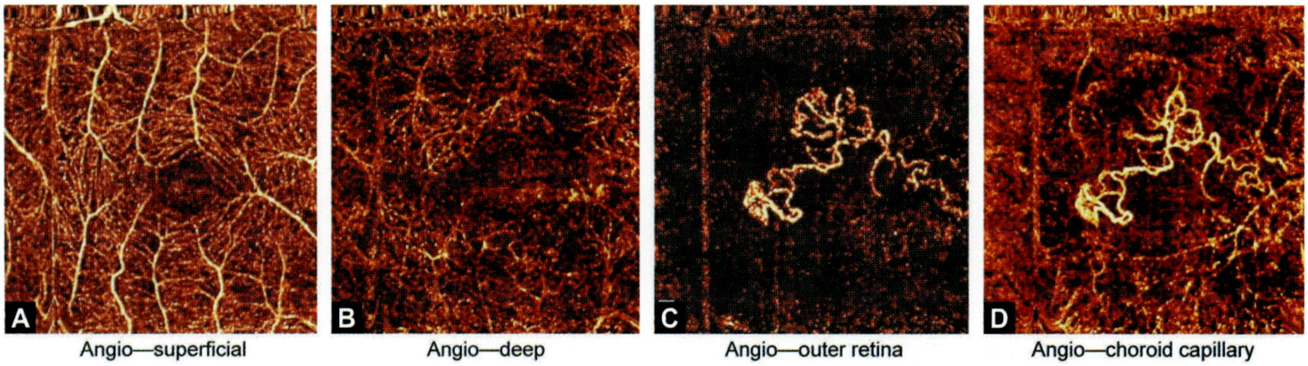

Figs. 4.11A to D: An OCTA SSADA protocol (3 × 3 mm) with en face angiograms of the superficial and deep vascular plexus, outer retina and choriocapillaris of the same eye. (A) The superficial vascular plexus seems to be regular in form but with sclerotic changes on the capillaries. Small vascular dropouts can also be seen in this plexus; (B) The deep vascular plexus is slightly irregular and the FAZ cannot be precisely observed; (C) Fine, active, thread-like neovascular change is seen in the outer retina as well as in the (D) choroidal layer. The capillaries are tangled and form a shape that resembles a knot-like structure. (FAZ: foveal avascular zone; OCTA: optical coherence tomography angiography)

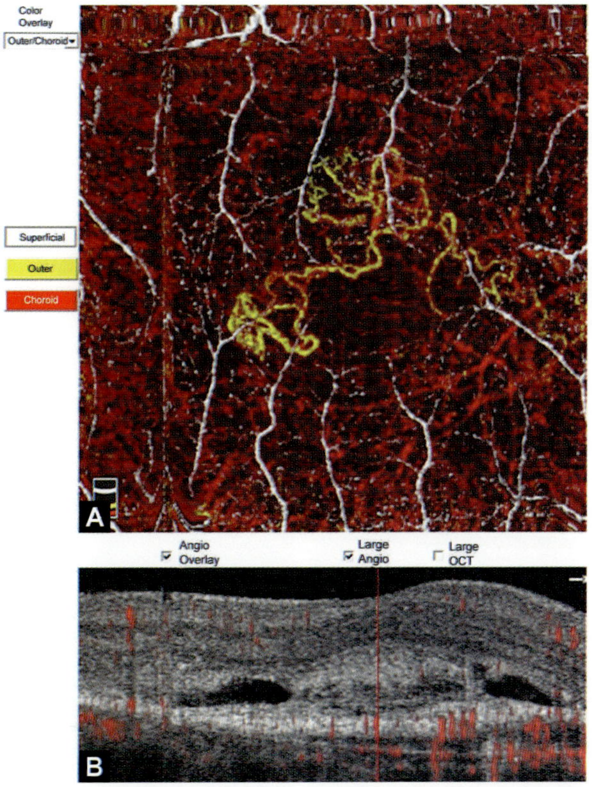

Figs. 4.12A and B: The OCTA software allows analytical approach, enabling the precise localization of the neovascular membrane. CNV is colored with yellow and red indicating its origin from the choroid part, followed by the perforation of the RPE and expansion into the outer retina. There is no dark halo zone around CNV so it is clearly active and rapidly becoming bigger and wider. (CNV: choroidal neovascular membrane; RPE: retinal pigment epithelium; OCTA: optical coherence tomography angiography)

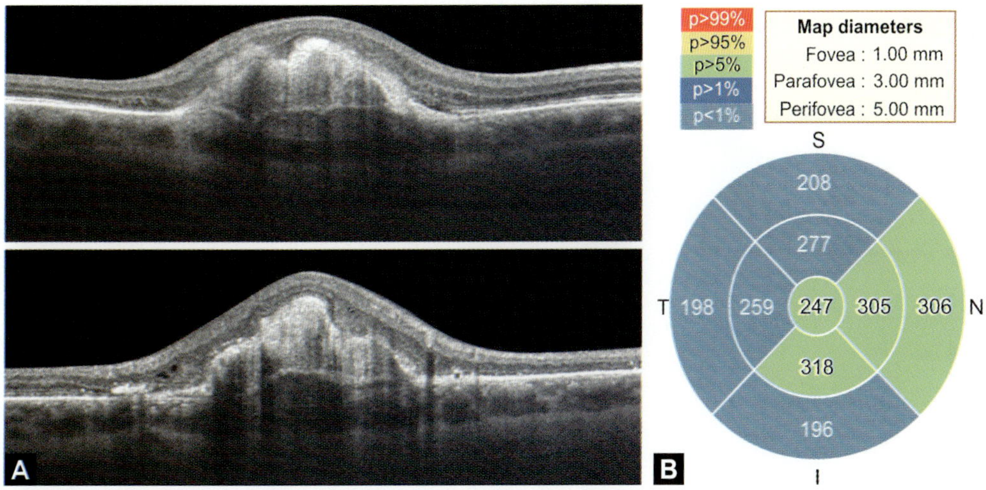

Figs. 4.13A and B: (A) An OCT B-scan of macular area in a 67-year-old patient. There is a large subretinal hyperreflective fibrous change that elevates the macula. The RPE, Bruch's membrane and outer layers of the retina are erased due to hyperreflectivity of the subretinal tissue. Subretinal fluid is visible in the very borders of the macular change, as well as an accumulation of intraretinal fluid; and (B) The retinal thickness map shows that a central macular thickness of 247 µm is physiological. However, superior, inferior and temporal parts of the macular area show decreased values of retinal tissue, which cannot be deemed physiological. (OCT: optical coherence tomography; RPE: retinal pigment epithelium)

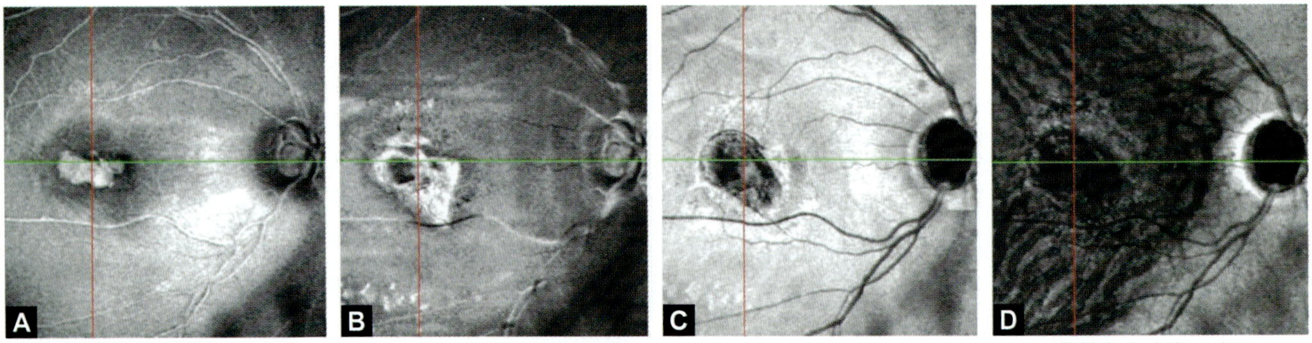

Figs. 4.14A to D: En face optical coherence tomography of retina layers of the same eye as in Figure 4.13 (12 × 9 mm), showing visible defect in the macula surrounded by a ring of hyperreflective tissue that corresponds to fibrous changes and the scar in the center.

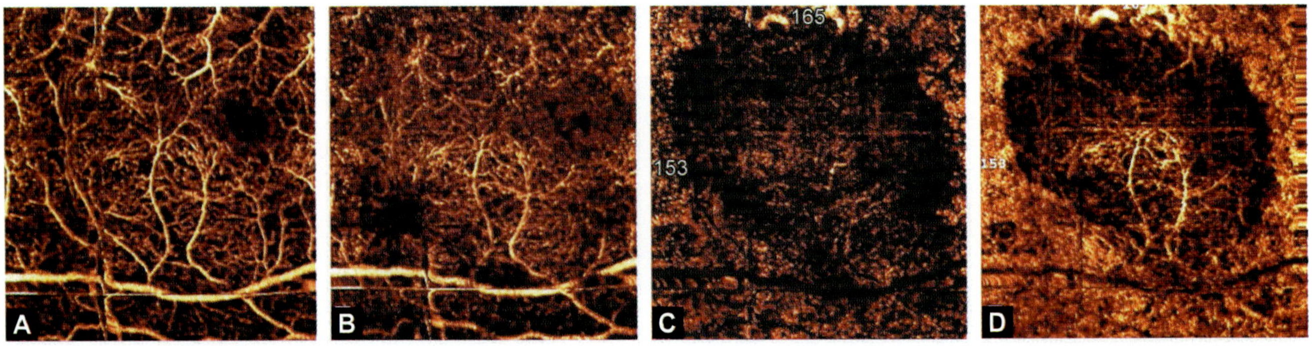

Figs. 4.15A to D: The OCTA SSADA protocol of retinal layers of the same patient (3 × 3 mm). (A and B) The superficial and deep vascular plexus show an irregular, sclerotically changed capillar network with many areas of vascular dropout, anastomoses, and small, irregular FAZ; and (C and D) A large, dark and dry area is seen in the outer retina and choriocapillaris. The change indicates a dried and no longer active old neovascular membrane. Little, blossoming active ends of capillary blood vessels are not visible. The big dark halo area shows that the change is old and inactive, and most likely a scar. (FAZ: foveal avascular zone; OCT: optical coherence tomography)

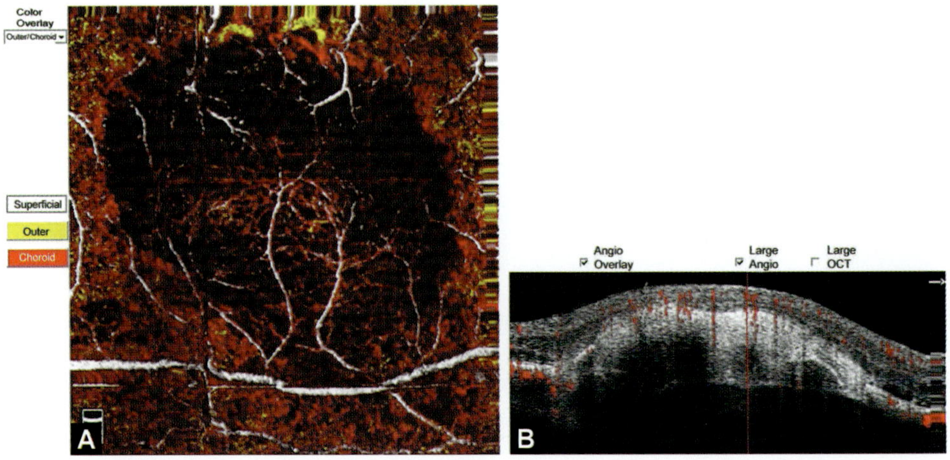

Figs. 4.16A and B: The optical coherence tomography angiography AngioAnalysis also presents a big dark halo with no active blood vessels. AngioAnalysis shows that the patient has a large cicatrix in the macular area and therefore must be regularly observed due to the risky edges of the central change. This figure also shows large central vessels in the dry central area, but no aggressive and new neovascularization can be seen. (B) Showing the corresponding B-scan with colored blood flow, in which no flow can be observed in the fibrous change elevating the macula.

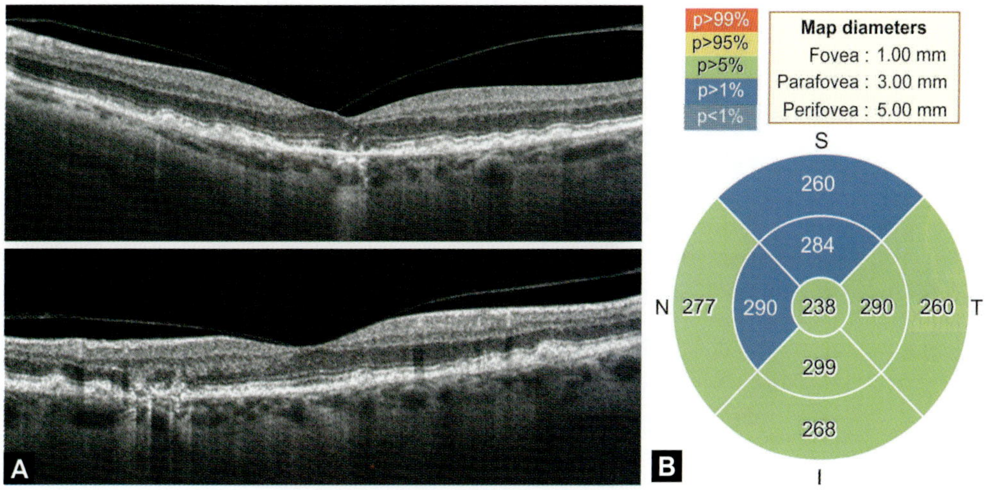

Figs. 4.17A and B: (A) An OCT B-scan of macular area in a 64-year-old patient. The scan shows a thin and changed retina with drusen, wavy and irregularly grouped RPE. The beginning of intraretinal fluid accumulation is visible in the central macula. The posterior hyaloid membrane can also be seen, as well as the posterior vitreous detachment; (B) Retinal thickness map. The thickness macular values seem to be normal although partially decreased. The central macular thickness is 238 µm. (OCT: optical coherence tomography; RPE: retinal pigment epithelium)

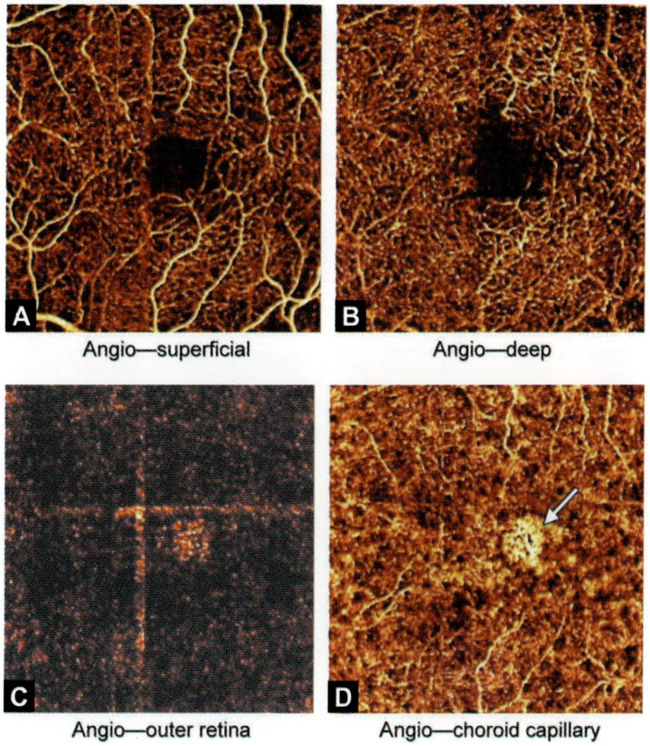

Figs. 4.18A to D: The OCTA SSADA protocol of the same eye as shown in Figure 4.17 (3 × 3 mm). (A) In the superficial capillary network no pathological changes are detected, the net is regular and symmetrical with a high capillar density. The FAZ size is regular; (B) The deep capillary network presents with a wider FAZ and a capillary net of expected density. There are several vascular dropout regions around the central FAZ; (C) A small, circular colored area is visible and highly indicative of suspected CNV; and (D) The choroidal layer (arrow) shows a small active circular neovascularization that spreads to the surrounding tissue, perforates the RPE and spreads into the outer retinal layer. (CNV: choroidal neovascular membrane; RPE: retinal pigment epithelium; FAZ: foveal avascular zone; OCTA: optical coherence tomography angiography)

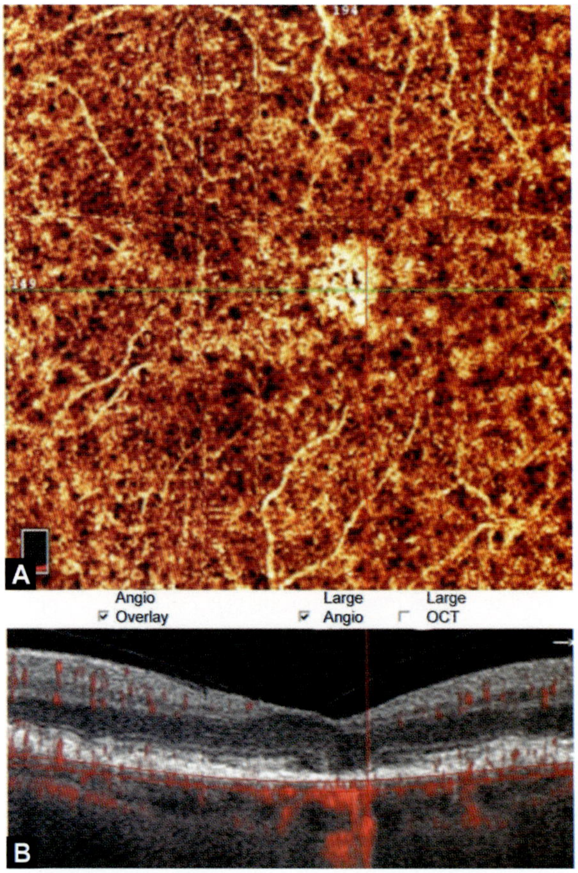

Figs. 4.19A and B: (A) An angiography of the choriocapillar layer with its corresponding B-scan. The round neovascular change is very easily seen; there is no dark halo around the CNV which means the change is active; (B) The choroidal layer in the macula on the B-scan is densely colored in red which corresponds to the higher blood flow of CNV. RPE seems to be partially lost in macula. (CNV: choroidal neovascular membrane; RPE: retinal pigment epithelium)

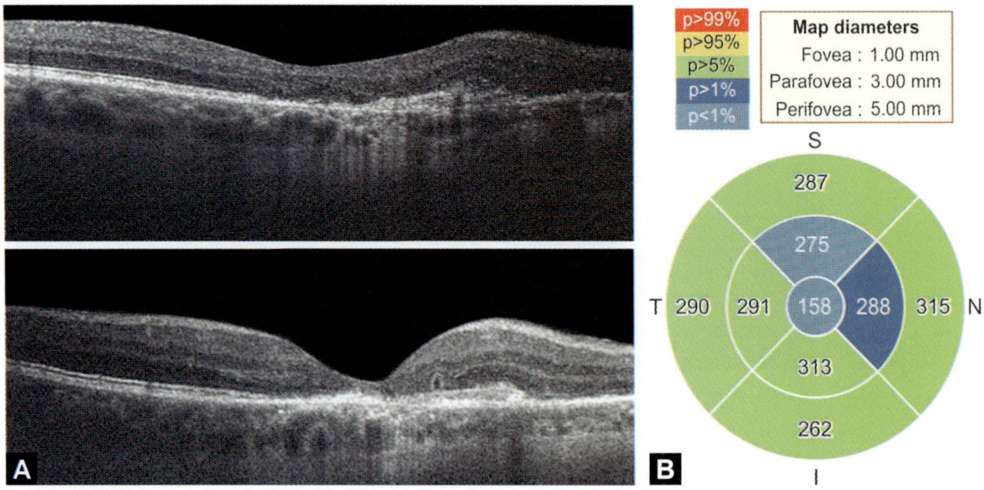

Figs. 4.20A and B: (A) An OCT B-scan of the macular area in a 68-year-old patient. There are subretinal hyperreflective tissue changes seen both in the macular and perimacular area. Along with incipient retinal edema, irregular RPE, in some places partially lost and in some partially thick and grouped, is visible; and (B) The retinal map shows decreased value of the central macular thickness as well as thinner values of other parts of the macula. (OCT: optical coherence tomography; RPE: retinal pigment epithelium)

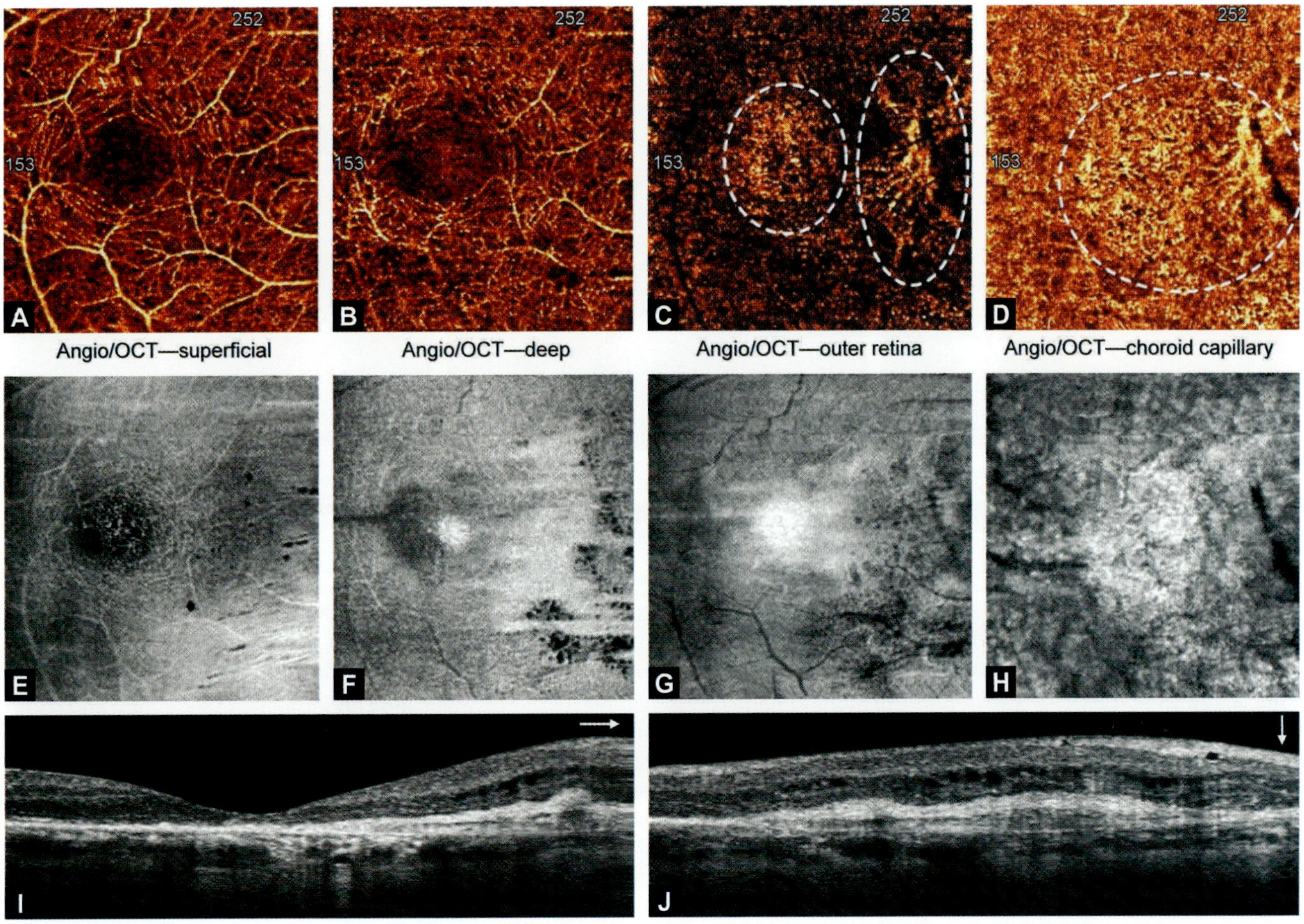

Figs. 4.21A to J: (A to D) The OCTA SSADA protocol 3 × 3 mm, en face OCT and OCT B-scan of the corresponding retinal layers of the same eye shown in Figure 4.20. From the point of view of angiography, there are no significant changes in the vascularization of the superficial plexus. (A) The FAZ is regular in shape and size and the capillary net is symmetrical and dense, however slightly sclerotically changed; (B) The deep vascular plexus of the inner retina does not present with significant abnormalities, disregarding the few rough anastomoses between the superficial and deep vascular net. The FAZ is slightly enlarged and very few vascular dropouts can be seen around it; (C) The outer retinal layer demonstrates subtle circular neovascularization in the very center, as opposed to the thicker one located in its close proximity. The appearance of CNV in the outer retina suggests that the membrane has actively spread from the choroidal layer and subsequently perforated the RPE (CNV type 2); (D) The changes are also shown in the choriocapillaris, in which the two neovascularizations seem to be joined and interconnected. That means that there is also a gentle neovascularization between the two CNV type 2 membranes in the choroidal layer. There is no black halo around CNV that would indicate its inactivity; (E to H) Demonstrating en face OCT of corresponding retinal layers. Even in the deep layer of the inner retina, a hyperreflective neovascular fibrous membrane is easily visible due to the thinner retina. In the outer retina and choroidea, the same fine hyperreflective membranous change is obvious; and (I and J) The OCT B-scans of the macular area show the hyperreflective subretinal changes, which partially elevate the retina, as well as the intraretinal fluid. (CNV: choroidal neovascular membrane; OCT: optical coherence tomography; RPE: retinal pigment epithelium; FAZ: foveal avascular zone; OCTA: optical coherence tomography angiography)

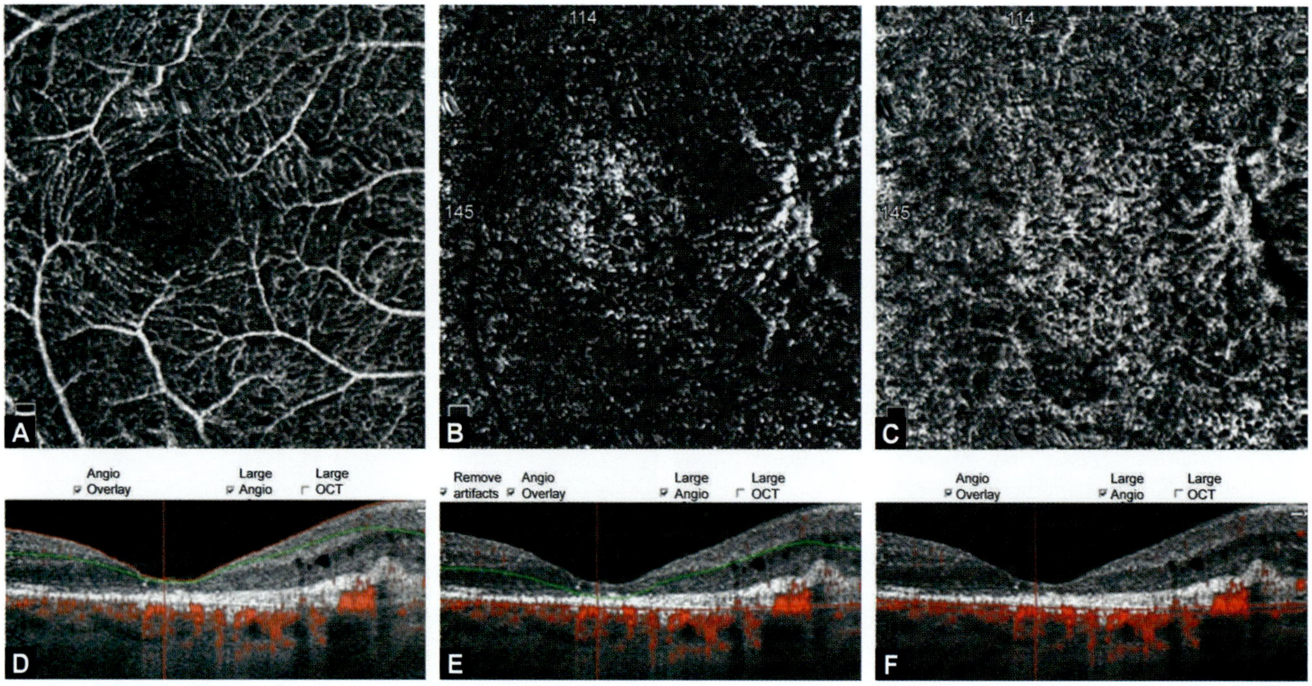

Figs. 4.22A to F: The OCTA SSADA protocol of the superficial vascular plexus, outer retina and choriocapillaris (3 × 3 mm) and corresponding findings of the OCT B-scan. The regular structure of the superficial vascular layer gives a misleading impression that the finding of retina and its vascularization is normal, but in the outer retinal layer and the choriocapillaris, there is clearly a classic neovascularization type 2 hiding. CNV corresponds to the hyperreflective subretinal cluster shown on the OCT B scan that elevates the upper layers of the retina. In the images above, a gentle, but larger and more elongated occult neovascular membrane type 1 (in fovea, under RPE), which connects two adjacent CNV types 2 in the choroidal layer, is much more visible. (CNV: choroidal neovascular membrane; OCT: optical coherence tomography; RPE: retinal pigment epithelium)

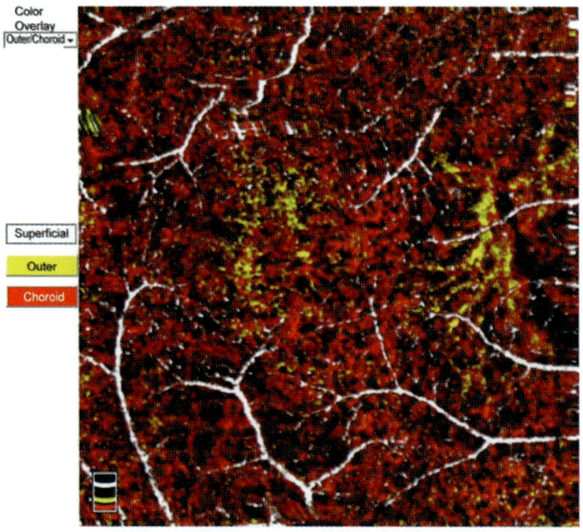

Fig. 4.23: The OCT angiography of the neovascularization shown in Figure 4.22. There are two neovascular membranes (CNV type 2) in the outer retina, both colored in yellow, and a red-colored CNV type 1 that connects the two membranes that have already perforated RPE and spread into the outer retina. This change can be labeled as a mixed neovascularization or CNV type 4. (CNV: choroidal neovascular membrane; OCT: optical coherence tomography; RPE: retinal pigment epithelium)

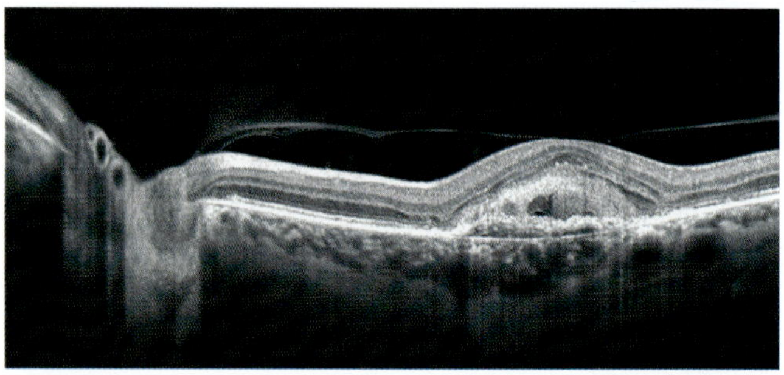

Fig. 4.24: An OCT B-scan of the macular area and papilla in a 77-year-old patient. Due to the accumulation of subretinal fluid, great elevation of the macular area is visible. An irregular and thicker RPE is also visible. The image shows posterior vitreous detachment and the posterior hyaloid membrane is also visible. (OCT: optical coherence tomography; RPE: retinal pigment epithelium)

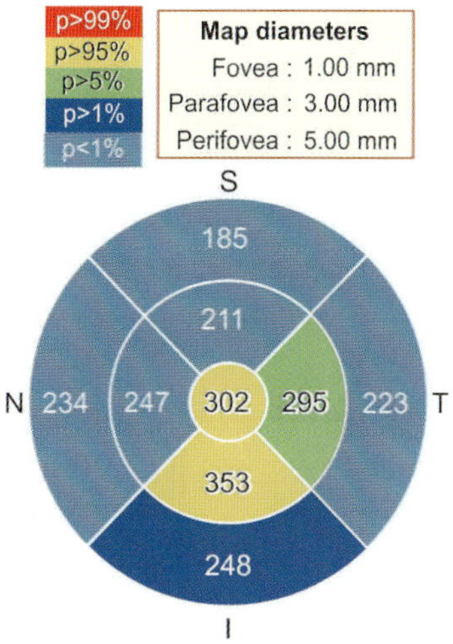

Fig. 4.25: Retinal map in which the central macular thickness is increased (302 μm), but the parafoveal and other parts of the retina are thinner.

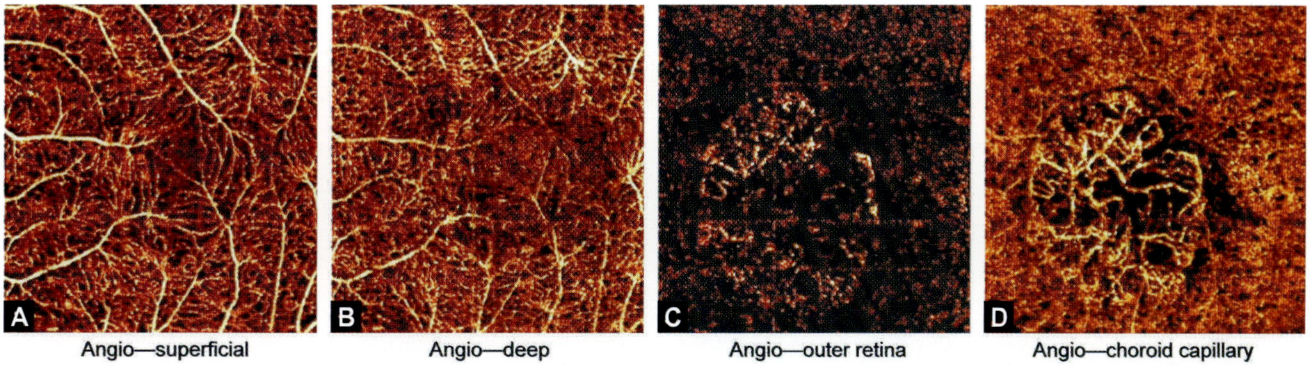

Figs. 4.26A to D: The OCTA SSADA protocol of the retinal layers of the same eye seen in Figure 4.25 (3 x 3 mm). (A and B) The superficial and deep vascular plexuses are changed, especially when taking into consideration the FAZ. In the superficial plexus, FAZ no longer has a normal shape, but an attenuated and trigonous one, with many vascular dropouts around it. The deep plexus presents itself wide in shape and unclear borders of the FAZ; and (C and D) In the outer retina and choriocapillaris, there is a fine round neovascularization that morphologically has the shape of a "bicycle wheel". It is characterized as CNV type 2 due to the fact that the RPE is perforated and that CNV has actively spread into the surrounding retinal tissue. (CNV: choroidal neovascular membrane; RPE: retinal pigment epithelium; FAZ: foveal avascular zone; OCTA: optical coherence tomography angiography)

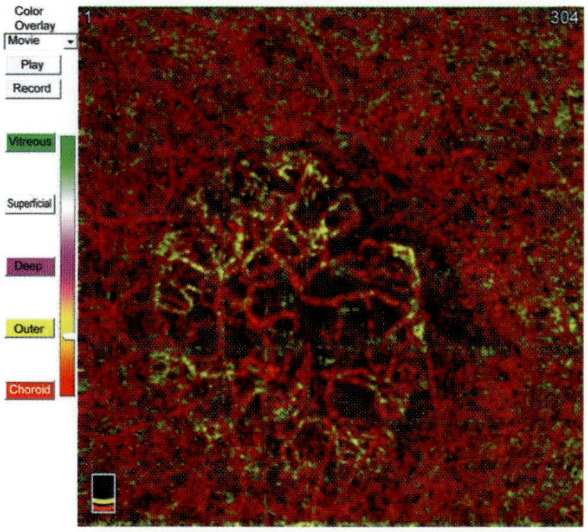

Fig. 4.27: The OCT angiography of the "bicycle wheel"––like neovascularization from Figure 4.26. Yellowish-red colors of the neovascularization show its exact localization, and there is no doubt that it is CNV 2 localized in the choroid and outer retinal layer. (CNV: choroidal neovascular membrane; OCT: optical coherence tomography)

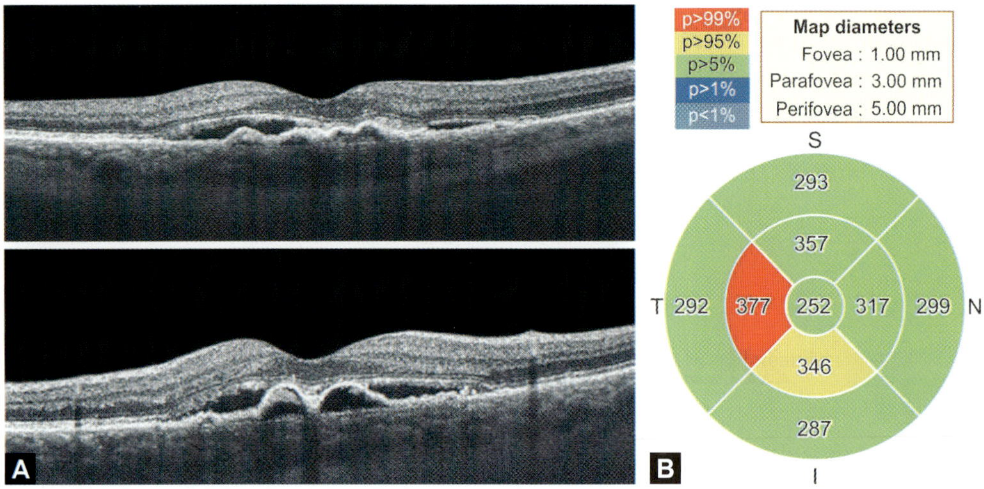

Figs. 4.28A and B: (A) An OCT B-scan of the macular area in a 73-year-old patient. In the margins of the confluent PEDs, subretinal edema and shallow sensory retinal detachment is visible. There are rough and irregular aggregations of the RPE on the edges of the PED; and (B) The retinal map is analogous to the mild thickening of the macula, especially in the temporal part. (OCT: optical coherence tomography; RPE: retinal pigment epithelium; FAZ: foveal avascular zone; PED: pigment epithelial detachment)

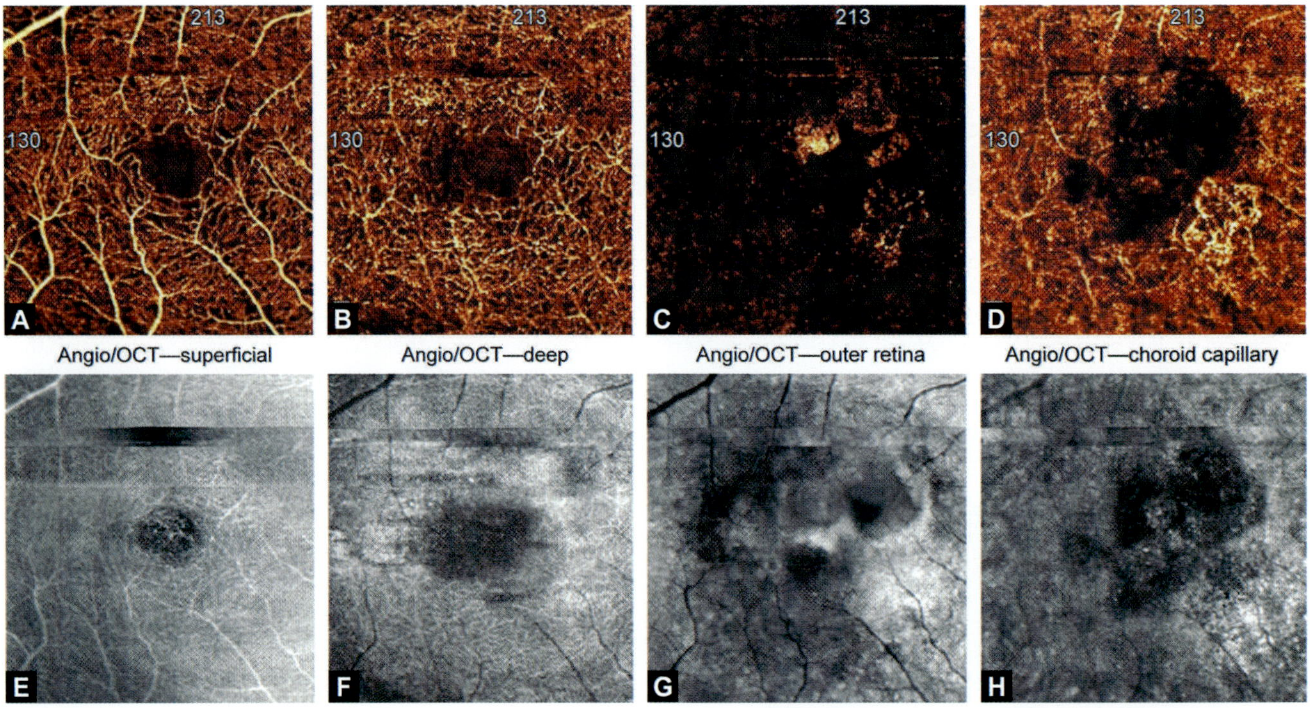

Figs. 4.29A to H: (A to D) The OCTA SSADA protocol of the same eye as shown in the previous image (3 × 3 mm). In the superficial and deep capillary plexuses, IRMA and a few anastomoses of these two vascular nets are visible. The FAZ is slightly enlarged and irregularly shaped in the deep vascular plexus. In the outer retina, there is precisely colored neovascularization with dark regions around it that match the area of the subretinal fluid on OCT B-scans. The neovascularization has an appearance resembling flourishing branches (CNV type 2). In the choroidal layer, another filamentous neovascularization is visible. However, it is softer and resembles a ball in form; and (E to H) En face OCT corresponds to the OCTA finding and shows hyporeflective areas in the outer retina and choroid (matches the cavities with subretinal fluid) with hyperreflective areas on the edges that match neovascular membranes. (IRMA, intraretinal microvascular abnormality; CNV: choroidal neovascular membrane; OCT: optical coherence tomography; FAZ: foveal avascular zone; OCTA: optical coherence tomography angiography)

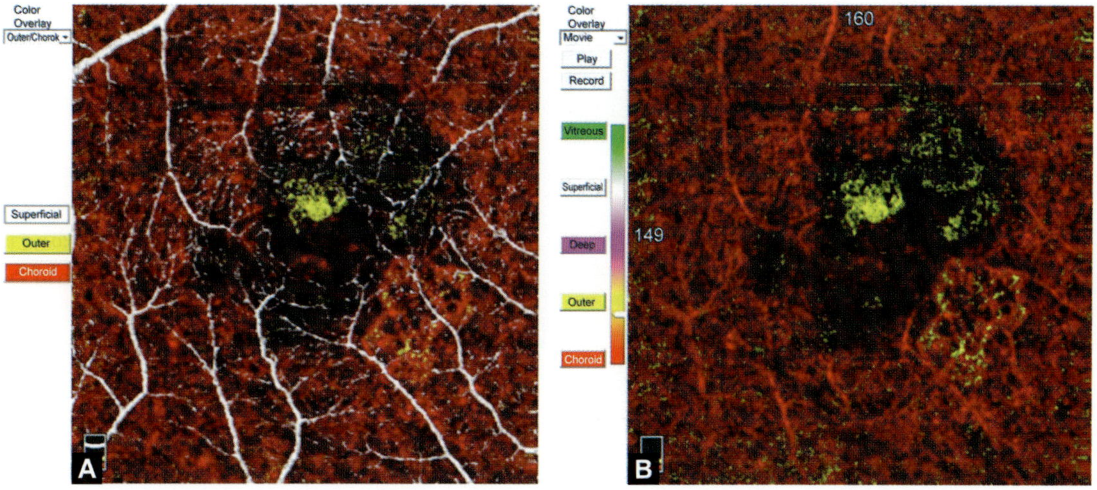

Figs. 4.30A and B: Two angiography image examples that show two fine neovascularizations different in shape. They have both perforated RPE and spread into the outer retina (CNV type 2). The yellow color marks the capillaries in the outer retina, while the red color marks the capillaries in the choroidal layer. (CNV: choroidal neovascular membrane; RPE: retinal pigment epithelium)

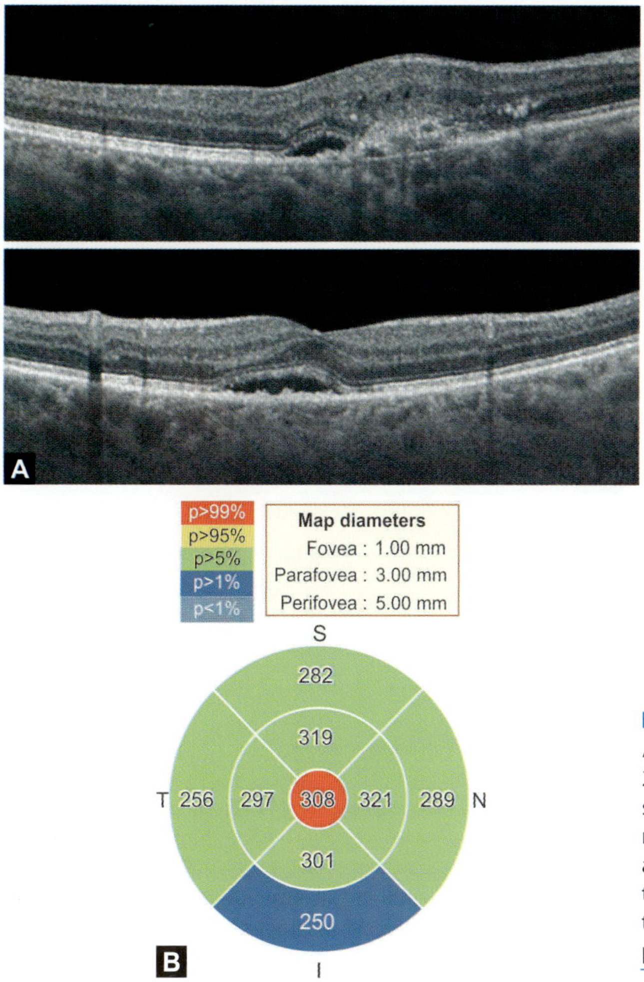

Figs. 4.31A and B: (A) An OCT B-scan of an eye with wet form of ARMD; female patient that has been suffering also from diabetes for 25 years. The B-scan shows an accumulation of subretinal fluid, a few small intraretinal cysts and the accumulation of hyperreflective subretinal tissue. RPE is irregular, granular and discontinued in places; and (B) The retinal thickness map shows an increased central macular thickness (308 μm). Other parts of the macular area display regular thickness values. (OCT: optical coherence tomography; RPE: retinal pigment epithelium; ARMD, age-related macular degeneration)

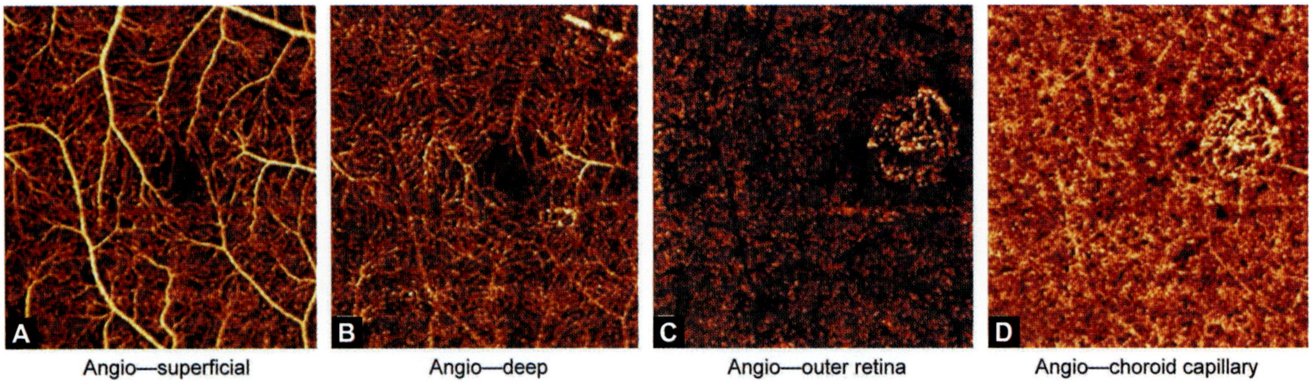

Figs. 4.32A to D: An OCTA SSADA protocol and angiography layers of the same eye as in Figure 4.31 (3 × 3 mm). (A) A superficial vascular layer shows a slightly changed vascular network, with irregularly shaped FAZ and many capillary dropouts; (B) A deep vascular plexus is presented with typical diabetical vascular changes. The net is completely irregular and asymmetrical, many microaneurysms can be seen, and capillaries show dilatations in places; (C) The outer retina should be without any flow, but there is a clear rounded vascular structure presenting itself in this layer; and (D) The choriocapillaris shows the same vascular structure in the same place. Neovascular capillaries are connected to the surrounding choroidal tissue and they are actively spreading. The neovascularization is classified as type 2, due to the fact that it has perforated the RPE and spread into the outer retina. (RPE: retinal pigment epithelium; FAZ: foveal avascular zone; OCTA: optical coherence tomography angiography)

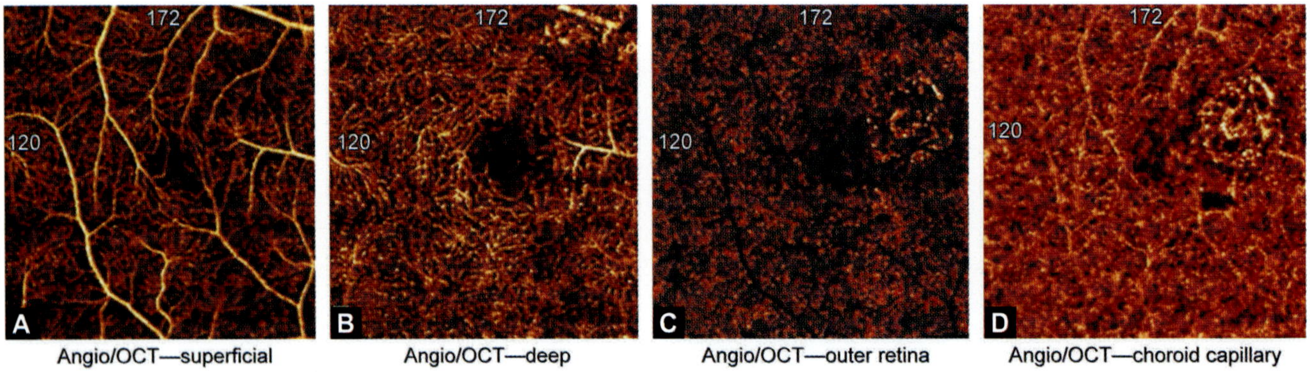

Figs. 4.33A to D: An OCTA SSADA protocol of the same eye as in Figure 4.32; a day after the first intravitreal ranibizumab injection (3 × 3 mm). Superficial and deep vascular plexus show no significant changes. The CNV is still visible in the outer retina and choriocapillaris, but it is definitely less dense. A dark halo around the neovascularization starts to appear, as a sign of decreased activity of the membrane. (CNV: choroidal neovascular membrane; OCTA: optical coherence tomography angiography)

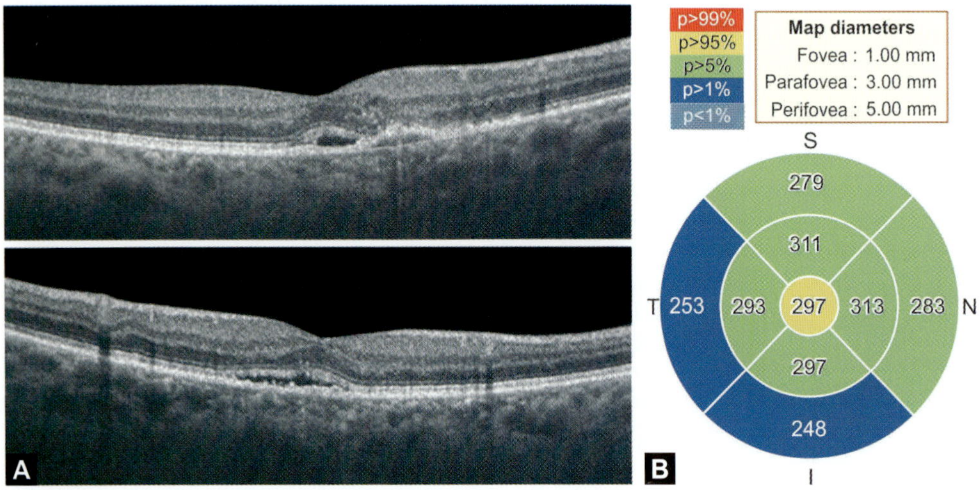

Figs. 4.34A and B: (A) An OCT B-scan of the same eye a day after the first intravitreal ranibizumab injection. The central sensory retinal detachment is shallower and the subretinal accumulated tissue is significantly smaller compared to the B-scan before the treatment. The RPE is still irregular and grouped in places; and (B) The retinal thickness map shows a less increased central macular thickness value after the treatment. (OCT: optical coherence tomography; RPE: retinal pigment epithelium)

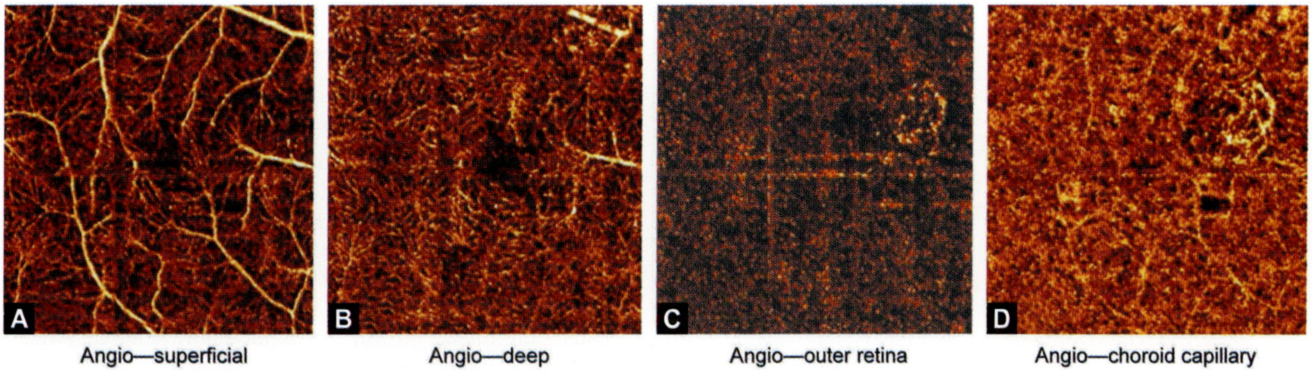

Figs. 4.35A to D: An OCTA SSADA protocol of the same eye shown in Figure 4.34; a day after the second ranibizumab injection. CNV is definitely less branchy and it is almost disappearing from the outer retina. The black halo is more visible in the outer retina and the membrane is less active. Inside the neovascularization, not many active small capillaries can be seen. This finding relates to the improvement and slow regression of the CNV. (CNV: choroidal neovascular membrane; OCTA: optical coherence tomography angiography)

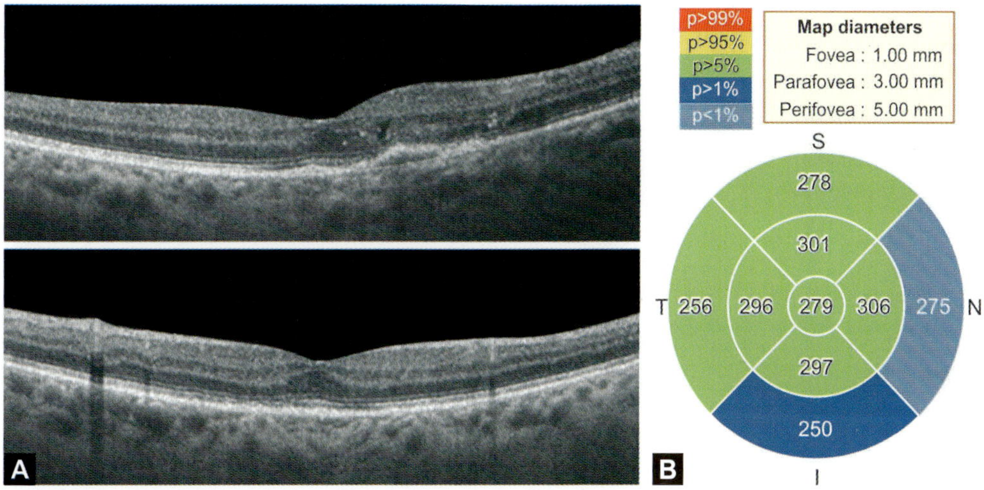

Figs. 4.36A and B: (A) An OCT B-scan of the same eye a day after the second intravitreal anti-VEGF injection. The finding is much better, compared to the one from the first visit. There is no subretinal fluid anymore, and the RPE is more flat. There are still a few places with a granular, irregular RPE, and with a shallow subretinal hyperreflective tissue; (B) The retinal thickness map shows regular, almost in all parts green colored segments, which correspond to a normal macular thickness. (OCT: optical coherence tomography; RPE: retinal pigment epithelium)

BIBLIOGRAPHY

1. Alten F, Clemens CR, Eter N. OCT angiography strengthens the theory of a purely serous pigment epithelium detachment in age-related macular degeneration. Graefes Arch Clin Exp Ophthalmol. 2016;254(8):1645-7.
2. Bressler NM, Bressler SB. Neovascular (Exudative or "Wet") Age-related macular degeneration. In: Ryan SJ, Schachat A, Wilkinson C, Hinton DR, Sadda SR, Wiedemann P (Eds). Retina, 5th edition. London: Elsevier Saunders; 2013. pp. 1183-212.
3. Brown DM, Kaiser PK, Michels M, et al. Ranibizumab versus verteporfin for neovascular age-related macular degeneration. N Engl J Med. 2006;355(14):1432-44.
4. de Carlo TE, Bonini Filho MA, Chin AT, et al. Spectral-domain optical coherence tomography angiography of choroidal neovascularization. Ophthalmology. 2015;122(6):1228-38.
5. Jia Y, Bailey ST, Wilson DJ, et al. Quantitative optical coherence tomography angiography of choroidal neovascularization in age-related macular degeneration. Ophthalmology. 2014;121(7):1435-44.

6. Kim KM, Kim JH, Chang YS, et al. Long-term outcomes in patients with neovascular age-related macular degeneration who maintain dry macula after three monthly ranibizumab injections. Semin Ophthalmol. 2016;14:1-6.
7. Kuehlewein L, Bansal M, Lenis TL, et al. Optical coherence tomography angiography of type 1 neovascularization in age-related macular degeneration. Am J Ophthalmol. 2015;160(4):739-48.
8. Lommatzsch A, Farecki ML, Book B, et al. OCT angiography for exudative age-related macular degeneration: Initial experiences. Ophthalmologe. 2016;113(1):23-9.
9. Marques JP, Costa JF, Marques M, et al. Sequential morphological changes in the CNV net after intravitreal anti-VEGF evaluated with OCT angiography. Ophthalmic Res. 2016;55(3):145-51.
10. Marques JP, Silva R. Optical coherence tomography angiography in wet age-related macular degeneration (AMD). Eye Sci. 2016;31(1):1-3.
11. Moult E, Choi W, Waheed NK, et al. Ultrahigh-speed swept-source OCT angiography in exudative AMD. Ophthalmic Surg Lasers Imaging Retina. 2014;45(6):496-505.
12. Pedrosa AC, Reis-Silva A, Pinheiro-Costa J, et al. Treatment of neovascular age-related macular degeneration with anti-VEGF agents: retrospective analysis of 5-year outcomes. Clin Ophthalmol. 2016;10:541-6.
13. Rosenfeld PJ, Brown DM, Heier JS, et al. Ranibizumab for neovascular age-related macular degeneration. N Engl J Med. 2006;355(14):1419-31.
14. Solomon SD, Lindsley K, Vedula SS, et al. Anti-vascular endothelial growth factor for neovascular age-related macular degeneration. Cochrane Database Syst Rev. 2014;(8):CD005139.
15. Taylor DJ, Hobby AE, Binns AM, et al. How does age-related macular degeneration affect real-world visual ability and quality of life? A systematic review. BMJ Open. 2016;6(12):e011504.
16. Yanoff M, Duker J. Ophthalmology, 3rd edition. London: Mosby Elsevier; 2009.

CHAPTER 5

Central Serous Retinopathy (Central Serous Chorioretinopathy, CSCR, CSR)

INTRODUCTION

Central serous chorioretinopathy (CSR) is an idiopathic disorder of the outer blood-retinal barrier, causing serous macular detachment.

EPIDEMIOLOGY AND ETIOLOGY

Central serous chorioretinopathy usually affects males who are exposed to psychological stress, mostly between 20 years and 50 years of age. The disease is associated with the type A personality with an incidence of 10 cases per 100,000 people. Females are six times less affected with CSR than males. This disease is usually unilateral with an unknown etiology. Risk factors include stress, pregnancy, local and systemic corticosteroid usage, hypertension, allergic diseases and Cushing's syndrome. The localized choroidal permeability allows the leakage of transudate through the retinal pigment epithelium (RPE) and its accumulation in the subretinal space. This condition usually resolves on its own, without any treatment.

SYMPTOMS AND SIGNS

Patients complain of decreased vision in one eye, blurred vision and changes in colors of observed objects. Relative central scotoma commonly occurs, described by patients as a spot in the center of the visual field. Other symptoms may include changes in the letter size, micropsia, and metamorphopsia. Previous episodes of decreased vision, constant changes of the refractive anomaly, frequent changes in glasses prescription and increased farsightedness are also often described.

All of these symptoms occur due to the serous detachment of the sensory retina in the macular region, with or without retinal pigment epithelial detachment (PED).

The disease can occur in an acute, chronic, or recurrent form with a possibility of relapse even months and years after the remission.

DIFFERENTIAL DIAGNOSIS

- Idiopathic polypoidal choroidal vasculopathy (IPCV)
- Retinal pigment epithelial detachment with choroidal neovascular membrane
- Optic disk pit
- Peripheral choroidal tumors
- Rhegmatogenous retinal detachment
- Age-related macular degeneration
- Choroidal inflammations.

DIAGNOSTICS

Amsler grid test is always positive. Ophthalmoscopy discloses a serous retinal elevation in the macular region. Previous episodes of the disease result in the atrophy of the

RPE that alters, incurves and elevates, forming granular formations. Visual acuity is reduced and choroidal layer thickened. Choroidal neovascularization (CNV) occurs in 3–4% of patients.

Optical coherence tomography (OCT) demonstrates subretinal fluid and an elevated retina with or without retinal PED. Fluorescein angiography (FAG) is not mandatory for the diagnosis of CSR, but it is helpful in detecting the areas that exhibit hyperfluorescence in the early stage, and in the late stage it identifies a sign known as a "smokestack". The changes in hyperfluorescence are known as "window" defects.

Optical coherence tomography B-scan shows a well-defined neurosensory retinal detachment with clearly seen fluid accumulation in the space between the outer retina and pigment epithelial layer. PED occurs simultaneously in 80% of cases. It seems that the retina is thickened, especially the choroidal part. Retinal thickening resolves as CSR spontaneously disappears.

The chronic form of the disease shows diffuse hyperfluorescence on FAG. OCT examination reveals hyperreflective material accumulation in the subretinal space, along with sensory retinal detachment. Cystoid retinal changes of the thinned retina may be seen in the regions with chronic form of the disease. Retinal thinning is associated with photoreceptor loss and changes in the pigment epithelial layer. Photoreceptors loss is related to a reduction in visual acuity, even when subretinal fluid is completely resorbed. As the outcomes of chronic form of

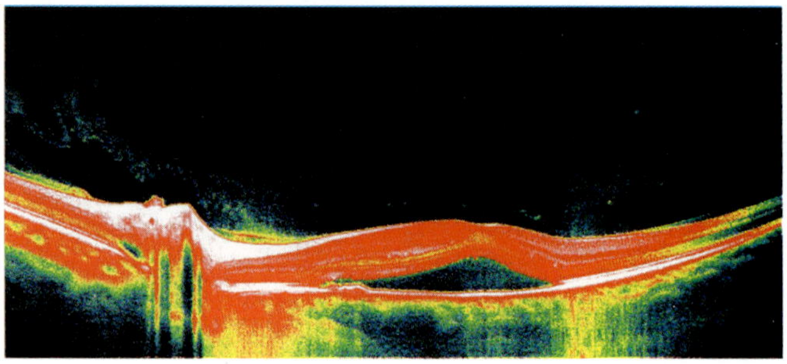

Fig. 5.1: An OCT B-scan of the macular region and optic nerve head in 40-year-old male patient. Sensory retinal detachment can clearly be detected. Accumulation of subretinal fluid is observed between the RPE and the outer retina. RPE is irregular and thickened in the part of the detachment that is closer to papilla. (OCT: optical coherence tomography; RPE: retinal pigment epithelium)

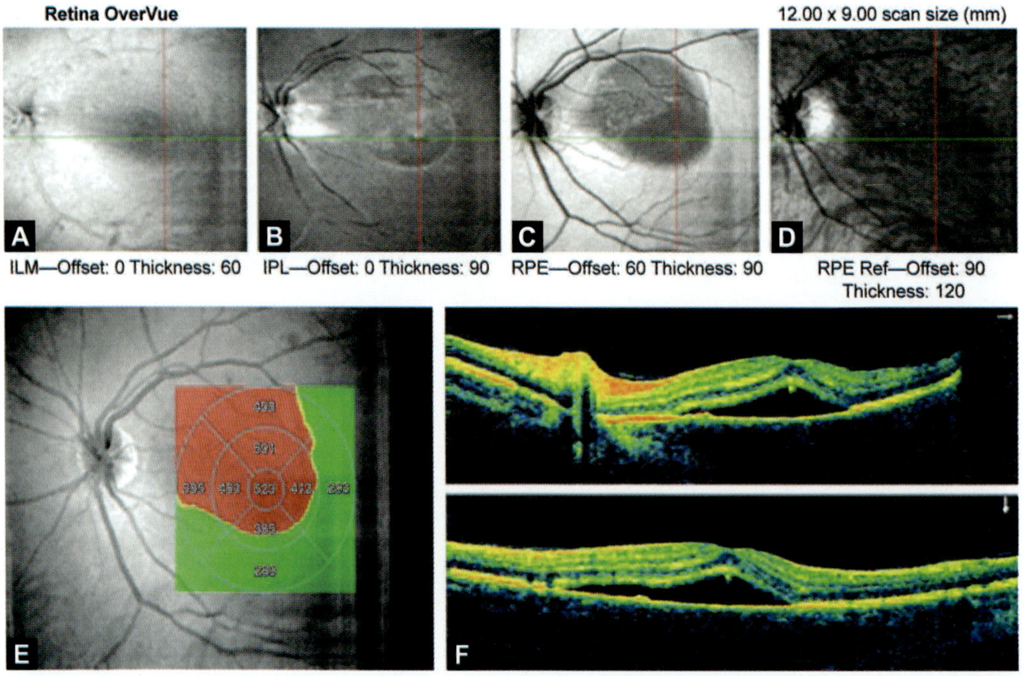

Figs. 5.2A to F: En face optical coherence tomography of the same eye. The superficial inner layer reveals a big shadow and a hyporeflective region corresponding to the surface area of sensory retinal detachment. A rounded hyporeflective region surrounded by a hyperreflective ring can be visualized in deep inner layer. Hyperreflective dots, which correspond to stretched and compressed photoreceptors of the outer retina, are observed. Large blood vessels and elongated photoreceptor reflexes are detected in the outer retina. Retinal thickness map reveals macular thickening.

the disease improve, a decrease in subretinal fluid can be observed on OCT. Regular follow-up regarding patients' recovery and status is necessary.

The example of an eye with an acute CSR presented by optical coherence tomography angiography (OCTA) is described in Figures 5.1 to 5.3.

The example of an eye with a chronic form of CSR presented by OCTA is described in Figures 5.4 to 5.8.

Focal choroidal excavation is local idiopathic cupping of the choroid, which can be associated with CSR, choroid neovascularization and polypoidal choroidal vasculopathy. OCT scans show excavated areas into the choroid, along the RPE/Bruch membrane complex line, without any history of prior trauma, infection, or inflammatory episode. Focal choroidal excavation can be classified by OCT as conforming (if photoreceptor tips are attached to the apical surface of the RPE), or as nonconforming (if there is a separation between the photoreceptor tips and the RPE).

A "pachychoroid" is defined as an abnormal and permanent increase in choroidal thickness often showing dilated choroidal vessels and other structural alterations of the normal choroidal architecture. Pachychoroid spectrum refers to a group of clinical entities that have a common characteristic--a pachychoroid. CSR, pachychoroid pigment epitheliopathy, pachychoroid neovasculopathy and polypoidal choroidal vasculopathy are entities of the pachychoroid clinical spectrum.

THERAPY

Most changes resolve spontaneously within 4 months. Visual acuity improves up to 1.0 in 85% of cases. However, 30–50% of patients develop chronic CSR. Both chronic and recurrent CSR lead to a poor prognosis. A treatment with oral steroids or steroid drops is not recommended. The treatment with argon laser and Iridex yellow laser shortens a recovery time without alteration of a long-term

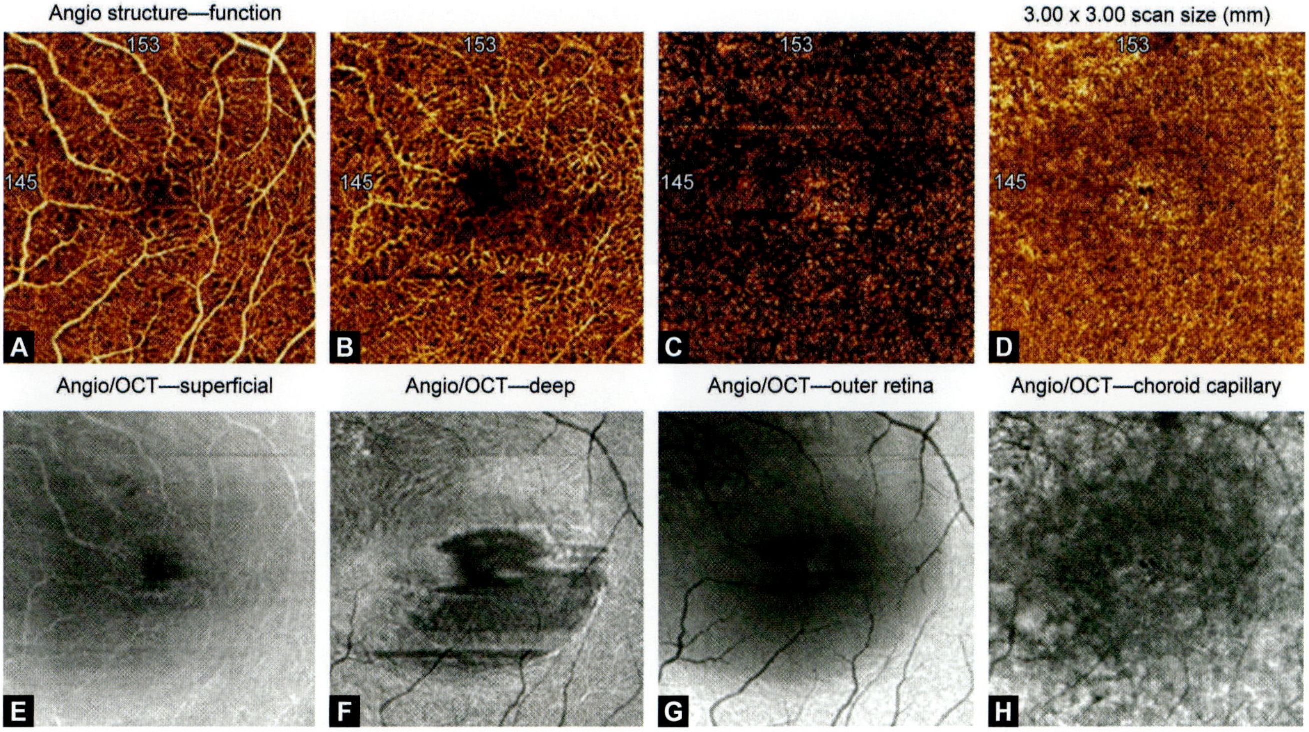

Figs. 5.3A to H: The OCTA SSADA imaging protocol and en face OCT of corresponding parallel macular layers of the same eye (3 × 3 mm). (A and B) Angiography demonstrated no changes in the superficial and deep retinal layer; whereas (E and F) en face OCT of the corresponding layers shows a round hyporeflective zone that correlates with sensory retinal detachment base; (C and G) Angiography revealed no neovascularization in the outer layer, while en face OCT still shows a dark shadow; (D and H) Changes of choroidal neovascularization are not detected by angiography, but a hyporeflective rounded region in this layer is seen on en face OCT as well. (OCT: optical coherence tomography; OCTA: optical coherence tomography angiography)

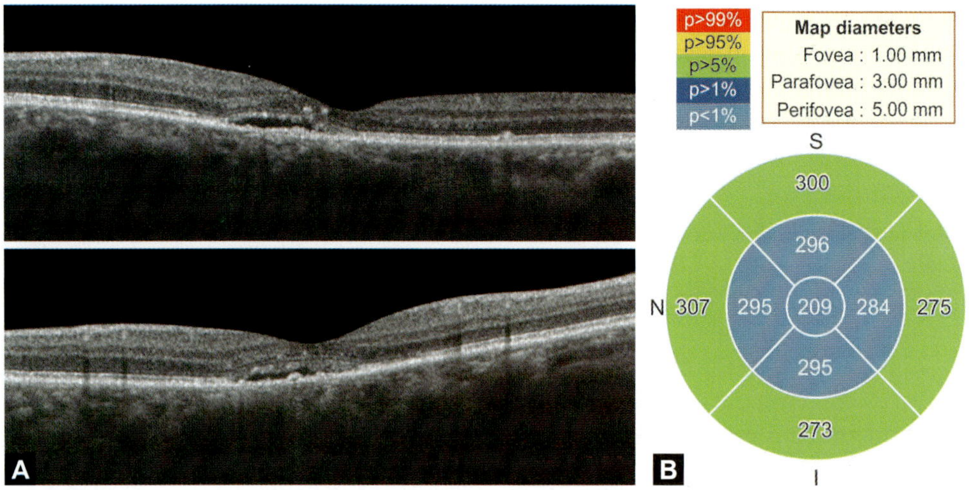

Figs. 5.4A and B: (A) An OCT B-scan of the macular region in 28-year-old male patient, who has been having chronic CSR treated for more than a year. A shallow sensory retinal detachment along with an irregular and hyperreflective RPE is seen. A shallow hyporeflective zone between the sensory retina and the RPE corresponds to the accumulated subretinal fluid; and (B) Retinal thickness map shows no thickening of the macular area. The values of the central region slightly below referential values are noted. (CSR: central serous chorioretinopathy; OCT: optical coherence tomography; RPE: retinal pigment epithelium)

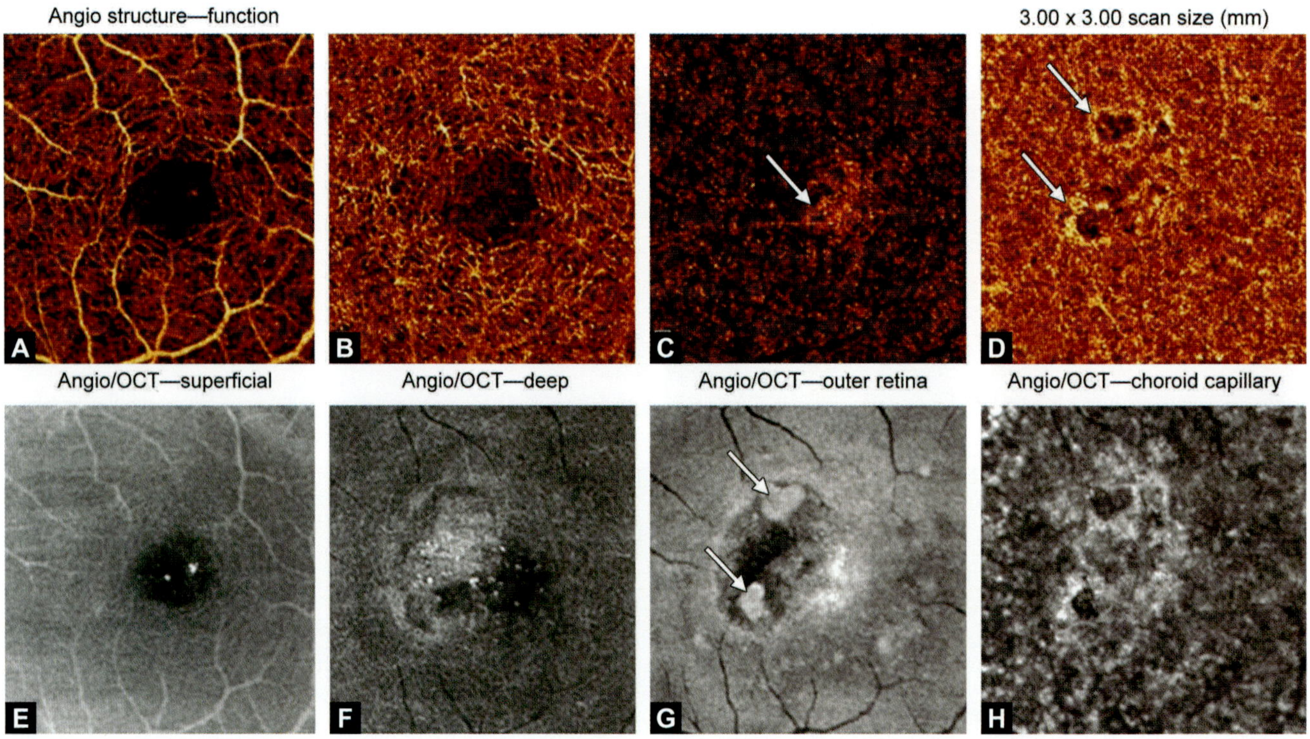

Figs. 5.5A to H: Parallel illustration of retinal layers using OCTA SSADA imaging protocol and en face OCT of the same eye as in Figure 5.4 (3 × 3 mm). (A and B) Superficial and deep vascular layer of the inner retina are without pathological changes, and show FAZ which is normal in size and shape; (E and F) Corresponding en face OCT images show a hyporeflective zone and a hyperreflective edge of sensory retinal detachment base, and numerous hyperreflective dots (stretched and elongated photoreceptors); (C and D) Showing an angiographic illustration of the outer retina and choriocapillaris. A delicate neovascularization, which corresponds to a fibrillar whitish membrane at the same location on en face OCT, is present; (G) Choriocapillaris angiography shows a few darker rounded lesions without the flow (detachment base), and along their edges active neovascularization can be seen; and (H) En face OCT of the choroidea corresponds to the angiography result and shows hyporeflective holes and along their edges delicate blossomed neovascularizations (hyperreflective whitish zones). (OCT: optical coherence tomography; OCTA: optical coherence tomography angiography)

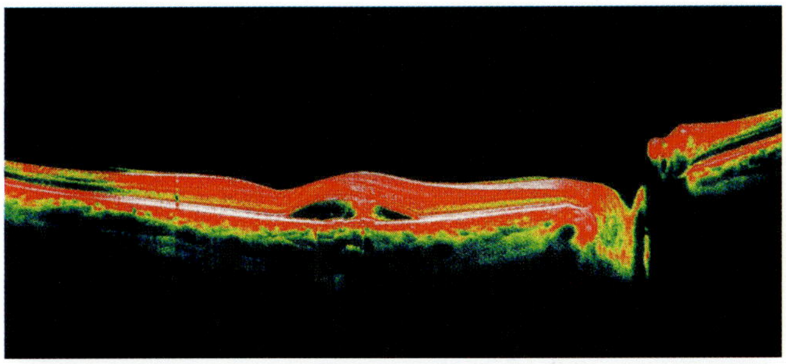

Fig. 5.6: The optical coherence tomography B-scan of the macula and optic nerve head in 36-year-old patient. In the nasal part of macular region, sensory retinal detachment and subretinal fluid can be seen. There is a small portion of preserved, "bridge-like" retinal tissue that connects choroidal part and deep part of inner, elevated retina.

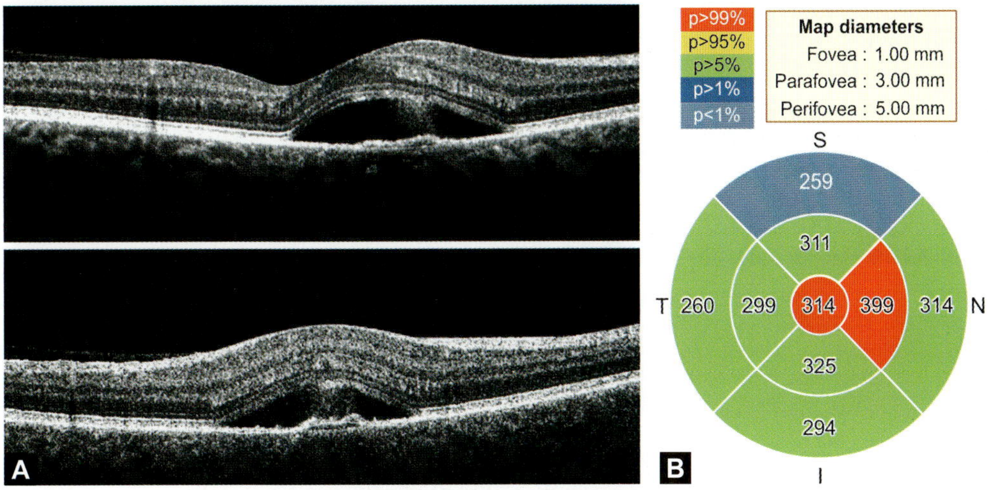

Figs. 5.7A and B: (A) The OCT B-scan of the same eye macula as in Figure 5.6. Sagittal cross-section of the macular region with a serous detachment of the sensory retina along with the RPE that is slightly elevated and irregular. A portion of retinal tissue pulls the RPE and forms a slight PED. The RPE is partially thinned; and (B) Illustration of retinal thickness map with a central and nasal thickening. (OCT: optical coherence tomography; RPE: retinal pigment epithelium; PED: pigment epithelial detachment)

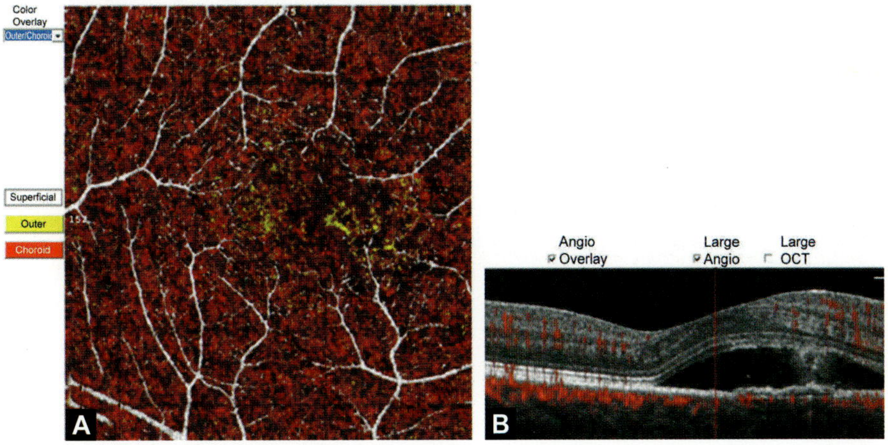

Figs. 5.8A and B: The OCTA AngioAnalytics of the same eye as in Figure 5.7. Colored neovascularization is illustrated on the retinal tissue "bridge" and on the site of elevation and RPE irregularities. It is an active neovascularization that forms a retino-retinal anastomosis, originating from deep vascular plexus and ending in a region below the RPE. The membrane has a renal glomerulus form as seen on en face angiogram of the choroidal layer. This is a distinct type of neovascularization, type 3 CNV. On the B-scan, focal choroidal excavation can be clearly seen. (CNV: choroidal neovascularization; OCTA: optical coherence tomography angiography; RPE: retinal pigment epithelium)

prognosis. Intravitreal anti-vascular endothelial growth factor treatment is recommended when the neovascularization appears, but is not advised as a therapy method in primary form of the disease. A treatment option including hormonal blockade, corticosteroid and mineralocorticoid inhibition is the subject of ongoing investigation. It is necessary to schedule regular medical check-ups and follow-up every 3–6 months.

BIBLIOGRAPHY

1. Abdallah A, Tsujikawa A, Ooto S, et al. Focal choroidal excavation in eyes with central serous chorioretinopathy. Am J Ophthalmol. 2013;156:673-83.
2. Agarwal A, Garg M, Dixit N, et al. Evaluation and correlation of stress scores with blood pressure, endogenous cortisol levels, and homocysteine levels in patients with central serous chorioretinopathy and comparison with age-matched controls. Indian J Ophthalmol. 2016;64(11):803-5.
3. Agrawal P. Increased choroidal vascularity in central serous chorioretinopathy quantified using swept-source optical coherence tomography. Am J Ophthalmol. 2017;174:176-7.
4. Arora S, Pyare R, Sridharan P, et al. Choroidal thickness evaluation of healthy eyes, central serous chorioretinopathy, and fellow eyes using spectral domain optical coherence tomography in Indian population. Indian J Ophthalmol. 2016;64(10):747-51.
5. Chan SY, Wang Q, Wei WB, et al. Optical coherence tomographic angiography in central serous chorioretinopathy. Retina. 2016;36(11):2051-8.
6. Daruich A, Matet A, Marchionno L, et al. Acute central serous chorioretinopathy: factors influencing episode duration. Retina. 2017;37(10):1905-15.
7. Ezuddin NS, Lanza NL, Weng CY. Subthreshold micropulse laser photocoagulation in the management of central serous chorioretinopathy. Int Ophthalmol Clin. 2016;56(4):165-74.
8. Feucht N, Maier M, Lohmann CP, et al. OCT angiography findings in acute central serous chorioretinopathy. Ophthalmic Surg Lasers Imaging Retina. 2016;47(4):322-7.
9. Islam QU, Hanif MK, Tareen S. Frequency of systemic risk factors in central serous chorioretinopathy. J Coll Physicians Surg Pak. 2016;26(8):692-5.
10. Kawada T. Shift Work: a risk factor for central serous chorioretinopathy. Am J Ophthalmol. 2016;171:151.
11. Lavinsky F, Lavinsky D. Novel perspectives on swept-source optical coherence tomography review. Int J Retina Vitreous. 2016;2:25.
12. Margolis R, Mukkamala SK, Jampol LM, et al. The Expanded Spectrum of Focal Choroidal Excavation. Arch Ophthalmol. 2011;129(10):1320-5.
13. Pang C, Freund B. Pachychoroid vasculopathy. Retina. 2015;35:1-9.
14. Regatieri CV, Novais EA, Branchini L, et al. Choroidal thickness in older patients with central serous chorioretinopathy. Int J Retina Vitreous. 2016;2:22.
15. Shin KH, Kim JH, Cho SW, et al. Efficacy of intravitreal bevacizumab for recurrent central serous chorioretinopathy in patients who had previously responded well to the same therapy. J Ocul Pharmacol Ther. 2016;32(7):425-30.
16. Shinojima A, Fujita K, Mori R, et al. Investigation of the etiology of central serous chorioretinopathy using en-face optical coherence tomography and indocyanine green angiography. Ophthalmologica. 2016;236(2):100-7.
17. Shinojima A, Kawamura A, Mori R, et al. Findings of optical coherence tomographic angiography at the choriocapillaris level in central serous chorioretinopathy. Ophthalmologica. 2016;236(2):108-13.
18. Shinojima A, Sawa M, Sekiryu T, et al. A multicenter randomized controlled study of antioxidant supplementation with lutein for chronic central serous chorioretinopathy. Ophthalmologica. 2017;237(3):159-66.
19. Tekin K, Sekeroglu MA, Cankaya AB, et al. Intravitreal bevacizumab and ranibizumab in the treatment of acute central serous chorioretinopathy: A single center retrospective study. Semin Ophthalmol. 2016. pp. 1-6.
20. Ünlü C, Erdogan G, Gezginaslan TA, et al. Subfoveal choroidal thickness changes after intravitreal bevacizumab therapy for central serous chorioretinopathy. Arq Bras Oftalmol. 2016;79(5):308-11.
21. Weng S, Mao L, Yu S, et al. Detection of choroidal neovascularization in central serous chorioretinopathy using optical coherence tomographic angiography. Ophthalmologica. 2016;236(2):114-21.
22. Yang D, Eliott D. Systemic mineralocorticoid antagonists in the treatment of central serous chorioretinopathy. Semin Ophthalmol. 2017;32(1):36-42.

CHAPTER 6

Polypoidal Choroidal Vasculopathy, Idiopathic Polypoidal Choroidal Vasculopathy

INTRODUCTION

Idiopathic polypoidal choroidal vasculopathy (IPCV) is a disease characterized by subretinal fluid accumulation, subretinal hemorrhage, retinal exudates, pigment epithelial detachment (PED), reddish-orange subretinal lesions, and/or retinal pigment epithelial atrophy.

EPIDEMIOLOGY AND ETIOLOGY

Idiopathic polypoidal choroidal vasculopathy, initially known as 'posterior uveal bleeding syndrome', was first described in African-American women. The highest prevalence is among heavily pigmented races. Women tend to be affected more often than men, and it usually occurs between 50 years and 65 years of age. The key factor of pathogenesis is a dilated network of inner choroid and leakage of fluid which leads to neurosensory retinal elevation and retinal pigment epithelium (RPE) detachment. The pathophysiological mechanism regarding the development of IPCV is not yet completely understood. It is believed that hypertension may also result in the development of choroidal vascular dilatation.

SYMPTOMS AND SIGNS

Patients report a reduction of vision over a period of time, along with the appearance of scotomas, with/without metamorphopsia. If the macula is spared, patients may be asymptomatic and not aware of being affected by the disease. The disease is usually bilateral, although unilateral cases have been described. Serosanguineous neurosensory and pigment epithelial detachment are the most prominent signs of the disease. Fundoscopic examination may reveal reddish and orange subretinal lesions, especially if the retinal atrophy is present. Those lesions are seen in the macular region, but also in peripapillary area. The absence of drusen and relatively minimal scarring helps in distinguishing IPCV from age-related macular degeneration (ARMD). Vitreous hemorrhage, retinal vascular disease, and signs of intraocular inflammation have also been reported.

DIFFERENTIAL DIAGNOSIS

- Central serous chorioretinopathy (CSCR),
- Neovascular ARMD,
- Choroidal hemangioma,
- Carcinoid metastasis, kidney cancer metastasis.

DIAGNOSIS

Idiopathic polypoidal choroidal vasculopathy can easily be discovered by an optical coherence tomography (OCT). Wavy and elevated RPE which interconnects forming a series of clearly defined elevations, with/without sharp notches can be seen. These types of polyps are described as PEDs on the OCT images.

Fluorescein angiography (FAG) is not required to establish the diagnosis of IPCV. Indocyanine green angiography (ICGA) is more useful. Pooling in the PED and areas of neurosensory detachment, and hyperfluorescence in the area of the choroidal plexus can be observed.

An early hyperfluorescence of the choroidal vascular network can be noted along with the late hyperfluorescence of the polyps at the edge of choroidal network that may leak. ICGA clearly detects the presence of polyps in the choroidal vasculature and it has been required for confirmation of the diagnosis until lately. Recently, OCT angiography (OCTA) has taken a very important role in diagnosing and monitoring polypoidal diseases. OCTA is a noninvasive imaging tool for detecting vascular changes in PCV.

An eye with IPCV presented by the OCTA is described in Figures 6.1 to 6.8.

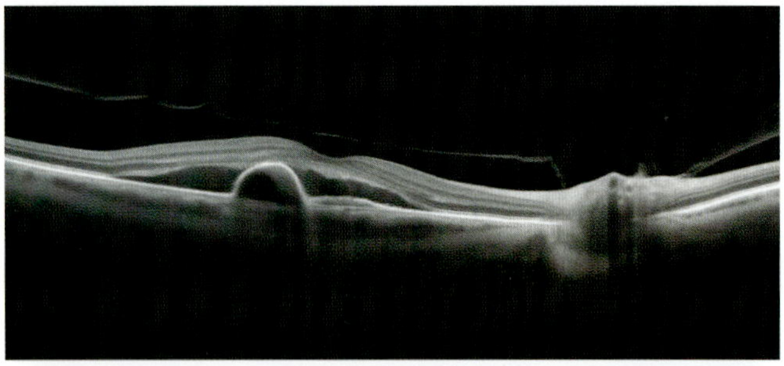

Fig. 6.1: An optical coherence tomography (OCT) B-scan of the macula and optic nerve head in a 58-year-old female patient. Retinal pigment epithelial detachment (PED) is illustrated along with a complete peripheral sensory retinal detachment and accumulated subretinal fluid.

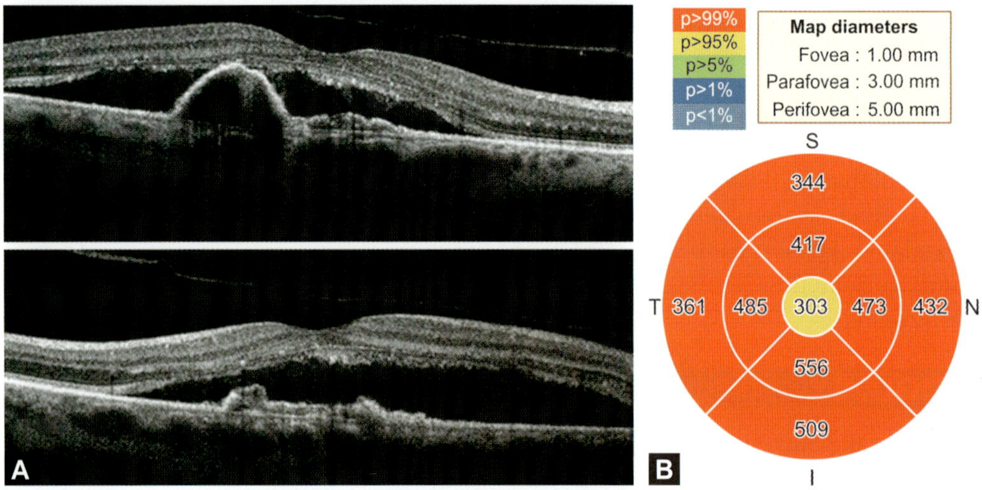

Figs. 6.2A and B: (A) The OCT B-scan of the macular area; the same eye as in previous image (3 × 3 mm). Macular cross-section images also show one large PED and several shallow irregular PEDs with granular surface that clusters and protrudes into subretinal hyporeflective fluid (suspected on the neovascularization); and (B) Retinal thickness map shows thickening in all macular segments. (OCT: optical coherence tomography; PED: pigment epithelial detachment)

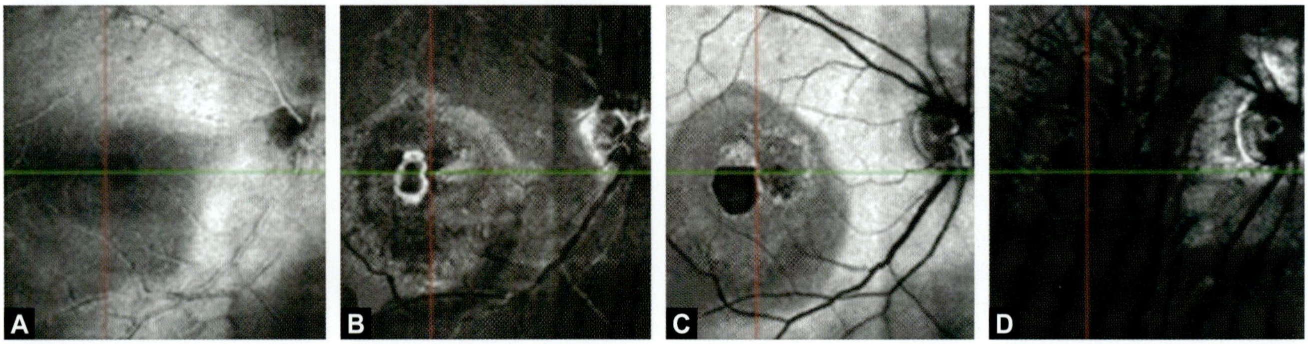

Figs. 6.3A to D: En face optical coherence tomography of retinal layers from superficial to choroidal (12 × 9 mm). (A) The superficial layer of the inner retina demonstrates a hyporeflective region and a hole in the foveal region. Deep layer of inner retina clearly shows a wide hyporeflective region which corresponds to the macular edema and subretinal fluid pooling; (B) In the middle of this region, a hyporeflective smaller zone with a hyperreflective sharp edge can be seen which matches the hole of the polyp cross section. Similar changes are visualized in the outer retina with the even better visualization of the polyp elevation base (the black hole in the center of hyporeflective region); (C) Hyperreflective dots correspond to changes in the photoreceptor layer; and (D) The choroidea shows a dark zone of the polyp base.

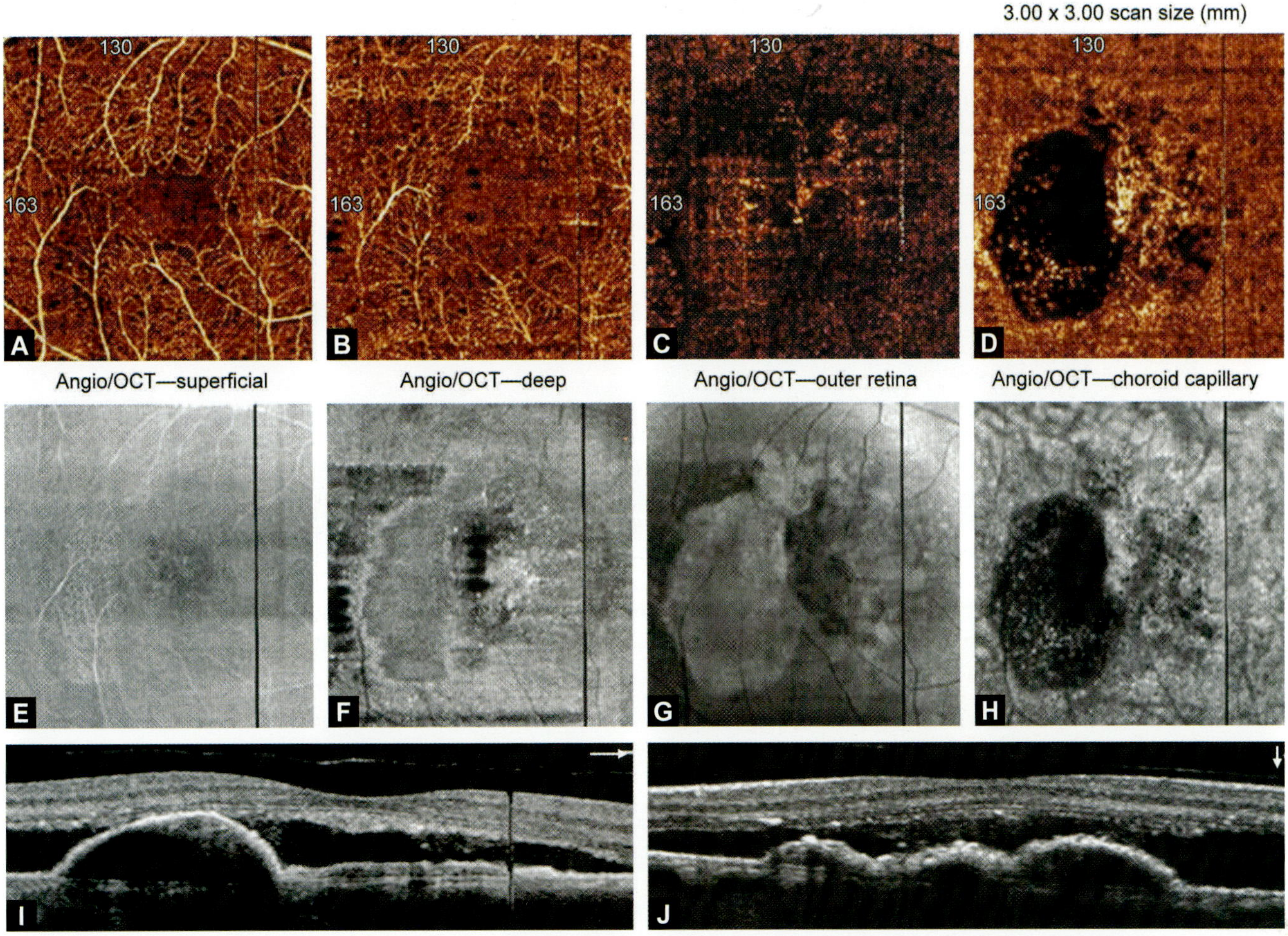

Figs. 6.4A to J: OCTA SSADA imaging protocol of the same eye as in the previous Figures (A to D) along with corresponding en face OCT images (E to H) and OCT B-scan (I and J). (A) In the superficial layer of inner retina a slightly enlarged FAZ can be seen, but without any other significant anomalies in the capillary network; (E) En face OCT of the corresponding layer correlates to the physiological finding; (B) Deep layer of inner retina demonstrates a significant FAZ enlargement with the disappearance of its regular, round configuration; (F) En face OCT of the deep inner retinal layer exhibits a hyporeflective region of the polyp base; (C) The angiogram of outer retina shows a delicate neovascular structure in the center; (G) En face OCT illustrates a hyporeflective region with hyperreflective membrane; (D) The choroidea shows a dark vascularization defect in the center, which corresponds to the flow disruption due to the polyp base, and an active and finely branched neovascularization on the edge of the defect; (H) En face OCT image corresponds to the angiography finding; and (I and J) A magnified image of the OCT B-scan shows a sequence of PEDs with sharply demarcated edges and sharp notches. A serous retinal detachment can also be seen. (OCTA: optical coherence tomography angiography; PED: pigment epithelial detachment)

THERAPY

Patients with IPCV have either a variant of wet ARMD or a completely isolated disorder. Differentiation between these two entities is very important, since each has a different prognosis, depending on responses to the treatment. Cases of IPCV without macular involvement are only observed. In patients with the involvement of the central portion as well, antivascular endothelial growth factor (anti-VEGF) treatment and/or photodynamic therapy are recommended. Patients with IPCV are more refractory to anti-VEGF therapy in comparison to patients with ARMD. The EVEREST trial showed that patients with IPCV variant of wet ARMD treated with combined anti-VEGF therapy (ranibizumab) and photodynamic therapy demonstrated significant polypoidal lesions regression than patients treated with anti-VEGF alone (Figs. 6.9A to H).

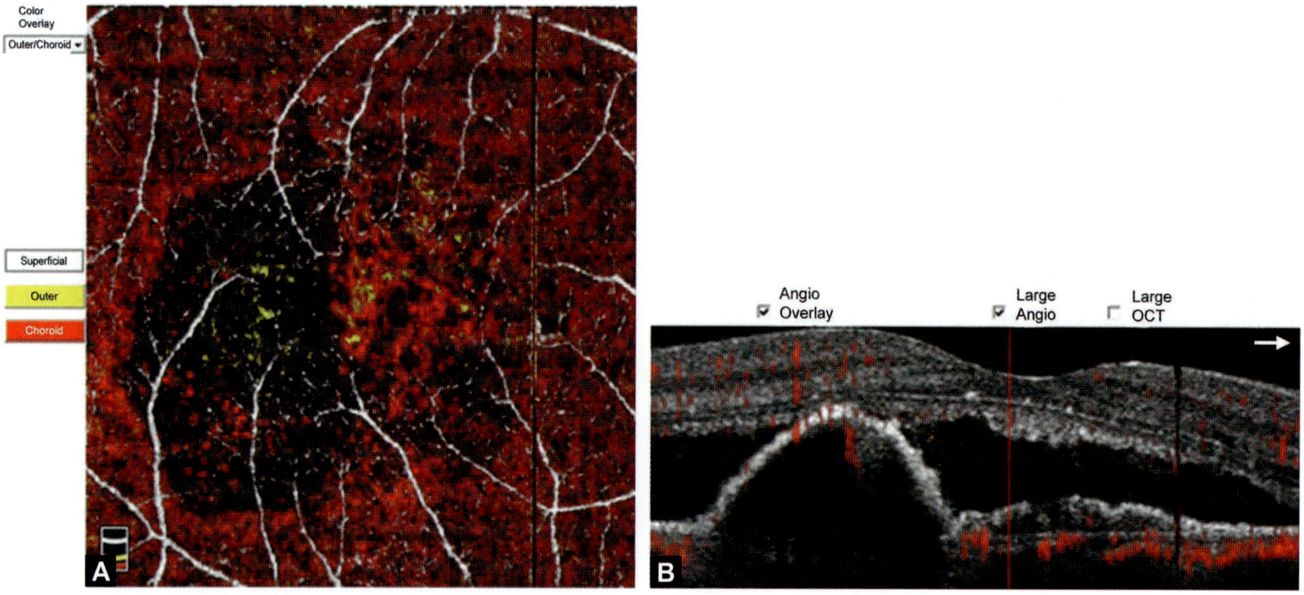

Figs. 6.5A and B: (A) AngioAnalytics shows the Type 2 neovascularization which is colored in red in the choroidal layer, and in yellow in the outer retina. A black region beside the neovascularization demonstrates an area without flow which matches the base of choroidal polyp; and (B) The optical coherence tomography B-scan of the region is processed by the AngioAnalytics.

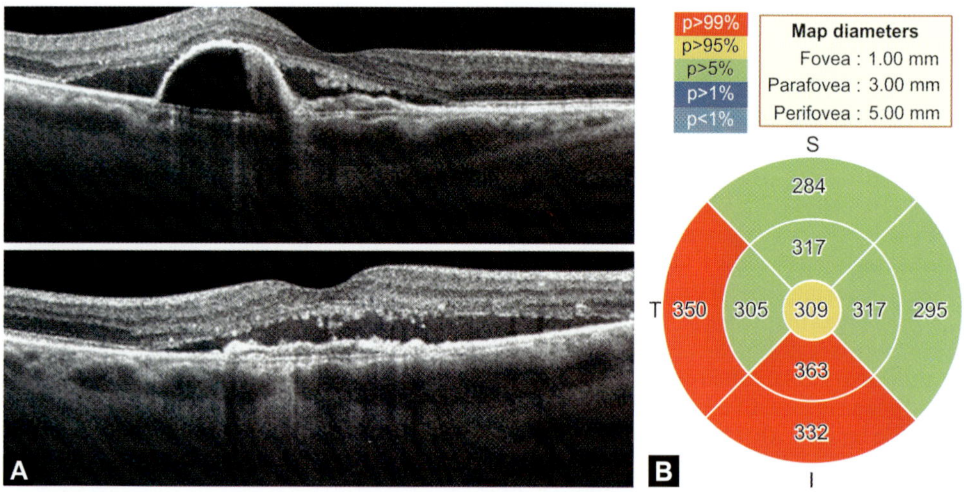

Figs. 6.6A and B: (A) The OCT B-scan of the same eye as in previous images, a day after intravitreal aflibercept injection. The size of PED is the same, but a hyporeflective subretinal fluid accumulation is significantly decreased; and (B) The finding is confirmed by a retinal thickness map which shows a significant decreasement in macular thickness, especially in the superior and nasal portion. (OCT: optical coherence tomography; PED: pigment epithelial detachment)

About a half of untreated patients have a rather satisfactory visual acuity with relatively good visual prognosis. In the other half of patients, visual acuity is significantly reduced over a short period of time. The best prognostic marker is the value of visual acuity at the time when patients present to an ophthalmologist.

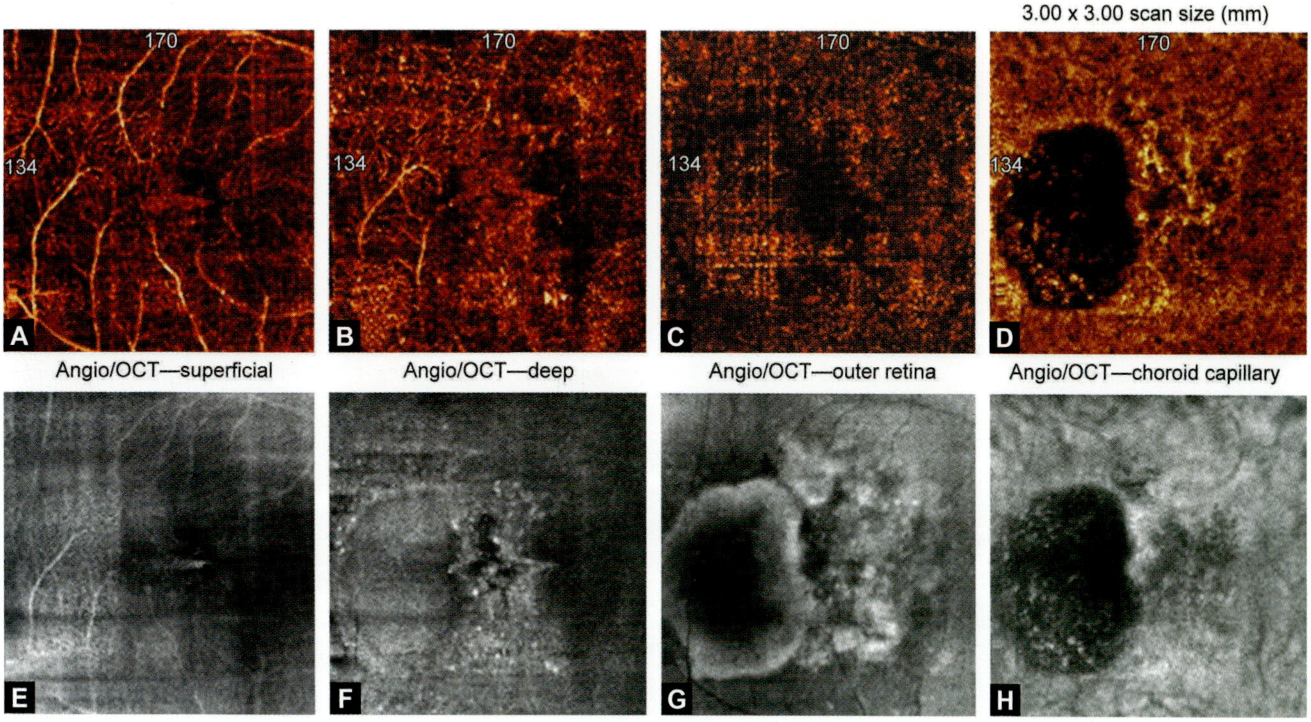

Figs. 6.7A to H: (A and B) The OCTA SSADA imaging protocol and en face OCT of outer and inner retinal layers of the same eye, a day after the first intravitreal aflibercept injection; (C and D) OCTA shows significantly lower activity of the CNV with a loss of tiny capillaries inside the neovascularization; (E and F) En face OCT images of superficial and deep part of inner retina show no significant changes when compared to the images before the treatment; and (G and H) The finding is also confirmed by the en face OCT, showing a significantly less visible hyperreflective membrane beside the base of PED. (CNV: choroidal neovascularization; OCTA: optical coherence tomography angiography; PED: pigment epithelial detachment)

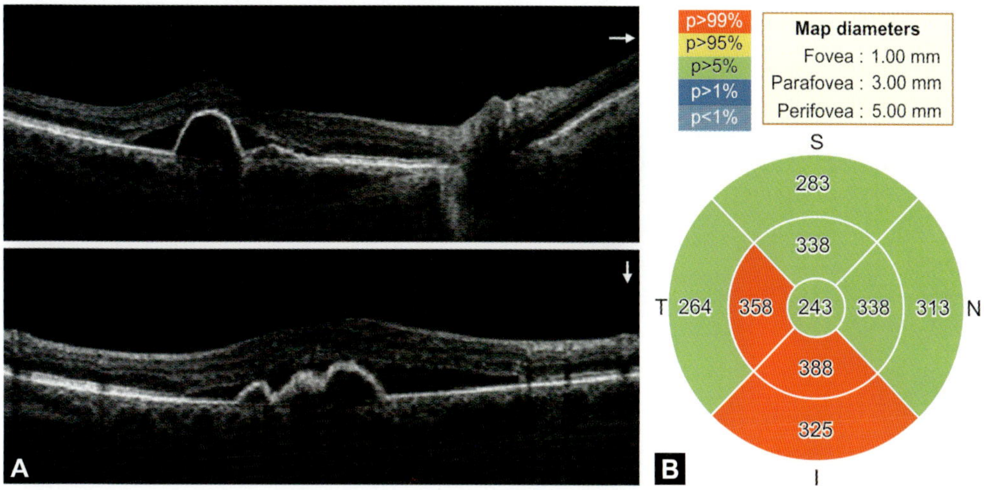

Figs. 6.8A and B: (A) An OCT B-scan of the same eye, a day after the second intravitreal aflibercept injection. PED is not changed in size, and the subretinal hyporeflective fluid is seemingly the same in size as after the first injection; and (B) Retinal thickness map reveals even lower and more referential values of the macular thickness, suggesting that the retinal detachment is even more shallow than after the first injection. (OCT: optical coherence tomography; PED: pigment epithelial detachment)

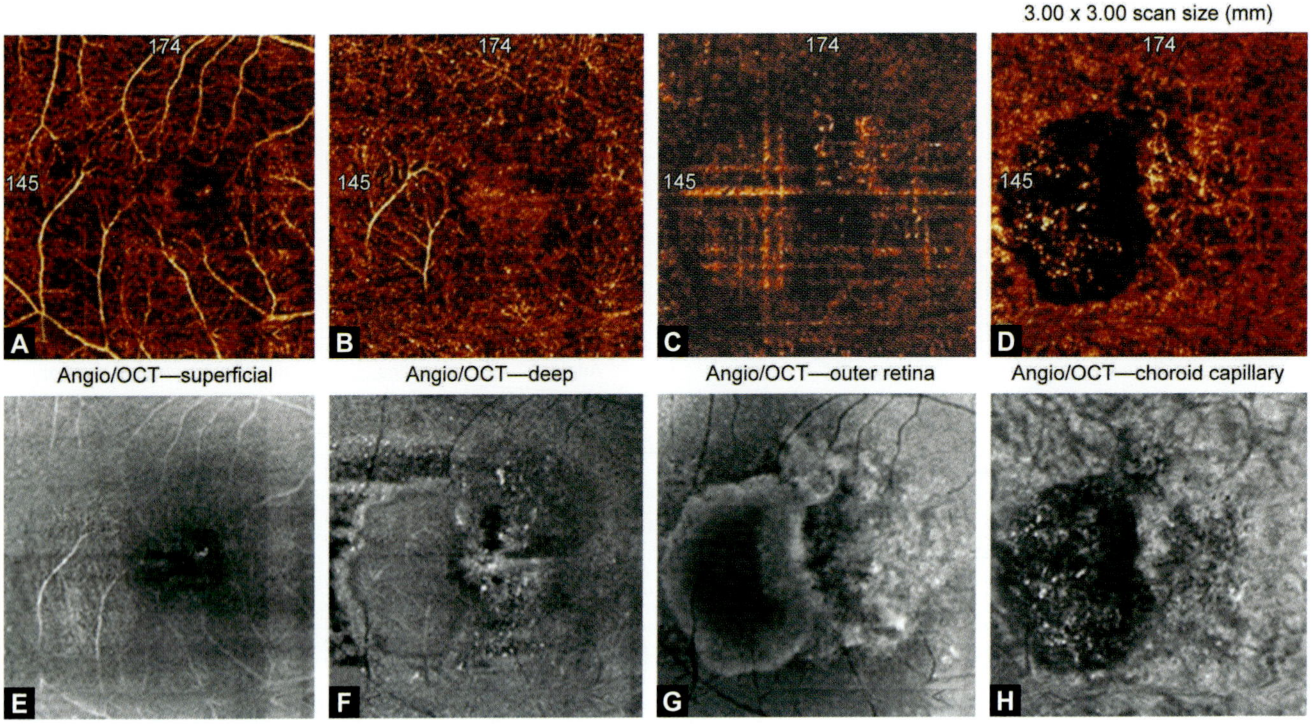

Figs. 6.9A to H: OCTA SSADA imaging protocol and en face OCT of inner and outer retinal layers, the same eye as in previous Figures, a day after the second intravitreal aflibercept injection. (A to D) Neovascular membrane is even more dry, less dense, and branchy. PED does not respond to anti-VEGF therapy; and (E to H) The finding is consistent with en face OCT showing a significantly smaller hyperreflective connective membrane along the edge of the hyporeflective region of the polyp basis. (OCT: optical coherence tomography; PED: pigment epithelial detachment; VEGF: vascular endothelial growth factor)

BIBLIOGRAPHY

1. Koh A, Lee WK, Chen LJ, et al. EVEREST Study: Efficacy and safety of verteporfin photodynamic therapy in combination with ranibizumab or alone versus ranibizumab monotherapy in patients with symptomatic macular polypoidal choroidal vasculopathy. Retina. 2012;32(8):1453-64.
2. Uyama M, Wada M, Nagai Y, et al. Polypoidal choroidal vasculopathy: Natural history. Am J Ophthalmol. 2002;133(5):639-48.
3. Wang M, Zhou Y, Gao SS, et al. Evaluating polypoidal choroidal vasculopathy with optical coherence tomography angiography. Invest Ophthalmol Vis Sci. 2016;57(9):OCT526-32.
4. Yannuzzi LA, Ciardella A, Spaide RF, et al. The expanding clinical spectrum of idiopathic polypoidal choroidal vasculopathy. Arch Ophthalmol. 1997;115(4):478-85.
5. Yannuzzi LA, Sorenson J, Spaide RF, et al. Idiopathic polypoidal choroidal vasculopathy (IPCV). Retina. 1990;10(1):1-8.

CHAPTER 7

Diabetic Retinopathy

INTRODUCTION

Diabetic retinopathy (DR) is an eye disease that affects the retina in people with diabetes mellitus (DM). It is the leading cause of vision impairment in adults between the ages of 20 years and 74 years. The main risk factors for the development of DR are the duration of diabetes and blood sugar levels. Due to the accumulation of glucose/fructose in blood, tiny, small blood vessels start being affected, and they start to develop microangiopathic changes. These microangiopathic changes lead to the occlusion and increased permeability of blood vessels, causing hypoxia, ischemia, and retinal edema.

EPIDEMIOLOGY AND ETIOLOGY

Diabetic retinopathy occurs only in patients with diabetes. Up to 84% of patients with type 1 diabetes develops retinopathy within 20 years, while about 50% with type 2 diabetes develop the disease in the same period. The longer a patient suffers from diabetes, the risk of developing DR increases. In the period from 1990 to 2010, DR was ranked as the fifth most common cause of the blindness that could be prevented, and the fifth most common cause of moderate or severe loss of visual acuity. One-third of 285 million DM patients worldwide, in 2010, had initial signs of DR and one-third had signs of vision-threatening diabetic retinopathy (VTDR), which was defined as a preproliferative diabetic retinopathy (PPDR), proliferative diabetic retinopathy (PDR), or DR with the presence of diabetic macular edema (DME). So far, many studies, affiliated with the frequency of the disease, its distribution and risk factors, have been published. They also include geographic and ethnic differences, but ultimately, epidemiological data on DME is relatively deficient. The review articles from 2012 indicate that 7% of patients with diabetes may have DME and that the risk factors for DME are similar to those for DR. The prevalence of DR is higher in patients with type 1 DM than in patients with type 2 DM. It is estimated that in the European countries and in the USA, the prevalence of DR among patients with DM type 1 is between 36.5% and 93.6%, while the prevalence of the VTDR is between 6.7% and 34.9%. The prevalence of the DME among patients with DM type 1 is between 4.2% and 7.9%, while in patients with DM type 2 it is between 1.4% and 12.8%. The prevalence of DME among patients with diabetes is generally lower than the prevalence of DR.

SYMPTOMS AND SIGNS

The disease is initially asymptomatic, however, when macular changes or a vitreous hemorrhage take place, a loss of visual acuity or visual scotomas can occur. According to the severity of the clinical picture, DR is divided into a mild, nonproliferative form [nonproliferative diabetic retinopathy (NPDR)] and into a more severe, proliferative form of the disease (PDR). Fundoscopical examination may reveal one or more signs of DR. NPDR can present with various fundoscopical changes, including microaneurysms, dot-and-blot or flame-shaped retinal hemorrhages, retinal edema (most commonly DME), soft (cotton-wool), and hard lipid exudates as well as arteriovenous anastomoses [intraretinal microvascular abnormalities (IRMAs)].

Disease progression leads to the obstruction of venules and arterioles and development of proliferative DR, which is manifested by the appearance of new blood vessels and growth of the glial tissue. Walls of new blood vessels have only endothelium, and no pericytes, so they tend to extravasate into the surrounding retinal tissue and vitreous. Neovascularization may occur anywhere in the retina [*new vessels elsewhere (NVE)*], in the area of the optic disk [*new vessels at disk (NVD)*], or on the iris [*new vessels at iris (NVI)*], and the process is completed by the development of neovascular blood vessels in the eye angle. Long-term neovascularization is followed by the proliferation of fibrous tissue and forming of the fibrovascular membrane, which retracts the surrounding tissue and causes a tractional retinal detachment.

Diabetic macular edema occurs in the preproliferative and proliferative DR due to increased vascular permeability. The loss of visual acuity appears due to the DME, macular capillary nonperfusion, vitreous hemorrhages, or retinal detachment.

INTERNATIONAL CLINICAL DIABETIC RETINOPATHY DISEASE SEVERITY SCALE ACCORDING TO THE AMERICAN ACADEMY OF OPHTHALMOLOGY

The International Clinical Diabetic Retinopathy Disease Severity Scale according to the American Academy of Ophthalmology is demonstrated in Table 7.1.

Table 7.1: International Clinical Diabetic Retinopathy Disease Severity Scale according to the American Academy of Ophthalmology.

Disease severity level	*Ophthalmoscopy findings*
No apparent retinopathy	No abnormalities
Mild NPDR	Microaneurysms (MA) only
Moderate NPDR	More than just microaneurysms, but less than severe NPDR. Additional findings can be: ▪ Dot and blot hemorrhages ▪ Soft (*cotton-wool*) exudates ▪ IRMA.
Severe NPDR	Any of the following: ▪ More than 20 intraretinal hemorrhages in each of four quadrants ▪ Definite venous beading in two or more quadrants ▪ Prominent IRMA in one quadrant or more No signs of PDR
PDR	One or more of the following: ▪ Neovascularization ▪ Vitreous or preretinal hemorrhage.

(NPDR: nonproliferative diabetic retinopathy; PDR: proliferative diabetic retinopathy)

DIFFERENTIAL DIAGNOSIS

- Radiation retinopathy
- Hypertensive retinopathy
- Retinal vein occlusion
- Ocular ischemic syndrome
- Vasculitis syndromes (sarcoidosis, lupus)
- Anemia, leukemia
- Coats' disease
- Sickle cell retinopathy
- Iatrogenic retinopathy (interferons, indomethacin, and chemotherapy).

DIAGNOSTICS

Dilated fundus examination can be performed by direct or indirect ophthalmoscopy. The fundus is analyzed along with its far periphery, with the aim of diagnosing DR and monitoring patients with pathological changes. In everyday clinical practice, the examination is performed using a biomicroscope and indirect noncontact slit-lamp lens, which allows the stereo-biomicroscopic examination of the fundus. Fundus photography is used as a document for monitoring the disease and therapy response. It is helpful in the proper assessment of the disease severity level. The analysis of stereoscopic fundus photographs is a very subjective method, almost like ophthalmoscopy, where interpretation of findings can vary largely among experts in the field.

Nowadays, the necessity for the early and objective diagnosis requires the use of a newer, automated image technology, primarily the optical coherence tomography (OCT). OCT is a noninvasive, noncontact diagnostic tool with high sensitivity and specificity for DR diagnosis and monitoring. It is actually a sort of optical biopsy, because it allows scanning in situ and in vivo, without the prescanning preparation of the patient. OCT quantifies the retinal thickening, monitors the macular edema development [cystoid macular edema (CME), DME], and visualizes vitreomacular tractions in patients with macular edema. It is unavoidable in monitoring the efficacy of therapy, it determines an optimal time for beginning the antivascular endothelial growth factor (anti-VEGF) therapy, shows the efficacy of the anti-VEGF therapy, and helps in deciding which kind of treatment is better for the patient—laser treatment or vitrectomy.

OPTICAL COHERENCE TOMOGRAPHY AND NONPROLIFERATIVE DIABETIC RETINOPATHY

Nonproliferative diabetic retinopathy stands for changes in the retinal blood capillaries, which may be occluded forming the regions without a flow or dilated and forming the edema. The OCT classifies and quantifies the existence of edema. The OCT can clearly show preretinal and intraretinal hemorrhage, epiretinal membrane, and soft and hard exudates. The OCT cannot visualize ischemia. Soft *(cotton-wool)* exudates are placed superficially, on the boundaries of the ischemic regions, due to the ischemic impairment of nerve fibers. The OCT can also show nodular, hyperreflective regions, or elongated lesions of nerve fibers, that can eventually make shadows on the deeper layers. The en face OCT can locate them in the nerve fiber layer.

Hard Exudates

Hard exudates are made of lipoproteins that precipitate in the retina, more precisely on the edges between the edema and normal retina. They are located in the deep retina and often occur around areas with vascular intraretinal abnormalities, from which the formation of the retinal edema begins. Hard exudates present as hyperreflective areas on OCT scans and they can be circular or star shaped. Those exudates can make a shadow on layers below, so they can sometimes be difficult for analyzing. If they develop furthermore, they can create macular fibrosis with many plaques, which can cause visual impairment.

Hemorrhages

Retinal hemorrhages are usually placed in the inner retina, and are usually flame-shaped. They are hyperreflective on the OCT and can also create shadows and cover up deeper layers. Small hemorrhages cannot be seen very easily.

Macular Edema

There are a few types of macular edema. It can be vascular macular edema, traction macular edema, and a mixed type. The OCT can clearly reveal the existence of retinal edema. It can show typical retinal thickening and the presence of hyperreflexive hard exudates in deeper retinal layers (outer plexiform, outer nuclear, and photoreceptor layer). Organization of the edema starts with the fluid leakage from the damaged capillary wall and from intraretinal microvascular changes. Hard exudates are always observed at the exact border between a healthy and edematous retina. The initial edema is focal, but in time it spreads into the surrounding tissue and forms a diffuse edema. Some authors assume that the spongy, edematous region appears due to the damage of Müller cells. The OCT shows a thickened retina with multiple cystoid spaces. The edema can be quantified precisely by measuring the retinal thickness.

Diffuse Edema

Diffuse edema is present in a majority of patients with DR. An OCT can show increased retinal thickness and the presence of numerous small irregular microcavities that give the retina a sponge-like appearance. Hyporeflective edema regions usually spread throughout the retina and are most commonly seen in the outer parts of the retina (outer plexiform and outer nuclear layer). After 5 years of progression, irregular microcavities can form pseudocysts.

Cystoid Macular Edema

After a longer period of time, diffuse macular edema can lead to the necrosis of Müller cells and the forming of cystoid cavitations within the retina. CME represents the initial stage, where many pseudocysts can be seen in the inner and outer retina. The cysts can merge into each other over time, and can form large cavitations. They begin to form in the inner and outer nuclear layer and then spread to the outer and inner plexiform layer. A severe form of CME can expand to the entire thickness of the retina, and cause atrophy of the entire surrounding tissue.

The en face OCT usually shows the CME as a honeycomb-shaped or a petal-shaped formation, depending on the depth and affected layer. A honeycomb-shaped CME on the en face image appears most commonly if the edema is localized in the outer plexiform and outer nuclear layer. If it has a petal-shape appearance, the edema is most commonly found in the inner retinal layers.

Serous Foveal Detachment

Serous retinal detachment is always placed in the macula and is related to the deterioration of the CME. Most commonly, it appears about 10 years after the onset of the disease. It is considered a normal path of diabetic edema progression. Serous detachment is less common in diffuse edema. It occurs in 10% of patients with DR. In many cases, the epiretinal membrane can be visualized on the OCT. A traction of the ERM on the retinal surface causes the deterioration of the edema and occurrence of folds, which can be accurately seen on en face OCT images. Neuroretina is thickened and a normal foveal depression disappears. It is very important to quantify the edema by measuring the thickness and volume of the macula. The retinal thickness is in direct correlation with visual acuity. Quantitative measurements of the macula and retinal edema are essential for the prognosis of the disease and making a decision about the method of treatment (they indicate either laser therapy or surgery).

THE PROGRESSION OF A NONPROLIFERATIVE INTO A PROLIFERATIVE FORM OF DIABETIC RETINOPATHY

When the DR initially begins to develop, retinal structures are usually physiological. An optical coherence tomography angiography (OCTA) can sometimes show small hyperreflective deposits, along with corresponding shadows in the deep retina (hard exudates). Edema can also often be visualized. Due to the disease progression, the number of exudates increases and they become more dense. Also, the serous elevation with the impairment of photoreceptors is possible.

If progression continues even after the laser treatment and anti-VEGF injections, the retina loses its normal structure. The layers of the retina cannot be easily recognized anymore and the number of hard exudates is significantly increased. Laser spots cause vertical shadows on the scans, which are seen through all layers of the retina. Progression of the disease in the macula causes the appearance of macular fibrous plaque. Usually, the central fibrous tissue can be seen as a central hyperreflective nodule, which is related to the atrophy and deformation of the entire macular area. The retinal thickness map can show central atrophic zones surrounded by edema.

Proliferative Diabetic Retinopathy

Proliferative diabetic retinopathy is characterized by the appearance of neovascularization and/or preretinal hemorrhages. Newborn blood vessels usually appear in the borders of ischemic regions and in the optical disk. On the OCT, retinal ischemic regions can present as a thickening of the inner retina along with the sponge-like edema. PDR is more common in younger people. New blood vessels are formed, preretinal vessels at first, and then prepapillar and intravitreal.

Preretinal blood vessels are new, young, and gentle blood vessels that appear on the edges of ischemic regions. The wall of those vessels consists of cells which have a very high permeability and are very fragile. An OCT can show the neovascular membrane only when enough fibrotic tissue is formed. Fibroglial membranes and deformations of the retinal profile can be clearly visualized in places where the traction causes a slight retinal elevation. The edema is usually present below the retinal elevation. Prepapillar blood vessels cause neovascularization on the papilla and usually fill the papillary pit.

The tractional retinal detachment can be precisely located and monitored by OCT, which is extremely important for determining the severity of DR and for monitoring the response to conservative or operative treatment. OCT can clearly demonstrate the progression of detachment in the area associated with the superior and inferior vascular arcade, as well as the location of the distortion caused by fibrovascular blood vessels.

OPTICAL COHERENCE TOMOGRAPHY ANGIOGRAPHY—SPLIT-SPECTRUM AMPLITUDE-DECORRELATION ANGIOGRAPHY PROTOCOL

Optical coherence tomography angiography—split-spectrum amplitude-decorrelation angiography (SSADA) protocol provides a detailed analysis of vascular anomalies throughout the entire retina. The thickness of the retina is split into four vascular layers, which are analyzed by the OCTA: (1) The superficial, (2) Deep vascular plexus, (3) The outer retina, and (4) The choriocapillary layer. OCTA can often show the pathological changes that cannot be seen by fundus examination or by OCT structural analysis.

The foveolar avascular zone (FAZ) in the DR usually expands, microaneurysms appear, and the number of intercapillary areas without flow increase (vascular dropouts). Changes in the FAZ are best seen in the superficial vascular plexus while vascular dilatation and changes in capillaries are best seen in the deep vascular plexus. Microaneurysms can be visualized only if the flow inside them is sufficient in speed, allowing the software to detect them. If capillaries are obliterated or thrombosed, microaneurysms cannot be visualized by the OCTA. Since the flow is usually very slow in microaneurysms, the SSADA protocol often does not detect nor show all of them. Expansion of the FAZ is directly related to the development of an ischemic maculopathy.

Fluorescein angiography (FAG) is no longer used for diagnosing minimal diabetic changes, but is recommended for patients in which retinal neovascularization and changes in the retinal periphery are suspected. FAG can show the appearance of hyperfluorescences with late dye leakage.

There are also some other diagnostic tools for DR. *Red-free* fundus photography demonstrates the presence of retinal hemorrhages, which are not visible in normal light, as well as the presence of microaneurysms and intraretinal microvascular abnormality (IRMA) that were not clearly seen during examination. Ultrasonography is also an inevitable diagnostic tool for retinal detachment, when other optical media are blurred (due to cataracts or vitreous hemorrhages), leaving no other diagnostic methods available.

NONPROLIFERATIVE DIABETIC RETINOPATHY

The nonproliferative diabetic retinopathy is shown in Figures 7.1 to 7.14.

PREPROLIFERATIVE DIABETIC RETINOPATHY

The preproliferative diabetic retinopathy is shown in Figures 7.15 to 7.19.

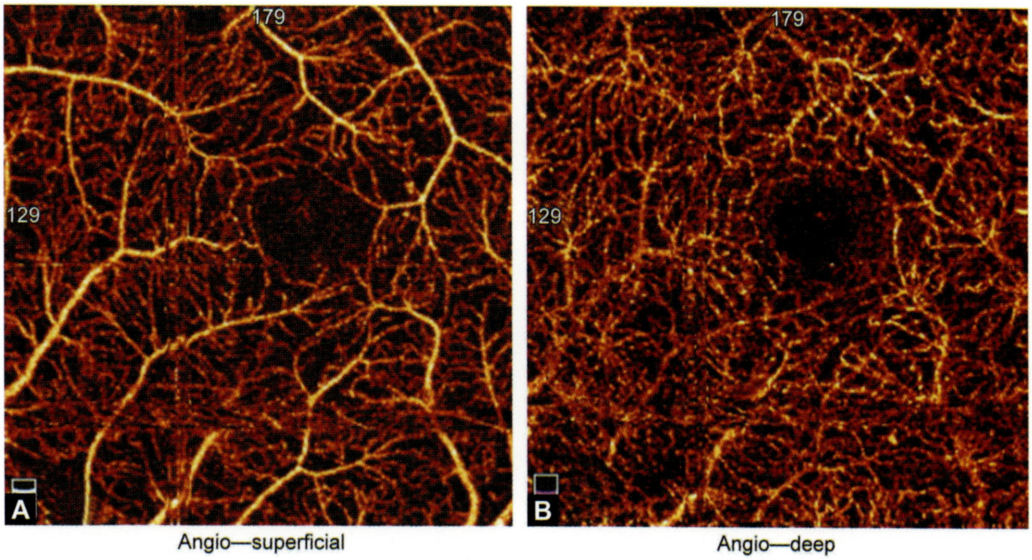

Figs. 7.1A and B: An OCTA SSADA protocol of the superficial and deep vascular plexus (3 × 3 mm). (A) An en face angiogram of the superficial vascular plexus with a gentle capillary net. There are a few slightly enhanced intercapillary areas without flow, especially around the FAZ (vascular dropouts). FAZ seems to be regular in size and very slightly changed in shape (on the right side of the FAZ). A few microaneurysms can be also visualized. They appear as tiny "hyperreflective" dots on the en face vascular scan; and (B) A deep vascular plexus, where a larger number of microaneurysms can be seen. Some capillaries seem to be dilated and irregular in this plexus, and the vascular structures are more harsh and asymmetrical. (FAZ: foveolar avascular zone; OCTA: optical coherence tomography angiography; SSADA: split-spectrum amplitude-decorrelation angiography)

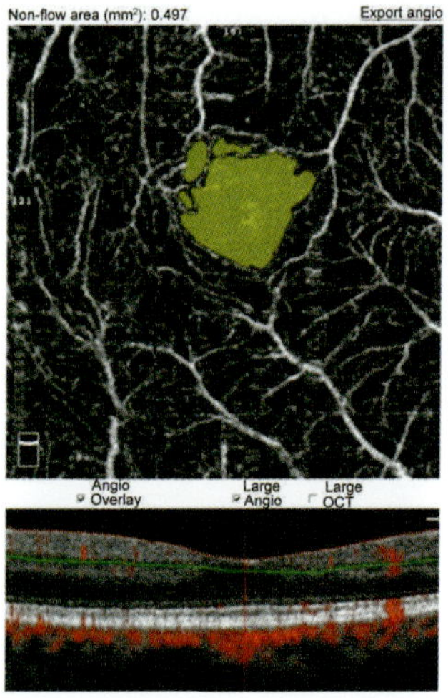

Fig. 7.2: OCT software allows the analysis of the foveal avascular zone (FAZ) and all the areas without flow (Angio analysis of non-flow areas); the same eye as in the previous image. Analysis is done in the superficial vascular plexus. Areas without flow are colored in yellow, and those areas can be quantified. FAZ is slightly enlarged and irregular in shape, which is one of the typical signs for the NPDR. The central foveal area, along with a few small capillary dropouts above it, measures 0.49 mm^2. In the lower part of the image, an OCT B-scan is shown, which signifies the superficial layer, where the analysis is performed. (NPDR: nonproliferative diabetic retinopathy; OCT: optical coherence tomography)

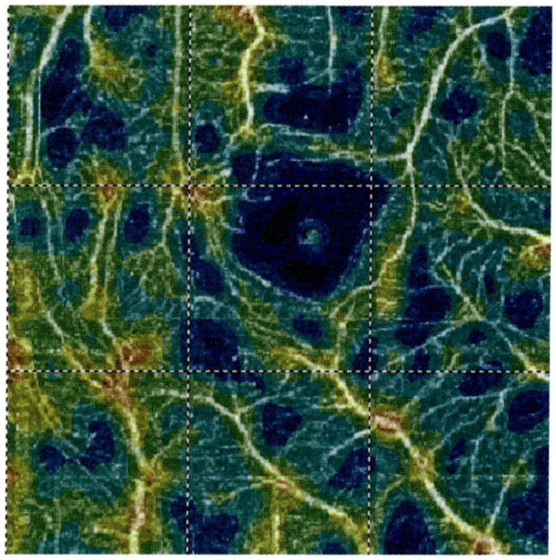

Fig. 7.3: Another type of Angio analysis that the software allows is the presentation of a vascular density map. Capillary density can be analyzed in the superficial or deep vascular plexus. In this image, the same eye as in the previous images is presented. Using cold and blue colors, the software presents areas with reduced flow or areas without any flow. The yellow and red colors are typical for areas with maintained and regular flow. In this image, the whole macular area has a reduced flow with many vascular dropouts (many blue areas, which are different in size and shape). This appearance of the macular density map is typical for nonproliferative diabetic retinopathy (NPDR).

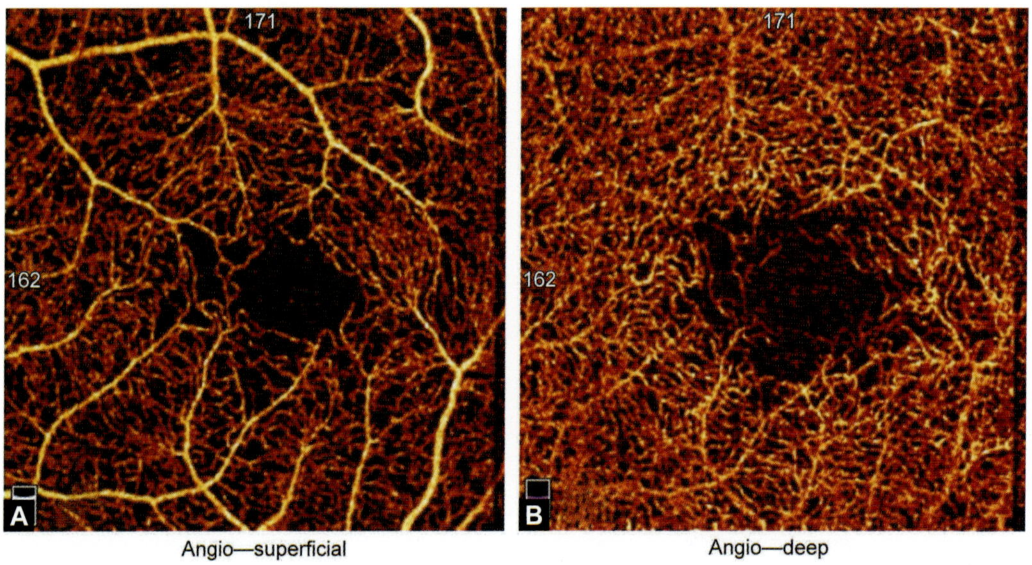

Figs. 7.4A and B: An OCTA SSADA protocol of the superficial and deep vascular plexus (3 × 3 mm). (A) The superficial vascular plexus shows typical changes that can be seen in the NPDR. FAZ is slightly changed in shape, and it looks oval. Around the FAZ, many nonflow areas can be seen (vascular dropouts). The ends of capillaries are tortuous and form loops. Vascular changes around the FAZ are irregular and asymmetrical; and (B) An OCTA en face angiogram of the deep vascular plexus shows significantly enlarged FAZ that is irregular in shape. It seems like it is connecting with surrounding dark nonflow zones. Many microaneurysms can be visualized, along with the capillary loops and other microvascular abnormalities. (FAZ: foveolar avascular zone; OCTA: optical coherence tomography angiography; SSADA: split-spectrum amplitude-decorrelation angiography)

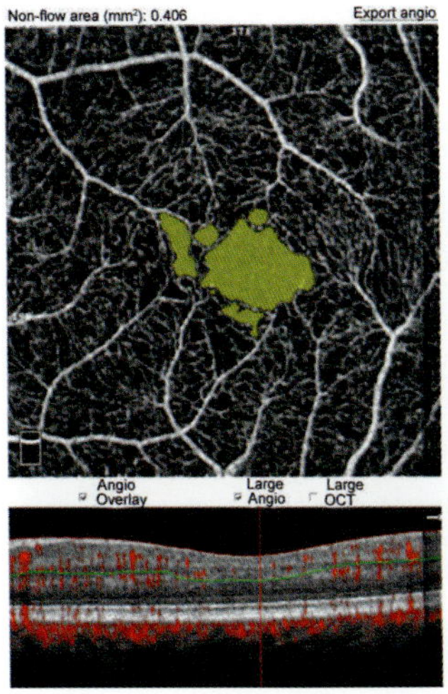

Fig. 7.5: Angio analysis of the superficial vascular plexus of the same eye as in Figures 7.4A and B. Foveolar avascular zone (FAZ) is colored in yellow and along with the few surrounding vascular dropout areas, it measures 0.406 mm^2. FAZ is irregular in shape and is surrounded with many dropout areas that are different in size and shape. In the lower part of the image, a corresponding B-scan can be seen, showing the flow with red dots, and the depth of the analyzed layer with the red and green horizontal line.

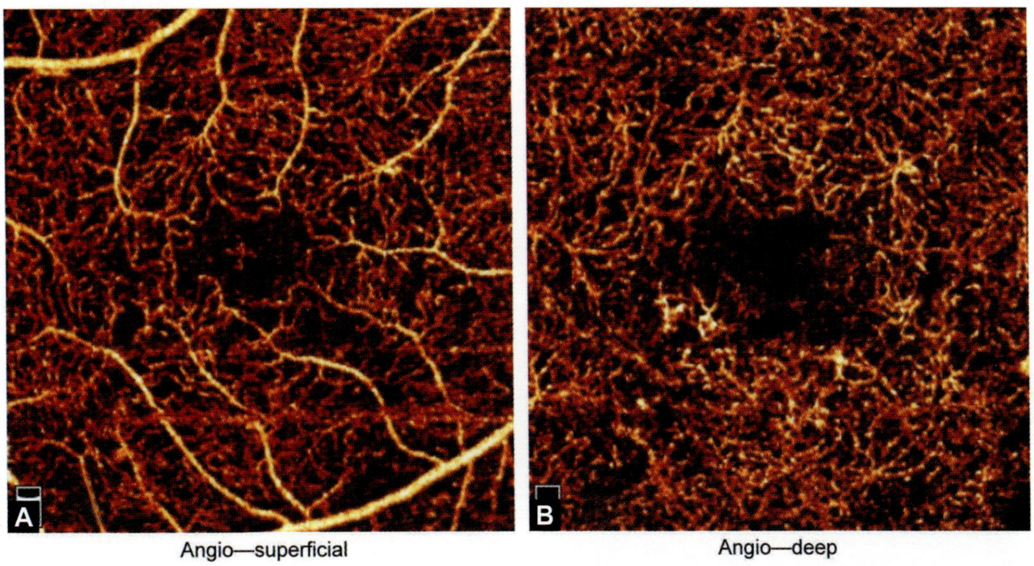

Figs. 7.6A and B: An OCTA SSADA protocol of the superficial and deep vascular plexus (3 × 3 mm). (A) The superficial vascular layer shows tortuous capillaries around the FAZ, many microaneurysms and vascular loops. The FAZ is irregular in shape and surrounded by numerous vascular dropouts; and (B) The deep vascular plexus shows typical signs of NPDR. Many microaneurysms, vascular loops, and anastomoses can be seen in this layer. Capillaries are dilated in places, and many small areas without flow can be seen. This finding of the deep vascular plexus is almost pathognomonic for the NPDR. (FAZ: foveolar avascular zone; NPDR: nonproliferative diabetic retinopathy; OCTA: optical coherence tomography angiography; SSADA: split-spectrum amplitude-decorrelation angiography)

THERAPY

A treatment plan for a patient with DR must include a diabetologist. Patients should be aware that a strict quarterly control of the hemoglobin A1c (HbA1c) glycolized hemoglobin is mandatory and that its value must be under 7. It is extremely important to maintain normal blood pressure. These factors significantly reduce the risk of development and progression of the DR.

Diabetic retinopathy can be treated with a focal or grid laser, intravitreal anti-VEGF injections, intravitreal corticosteroid injections, or with surgical procedures. Vitrectomy is indicated in cases of a vitreous detachment and traction, but also in cases where the traction pulls the

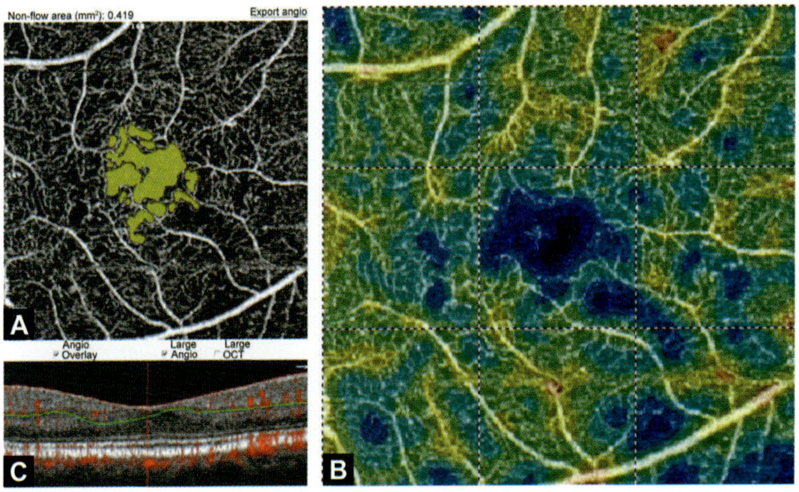

Figs. 7.7A to C: (A) Angioanalysis of the same eye as in the previous image. The FAZ, which is colored in yellow, has an irregular and bizarre shape. It seems like it is sparsed in a few smaller and larger parts. Although the size of FAZ is normal in range, this appearance of FAZ is surely pathological; (B) A capillary density map of the superficial vascular plexus. There is a clear domination of bluish colors, which represent an increased number of areas with reduced or without any flow; and (C) An OCT B-scan indicating the depth of the analyzed layer (superficial vascular layer). (FAZ: foveolar avascular zone; OCT: optical coherence tomography)

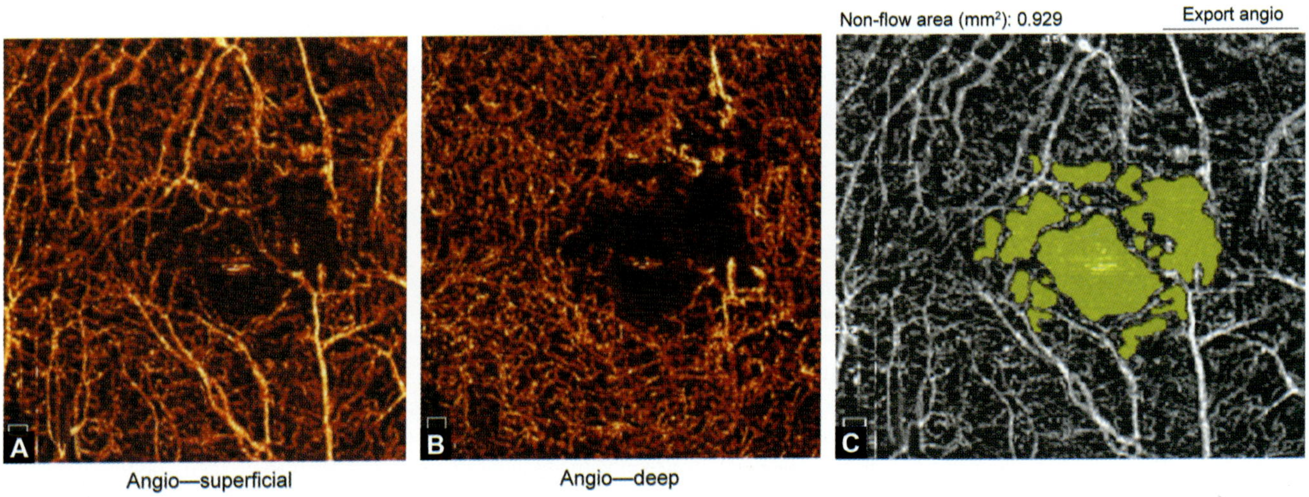

Figs. 7.8A to C: (A) An en face angiogram of the superficial vascular plexus in a patient with NPDR. The very first thing that can be detected is a bizarre foveal zone. It is changed in size and shape, and surrounded with very large dropout areas. Microaneurysms can also be visualized. The whole vascular net seems to be unsymmetrical and irregular. There are also a few larger, straight blood capillaries that seem to be very harsh. A fine, gentle net is completely lost; (B) An OCTA SSADA protocol of the deep vascular plexus where the macular area is significantly changed. It seems like the FAZ merged with the surrounding vascular dropout areas, now forming a large central nonflow area. Anastomoses, microaneurysms, and capillary dilatations can also be seen in this scan; and (C) An OCTA Angioanalysis of the superficial vascular plexus. The size of the FAZ and surrounding vascular dropouts is 0.929 mm^2, which is significantly above physiological sizes. The enlargement of the few vascular dropout areas is emphasized with yellow. (FAZ: foveolar avascular zone; NPDR: nonproliferative diabetic retinopathy; OCTA: optical coherence tomography angiography; SSADA: split-spectrum amplitude-decorrelation angiography)

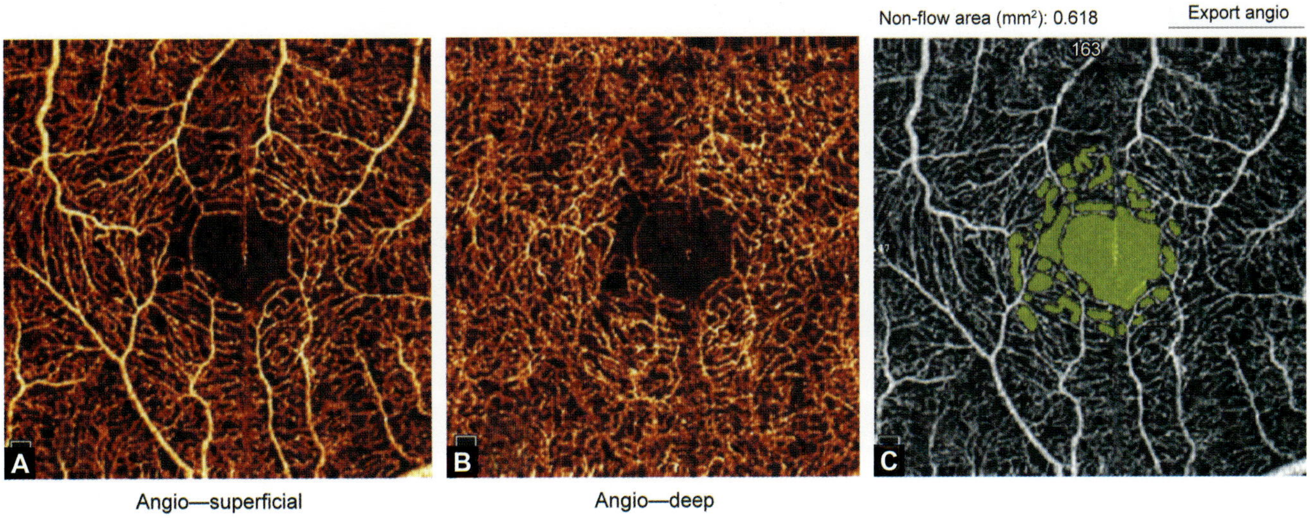

Figs. 7.9A to C: (A) An OCTA SSADA protocol of the superficial vascular plexus in a patient with NPDR. The capillary net is slightly changed. FAZ seems to be regular in size and shape. There are only a few intercapillary areas without flow that can be visualized around the FAZ. In other terms, the vascular network seems to be regular and symmetrical; (B) An en face angiogram of the deep vascular plexus, where many microaneurysms and vascular loops can be seen. Asymmetry is slightly present. The FAZ is slightly wider than in the superficial plexus, however, this is a regular finding. Very few capillary dropouts can still be seen around the FAZ; and (C) An Angio analysis of the FAZ and surrounding vascular dropouts measures the size of these changes, and their value in this eye is 0.618 mm^2. (FAZ: foveolar avascular zone; NPDR: nonproliferative diabetic retinopathy; OCTA: optical coherence tomography angiography; SSADA: split-spectrum amplitude-decorrelation angiography)

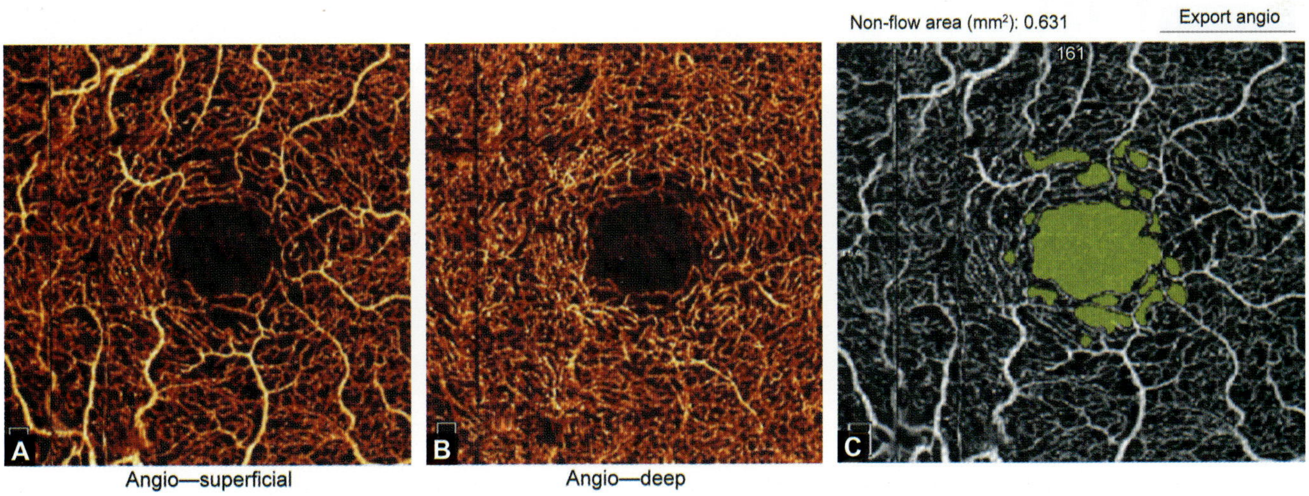

Figs. 7.10A to C: (A) An OCTA SSADA protocol of the superficial vascular plexus in the eye with NPDR. FAZ seems to be slightly enlarged, and there are a lot of parafoveal vascular dropout areas; (B) An angiography image of the deep vascular plexus with typical changes on the ends of the capillaries; and (C) The FAZ and vascular dropouts presented by Angioanalysis. FAZ is enlarged and slightly irregular in shape. The size of those marked areas is 0.631 mm^2. (FAZ: foveolar avascular zone; NPDR: nonproliferative diabetic retinopathy; OCTA: optical coherence tomography angiography; SSADA: split-spectrum amplitude-decorrelation angiography)

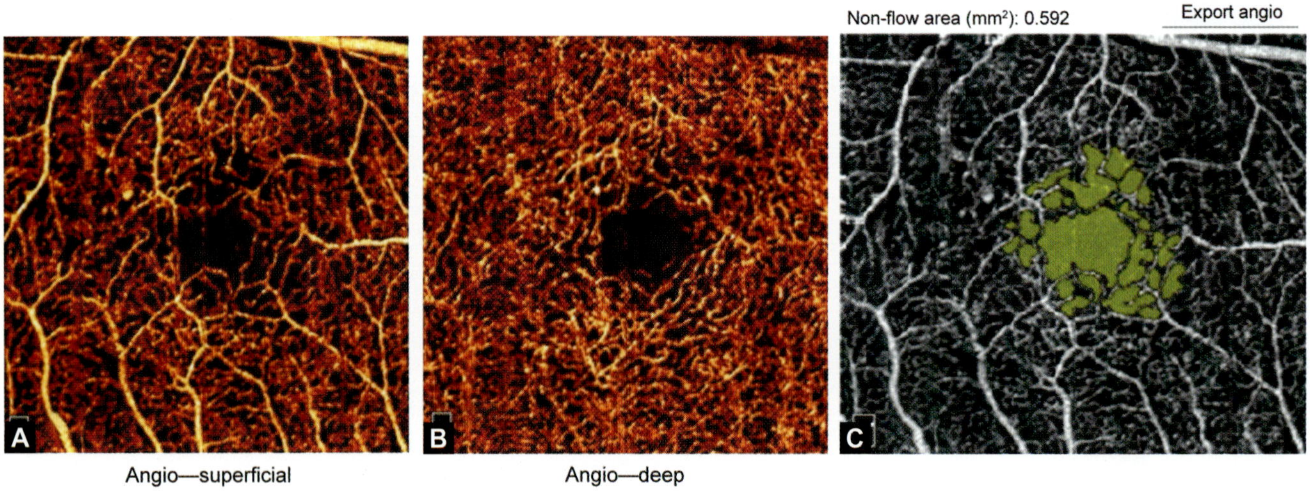

Figs. 7.11A to C: (A) An OCT angiography of the other eye of the same patient as in the Figures 7.10A to C. The NPDR presents with the more severe changes in this eye. Superficial vascular plexus shows the irregular and enlarged FAZ. Microaneurysms, vascular loops, and many capillary dropouts around the FAZ can also be seen; (B) Deep vascular plexus shows also a more significant changes. There are many tiny capillary dropouts in big area around the FAZ, many microaneurysms, and loops; and (C) An Angio analysis of the superficial vascular plexus demonstrates the yellow-colored FAZ and surrounding dropout areas that measure 0.59 mm^2. (FAZ: foveolar avascular zone; NPDR: nonproliferative diabetic retinopathy; OCT: optical coherence tomography)

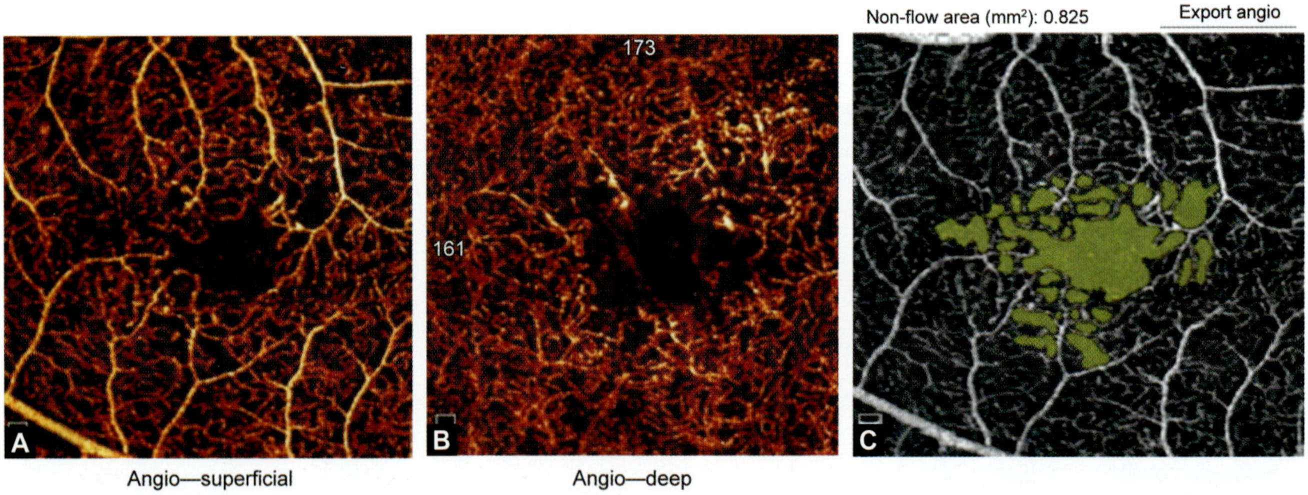

Figs. 7.12A to C: (A) An OCTA SSADA protocol of the superficial vascular plexus in an eye with NPDR. Vascular changes and an unsymmetrical capillary network are emphasized. FAZ is irregular in shape and there are many capillary dropouts around it. The vascular profile seems to be very harsh and rigid. There are also a few vascular loops as well as many microaneurysms seen in this plexus; (B) An angiography image of the deep vascular plexus. Similar changes are presented in this plexus as well. FAZ is much wider and it seems like it is merging with the vascular dropout areas, and is forming a large central area without any flow. Microaneurysms, vascular loops, and anastomoses are very significant in this layer; and (C) Angio analysis of the FAZ and vascular dropouts in the superficial vascular plexus shows the nonflow area size of 0.825 mm^2. It is more clearly shown that the FAZ is irregular and elongated in shape. (FAZ: foveolar avascular zone; NPDR: nonproliferative diabetic retinopathy; OCTA: optical coherence tomography angiography; SSADA: split-spectrum amplitude-decorrelation angiography)

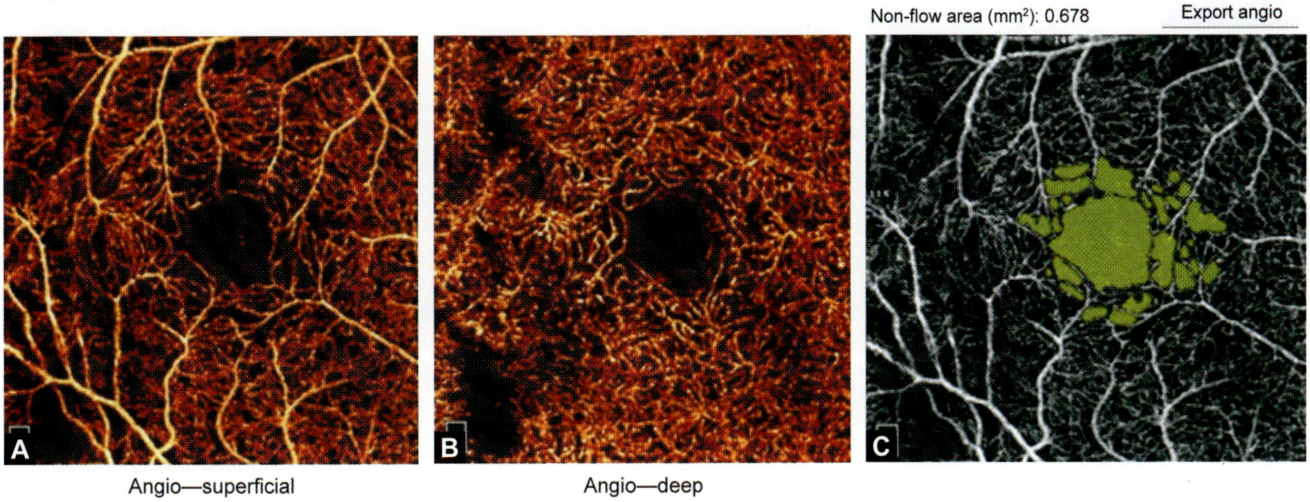

Figs. 7.13A to C: (A) An OCTA SSADA protocol of the superficial vascular plexus in an eye with NPDR. The macular area has reduced vascular flow. FAZ is regular in size and shape, but there are many dropout areas around it. The vascular network is asymmetrical due to the many vascular loops and hooked capillary ends. The left part of the image shows a few larger intercapillary areas without the flow, that are situated one above the other; (B) The deep vascular network shows also many vascular loops, microaneurysms, and capillary dropouts. Same ischemic regions can be seen in the left part of the image in this layer; and (C) Angio analysis confirms the existence of many capillary dropouts, also showing that the size of the FAZ and those regions in this eye is 0.678 mm^2. (FAZ: foveolar avascular zone; NPDR: nonproliferative diabetic retinopathy; OCTA: optical coherence tomography angiography; SSADA: split-spectrum amplitude-decorrelation angiography)

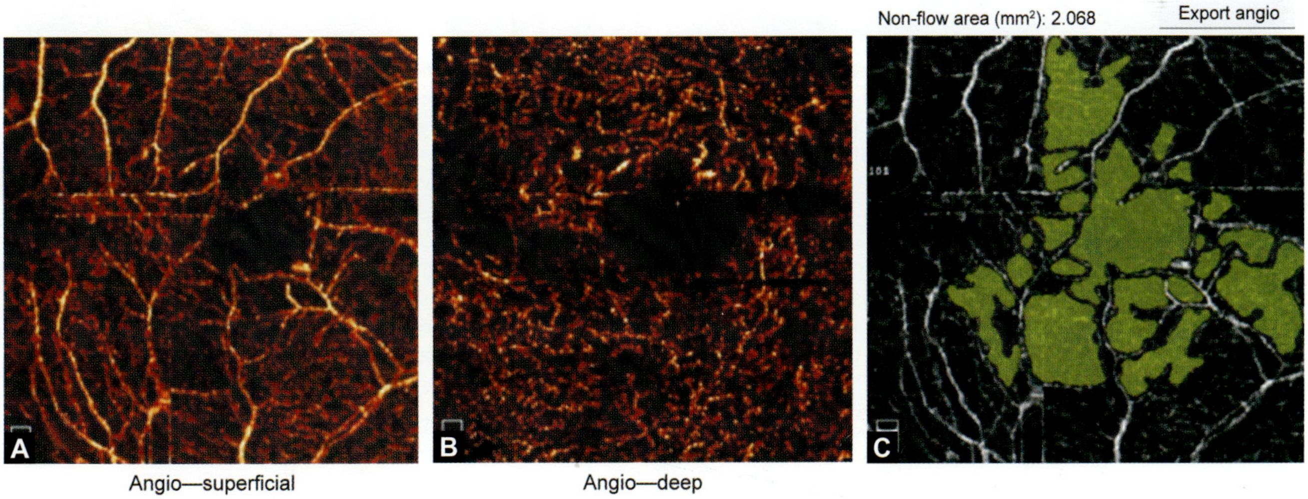

Figs. 7.14A to C: (A) OCTA SSADA protocol of the superficial vascular plexus in the eye with the ischemic form of NPDR. This plexus shows many dark regions without any flow in all parts of the image, not just around the FAZ. A fine, gentle vascular structure is completely lost; (B) An OCTA of the deep vascular plexus shows a pathognomonic appearance of this layer in diabetic retinopathy (DR). It shows many microaneurysms, anastomoses, and vascular dropouts. The region is almost completely ischemic; and (C) The software of the Angio analysis colors big dropout areas in the superficial vascular layer is yellow. The FAZ is completely bizarre in shape and very enlarged. Capillaries seem to be very straight and dried. This eye suffers from a severe form of ischemic DR. (FAZ: foveolar avascular zone; NPDR: nonproliferative diabetic retinopathy; OCTA: optical coherence tomography angiography; SSADA: split-spectrum amplitude-decorrelation angiography)

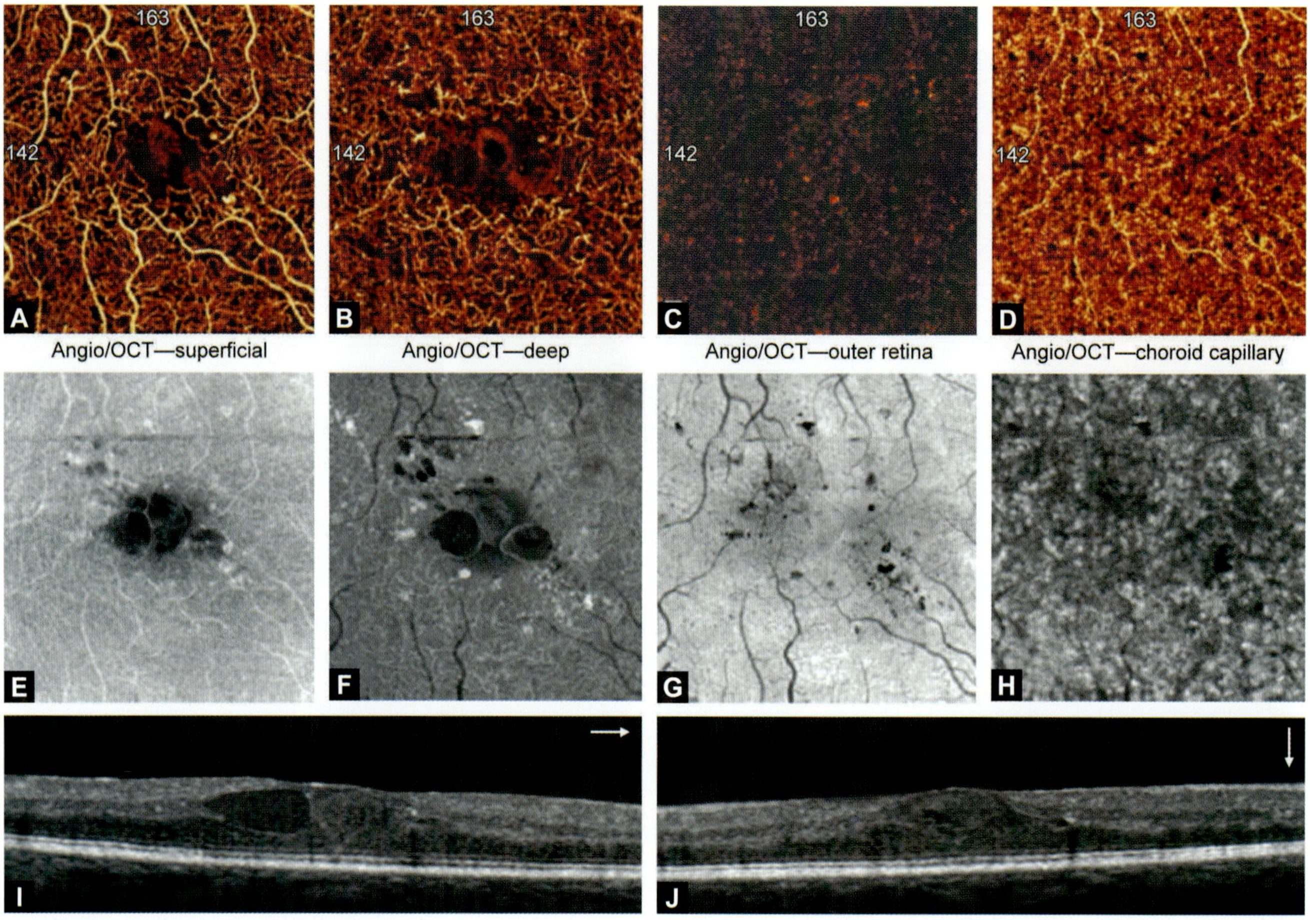

Figs. 7.15A to J: An OCTA SSADA protocol and en face OCT of corresponding retinal vascular layers, along with matching OCT B-scans (3 × 3 mm). (A to D) En face angiograms in an eye with the preproliferative form of DR. The superficial and deep vascular plexus show many microaneurysms, vascular loops, anastomoses and capillary tortuosity. The vascular networks are unsymmetrical and show many vascular dropouts. FAZ is irregular in size and shape. The deep vascular plexus shows a central circular space, like a defect, that matches the cystoid edema in the inner part of the retina. The same cystoid changes are presented in the corresponding en face OCT image (F). Edema is still best visualized on B-scans (I and J). The outer retina is avascular and does not show signs of the neovascularization. Choriocapillaris also has a harsh, but regular appearance; (E to H) An en face OCT of the corresponding retinal layers. Superficial and deep vascular plexuses show central cystoid changes (edema) and many hard exudates (hyperreflective spots). The RPE and Bruch's membrane are intact. Hyporeflectivity in the outer retina matches the edema. The choroidal layer is regular and shows no signs of neovascularization; and (I and J) An OCT B-scan shows a thickened retina with the central macular edema. RPE and Bruch's membrane are regular. Hard exudates are hyperreflective on the scans and they make shadows on deeper parts of the retina. Scans correspond to the preproliferative DR. (DR: diabetic retinopathy; FAZ: foveolar avascular zone; OCTA: optical coherence tomography angiography; RPE: retinal pigment epithelium; SSADA: split-spectrum amplitude-decorrelation angiography)

macula causing the type of DME that does not respond to medicamentous therapy.

The PDR as well as a severe nonproliferative retinopathy are treated by panretinal photocoagulation (PRP). If PRP is planned on an eye with macular edema, including anti-VEGF therapy or focal photocoagulation first is advised, due to the fact that PRP may lead to the deterioration of the macular edema in some cases.

If the DR is very severe, and presents itself with disk neovascularization or repeated vitreous hemorrhages and preretinal bleedings, both anti-VEGF therapy and PRP are recommended. For patients with untreated PDR and vitreous hemorrhages, a very early vitrectomy is recommended, especially if there are any signs of neovascularization of the iris (rubeosis iridis).

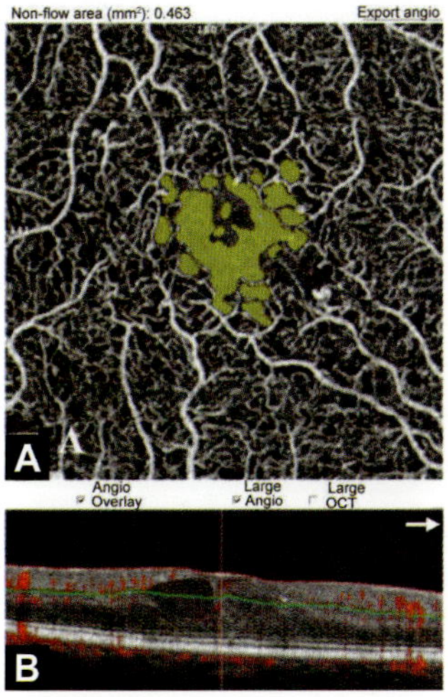

Figs. 7.16A and B: (A) An Angio analysis of the superficial vascular layer of the same eye shown in the previous image. Regions without flow are colored in yellow, while the grayish central part, that cannot be colored, matches the edema spreading to the superficial layer. The area of nonflow measures 0.463 mm^2; and (B) An optical coherence tomography (OCT) B-scan with the horizontal lines pinpointing the depth of the analyzed layer (superficial vascular layer).

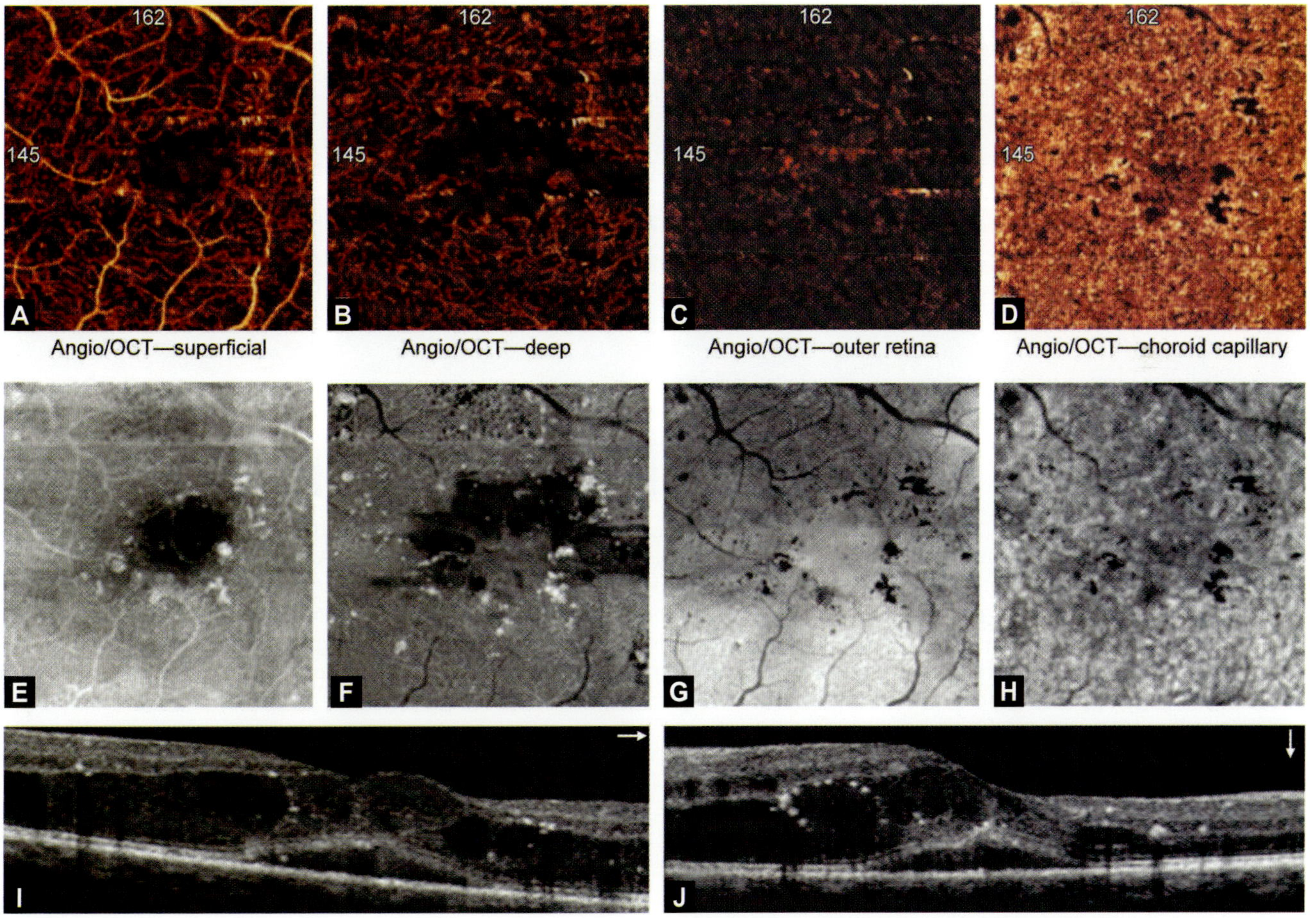

Figs. 7.17A to J: An OCTA SSADA protocol and en face OCT of the corresponding vascular layers, along with the OCT B-scan of the other eye of the same patient (3 × 3 mm). (A to D) An angiography presenting an eye with advanced preproliferative diabetic retinopathy. Superficial and deep vascular plexuses show an enlarged FAZ, irregular in shape, and surrounded with many microaneurysms and vascular dropouts. The outer retina is avascular, without significant changes. Choriocapillaris shows a few dark breakups, which are caused by shadows due to hard exudates; (E to H) The en face OCT clearly shows central cystoid spaces in the inner retina, along with many hyperreflective granular changes (hard exudates) around them. There are no neovascularizations or perforations of the RPE; and (I and J) OCT B-scans. CME along with the serous foveal detachment is presented. Also, there are many hard exudates surrounding the edematous cysts. (CME: cystoid macular edema; FAZ: foveolar avascular zone; OCTA: optical coherence tomography angiography; RPE: retinal pigment epithelium; SSADA: split-spectrum amplitude-decorrelation angiography)

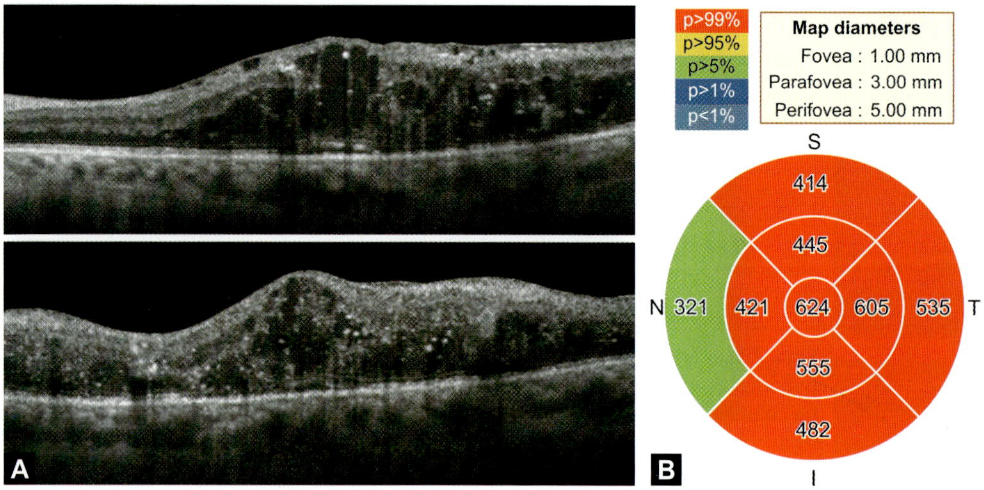

Figs. 7.18A and B: (A) An OCT B-scan of an eye with preproliferative diabetic retinopathy. It shows the CME, shallow serous foveal detachment, RPE that is thickened in places, and numerous hard exudates (hyperreflective spots); and (B) The retinal thickness map shows increased thickness in macular area, measuring 624 µm in its center. (CME: cystoid macular edema; OCT: optical coherence tomography; RPE: retinal pigment epithelium)

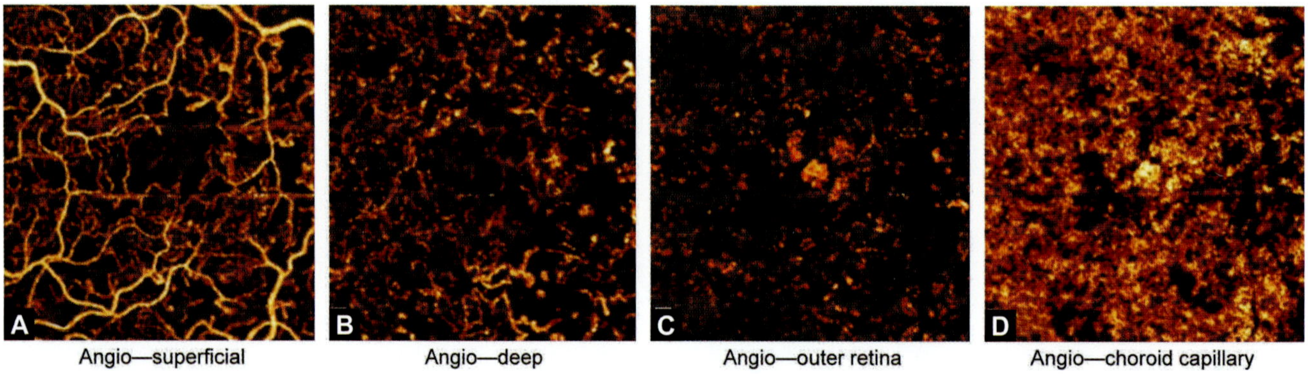

Figs. 7.19A to D: An OCTA SSADA protocol of vascular retinal layers, of the same eye as in Figures 7.18A and B (3 × 3 mm). The superficial vascular plexus shows an irregularly-shaped FAZ, numerous areas of vascular dropout, many microaneurysms, and a significant tortuosity of capillaries. The deep vascular plexus shows similar changes, along with a few central cystoid areas. The outer retina shows a few central circular vascular structures, which should not be seen in this layer. Choriocapillaris has an irregular vascular appearance, with a central blossoming vascular structure suspected on CNV. (CNV: choroidal neovascularization; FAZ: foveolar avascular zone; OCTA: optical coherence tomography angiography; SSADA: split-spectrum amplitude-decorrelation angiography)

If the patient has a NPDR or minimal changes in blood vessels, regular checkups every 6–12 months are obligatory. Patients with DME and severe nonproliferative or proliferative changes need the checkup every 2–4 months.

BIBLIOGRAPHY

1. American Academy of Ophthalmology Vision Rehabilitation Committee. Preferred Practice Pattern Guidelines: Vision Rehabilitation for Adults. San Francisco: American Academy of Ophthalmology; 2007.
2. Bandello F, Corbelli E, Carnevali A, et al. Optical coherence tomography angiography of diabetic retinopathy. Dev Ophthalmol. 2016;56:107-12.
3. Barham R, El Rami H, Sun JK. Evidence-based treatment of diabetic macular edema. Semin Ophthalmol. 2017;32(1):56-66.
4. Bertelsen G, Peto T, Lindekleiv H, et al. Tromso eye study: prevalence and risk factors of diabetic retinopathy. Acta Ophthalmol. 2013;91(8):716-21.
5. Bourne RR, Stevens GA, White RA, et al. Causes of vision loss worldwide, 1990–2010: a systematic analysis. Lancet Glob Health. 2013;1(6):e339-49.

6. Chalam KV, Sambhav K. Optical coherence tomography angiography in retinal diseases. J Ophthalmic Vis Res. 2016;11(1):84-92.
7. Cheung N, Mitchell P, Wong TY. Diabetic retinopathy. Lancet. 2010;376(9735):124-36.
8. Chew EY, Klein ML, Ferris FL, et al. Association of elevated serum lipid levels with retinal hard exudate in diabetic retinopathy. Early treatment diabetic retinopathy study (ETDRS) Report 22. Arch Ophthalmol. 1996;114(9):1079-84.
9. Chew EY, Mills JL, Metzger BE, et al. Metabolic control and progression of retinopathy. The Diabetes in Early Pregnancy Study. National Institute of Child Health and Human Development Diabetes in Early Pregnancy Study. Diabetes Care. 1995;18(5):631-7.
10. Davis MD, Fisher MR, Gangnon RE, et al. Risk factors for high-risk proliferative diabetic retinopathy and severe visual loss: early treatment diabetic retinopathy study report number 18. Invest Ophthalmol Vis Sci. 1998;39(2):233-52.
11. Dedov I, Maslova O, Suntsov Y, et al. Prevalence of diabetic retinopathy and cataract in adult patients with type 1 and type 2 diabetes in Russia. Rev Diabet Stud. 2009;6(2):124-9.
12. Hautala N, Hannula V, Palosaari T, et al. Prevalence of diabetic retinopathy in young adults with type 1 diabetes since childhood: the Oulu cohort study of diabetic retinopathy. Acta Ophthalmol. 2014;92(8):749-52.
13. Heier JS, Bressler NM, Avery RL, et al. Comparison of aflibercept, bevacizumab, and ranibizumab for treatment of diabetic macular edema: Extrapolation of data to clinical practice. JAMA Ophthalmol. 2016;134(1):95-9.
14. Hwang TS, Jia Y, Gao SS, et al. Optical coherence tomography angiography features of diabetic retinopathy. Retina. 2015;35(11):2371-6.
15. Ishibazawa A, Nagaoka T, Takahashi A, et al. Optical coherence tomography angiography in diabetic retinopathy: A prospective pilot study Am J Ophthalmol. 2015;160(1):35-44.
16. Lee J, Rosen R. Optical coherence tomography angiography in diabetes. Curr Diab Rep. 2016;16(12):123.
17. Matsunaga DR, Yi JJ, De Koo LO, et al. Optical coherence tomography angiography of diabetic retinopathy in human subjects. Ophthalmic Surg Lasers Imaging Retina. 2015;46(8):796-805.
18. Mrugacz M, Krajewska M, Bryl A, et al. Evaluate the effectiveness of laser therapy in the treatment of diabetic maculopathy. Pol Merkur Lekarski. 2013;34(204):351-4.
19. Nicholson BP, Schachat AP. A review of clinical trials of anti-VEGF agents for diabetic retinopathy. Graefes Arch Clin Exp Ophthalmol. 2010;248(7):915-30.
20. Roy MS, Klein R, O'Colmain BJ, et al. The prevalence of diabetic retinopathy among adult type 1 diabetic persons in the United States. Arch Ophthalmol. 2004;122(4):546-51.
21. Salz DA, Witkin AJ. Imaging in diabetic retinopathy. Middle East Afr J Ophthalmol. 2015;22(2):145-50.
22. Stanga PE, Papayannis A, Tsamis E, et al. New findings in diabetic maculopathy and proliferative disease by swept-source optical coherence tomography angiography. Dev Ophthalmol. 2016;56:113-21.
23. Thomas BJ, Shienbaum G, Boyer DS, et al. Evolving strategies in the management of diabetic macular edema: Clinical trials and current management. Can J Ophthalmol. 2013;48(1):22-30.
24. Thomas BJ, Yonekawa Y, Wolfe JD, et al. Contralateral eye-to-eye comparison of intravitreal ranibizumab and a sustained-release dexamethasone intravitreal implant in recalcitrant diabetic macular edema. Clin Ophthalmol. 2016;10:1679-84.
25. Thomas RL, Dunstan FD, Luzio SD, et al. Prevalence of diabetic retinopathy within a national diabetic retinopathy screening service. Br J Ophthalmol. 2015;99(1):64-8.
26. Villena JE, Yoshiyama CA, Sanchez JE, et al. Prevalence of diabetic retinopathy in Peruvian patients with type 2 diabetes: Results of a hospital-based retinal telescreening program. Rev Panam Salud Publica. 2011;30(5):408-14.
27. World Health Organization (WHO). (2016). Global report on diabetes. [online] Available from www.who.int/diabetes/global-report/en/. [Accessed December, 2017].
28. Yau JW, Rogers SL, Kawasaki R, et al. Global prevalence and major risk factors of diabetic retinopathy. Diabetes Care. 2012;35(3):556-64.

CHAPTER 8

Degenerative Myopia

INTRODUCTION

Degenerative myopia is a type of short-sightedness, which is always associated with the process of axial elongation and characterized by posterior staphyloma formation and macular complications.

EPIDEMIOLOGY AND ETIOLOGY

Degenerative myopia occurs in patients with prescriptions from -6 diopters of myopia. Not every eye with high myopia develops degenerative changes in fundus. The prevalence is 2.1%, and women are affected twice as commonly as men. The exact pathophysiological mechanism of neovascular membrane development in the high myopic eye is still unknown. Malignant myopia could be associated with various systemic disorders, including Ehlers-Danlos syndrome, Marfan syndrome, and Stickler syndrome, or it can appear as a separate entity. Degenerative myopia causes the visual impairment and always significantly earlier in life than the age-related macular degeneration (ARMD).

SYMPTOMS AND SIGNS

Patients are mostly asymptomatic until they present with symptoms of distorted vision (metamorphopsia) and photopsy, which are caused by the perforation of Bruch's membrane or occurrence/growth of a neovascular membrane. Patients who are suffering from high myopia have a significant risk of cataract development, glaucoma, retinal detachment, and vitreous detachment at younger age. A posterior staphyloma can be often found in patients with degenerative myopia, along with scleral ectasia, which is located most frequently in the superior-temporal quadrant. Stretching of the posterior sclera leads to progressive thinning of all retinal layers, including retinal pigment epithelium and choroid. Bruch's membrane is acellular, elastic, and has limited capacity to stretch. At one point, stretching can lead into the ruptures of Bruch's membrane (*lacquer* cracks). Acute macular hemorrhage is very frequent in cases where choroidal neovascular membrane invades the crack. The hemorrhage is restrictive and could be absorbed resulting in small scars (*Forster-Fuchs'* spots). Fuchs' spot is the scar which may lead to a permanent and irreversible scotoma in the visual field. It is also possible to detect multiple cracks and breaks of Bruch's membrane, which can lead to the progressive scarring and atrophy. In later stages, the central macular part may appear like geographic atrophy, and changes can resemble of dry form of ARMD.

DIFFERENTIAL DIAGNOSIS

- Age-related macular degeneration
- Ocular histoplasmosis.

DIAGNOSTICS

The diagnosis is based on specific findings of the posterior ocular segment, optical coherence tomography (OCT), and OCT angiography, which proves the existence of the neovascularization. The fundoscopic examination reveals large choroidal blood vessels, focal or diffuse regions of retinal atrophy, posterior staphyloma, posterior vitreous detachment, and small, pale myopic optic nerve head surrounded by typical myopic conus. Peripapillar atrophy, which appears as degenerative myopic conus, is always present in degenerative myopic fundus.

An OCT is useful diagnostic tool for the detection of choroidal neovascularization (CNV) and associated tears of retina (myopic macular schisis). CNV is shown as an elevated, hyperreflective lesion in subretinal space. The pooling of subretinal and intraretinal fluid is not usually present in cases of myopic vascular membrane, which makes difference when compared with the CNV lesions in ARMD.

Fluorescein angiography (FAG) helps in diagnosing the myopic CNV by showing the focal area of higher hyperfluorescence. It can also detect small, almost invisible myopic neovascularizations. Indocyanine green (ICG) is not useful in diagnosing. OCT angiography offers easy detection of myopic type 2 small CNV in myopic eyes.

The example of myopic eye (–19.0 diopters) in a 52-year-old patient with corrected visual acuity 20/40 is described in Figures 8.1 to 8.3.

The example of myopic eye (–16.0 diopters) in a 48-year-old patient with corrected visual acuity 20/70 is given in Figures 8.4 to 8.9.

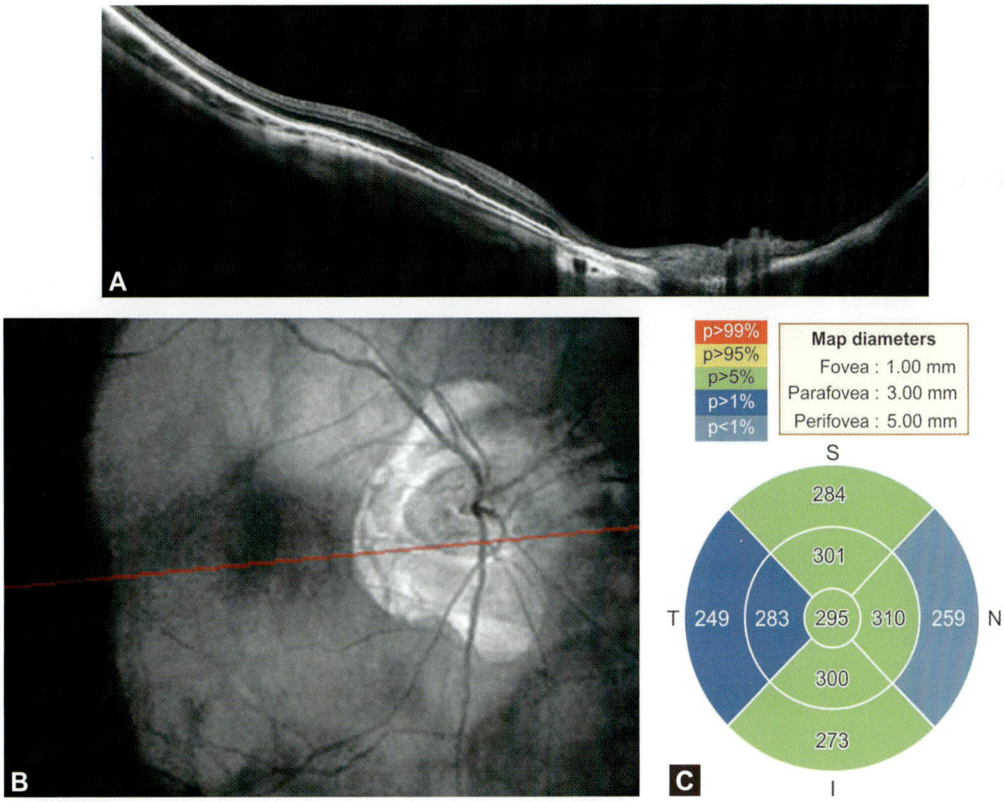

Figs. 8.1A to C: (A) An optical coherence tomography (OCT) B-scan of the macula and optic disk. The posterior staphyloma, thinned retina, and regular macular structure can be seen; (B) Fundus photography shows a small, oval, and pale optic disk, which is horizontally stretched and surrounded with wide peripapillar myopic conus. Blood vessels are thin and straight with decreased tortuosity. Central macular is blurry; and (C) Macular thickness map shows thinning of retina, which is caused by the elongation of eyeball.

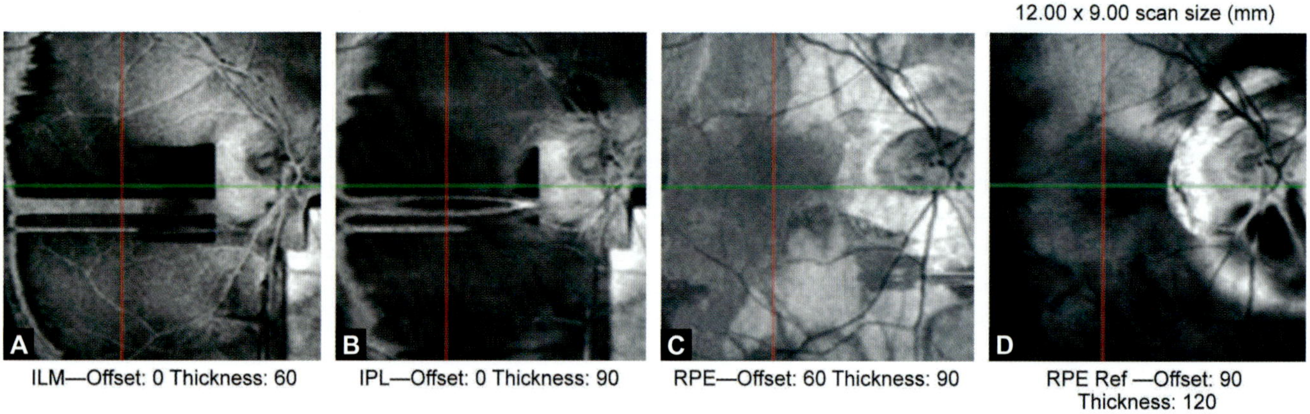

Figs. 8.2A to D: En face optical coherence tomography (OCT) images of the retina, the same eye as in Figures 8.1A to C (12 × 9 mm). Many horizontal artifacts are present, but major changes can be clearly seen. (A and B) Superficial and deep layer of inner retina show a pale and horizontally elongated disk with hyperreflective peripapillar myopic conus. Blood vessels are thin and straight; and (C and D) Hyporeflective and hyperreflective areas of atrophy are visualized in the outer part of the retina and choroid.

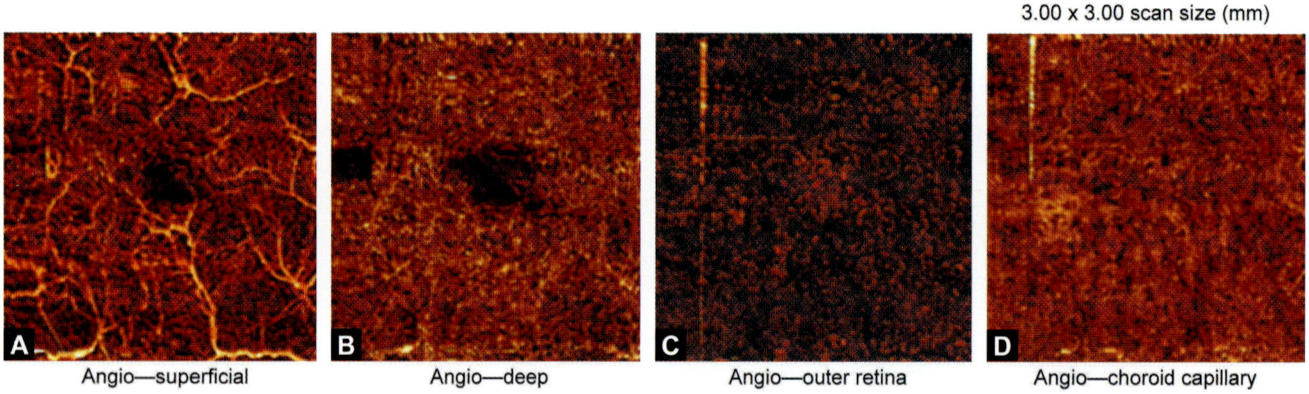

Figs. 8.3A to D: Optical coherence tomography angiography (OCTA) SSADA protocol of retinal layers, the same eye as in previous figures (3 × 3 mm). (A and B) The superficial and deep vascular plexus show no specific changes, although a few small areas with reduced blood flow and rarefied tenuous vascular network, which is caused by elongation of the posterior ocular pole, are visualized; (C) The outer part of retina is avascular and shows no pathological changes; and (D) Rough granular structure of the choroid is observed. Neovascularization cannot be seen.

The example of myopic eye (–14.0 diopters) in a 42-year-old patient with corrected visual acuity 20/200 is illustrated in Figures 8.10 to 8.12.

The example of myopic eye (–14.0 diopters) in a 55-year-old patient with corrected visual acuity 20/200 is given in Figures 8.13 and 8.14.

The example of myopic eye (–15.0 diopters) in a 48-year-old patient with corrected visual acuity 20/400 is described in Figures 8.15 to 8.17.

TREATMENT

There is no proven treatment for prevention or reducement of risk from progressive myopic neovascular membrane growth in young myopic eyes. Neovascular membrane is a complication of degenerative myopia and it is treated with antivascular endothelial growth factor (anti-VEGF) therapy, as any other CNV. The prognosis of visual acuity recovery in patients with myopic degenerative changes is

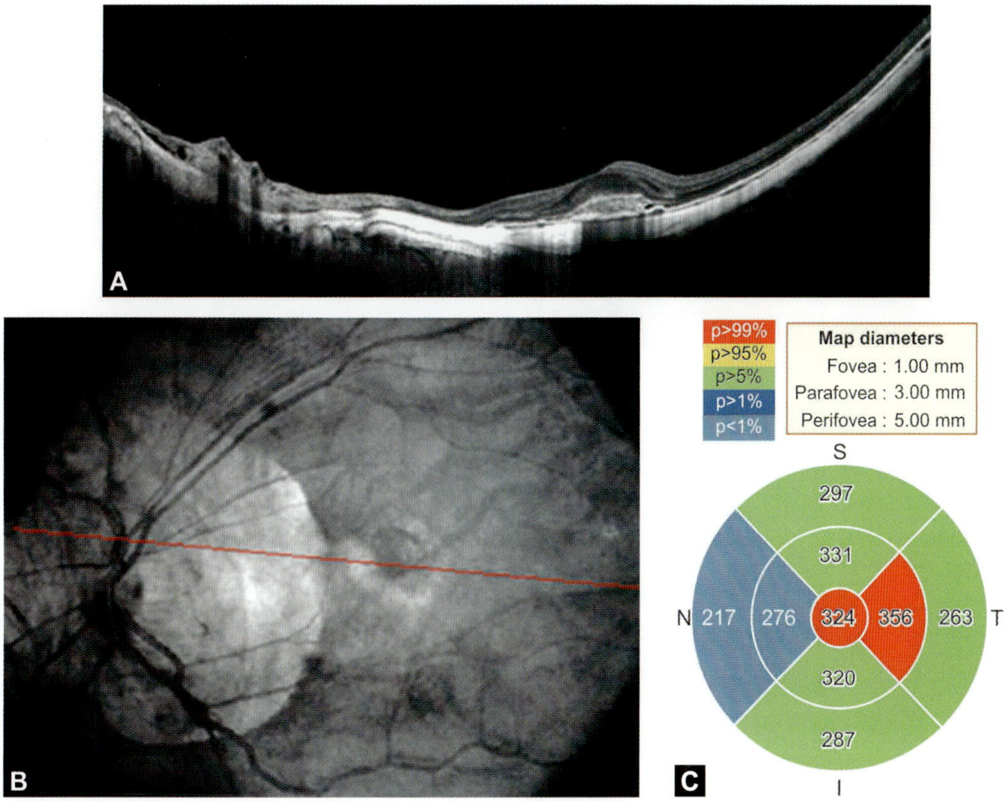

Figs. 8.4A to C: (A) An OCT B-scan of the macula and optic disk. The posterior staphyloma, thinner retina, and subretinal hyperreflective tissue, which correspond to CNV, can be visualized. A flat RPE detachment and a few PEDs can also be seen, along with the choroidal thickening; (B) The optic disk shows indistinct margins and large myopic conus. Blood vessels are thin and straight, typical of degenerative myopia. The macula is hyporeflective, and shows hyperreflective margins; and (C) The macular thickness map shows central and temporal thickening, which corresponds to the CNV location. Retinal thinning in nasal segments is associated with the eyeball elongation. (CNV: choroidal neovascularization; OCT: optical coherence tomography; PED: pigment epithelial detachment; RPE: retinal pigment epithelium)

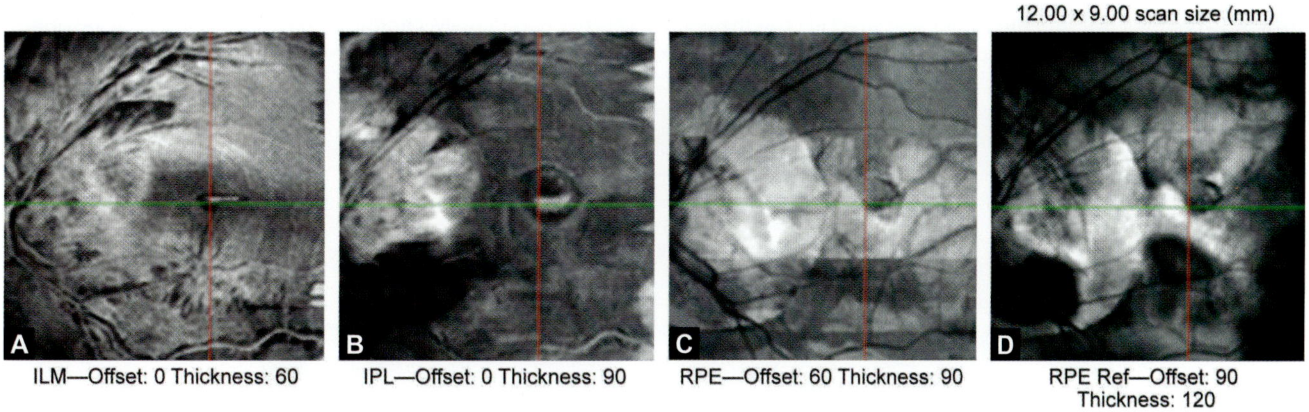

Figs. 8.5A to D: En face optical coherence tomography (OCT) images of the same eye (12 × 9 mm). (A) There is a hyporeflective macular area with retraction of the ILM and wrinkling of surrounding retinal tissue in the superficial retinal layer; (B) Deep layer of inner retina shows a hyporeflective space with hyperreflective edge, due to the fibrosis. The myopic conus and atrophic optic disk are clearly visible; and (C and D) In the outer retina and choroid, a hyperreflective tissue which covers hyporeflective zones of atrophy is seen.

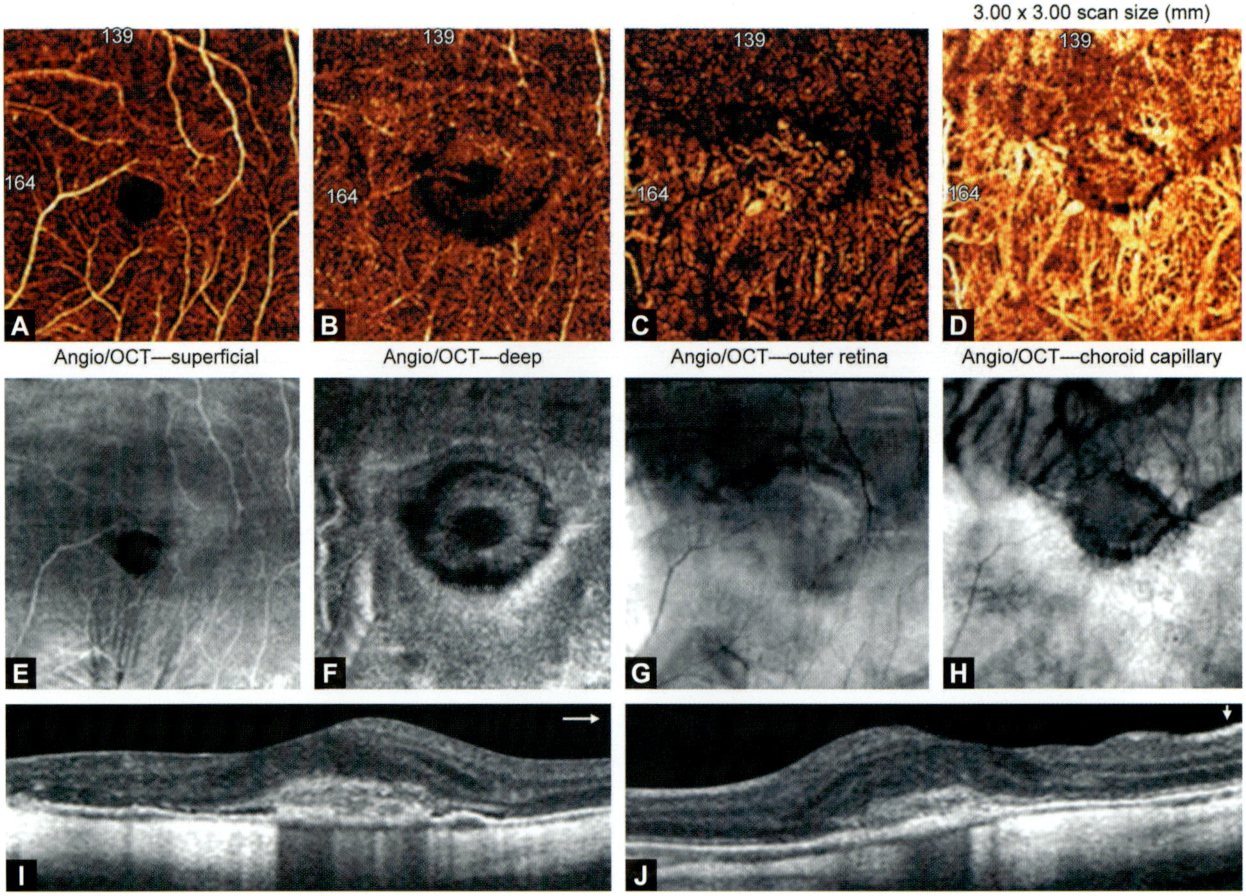

Figs. 8.6A to J: Images of retinal layers presented by the OCTA SSADA protocol, en face OCT and OCT B-scan (3 × 3 mm). (A to D) Superficial vascular plexus shows no significant changes. Deep vascular plexus shows the central dark defect. Outer retina and choroid clearly show a new glomerular neovascular membrane, which perforates the RPE and creates the type 2 CNV; (E to H) En face OCT shows the superficial part of inner retina with no significant changes. Only the retraction of ILM can be seen in the inferior part of image. A hyporeflective and sharply delineated central change in the form of a hole or cavity is clearly visualized in other layers. Deep part of inner retina shows a hyperreflective ring around the central defect; and (I and J) OCT B-scan illustrates an irregular and wavy RPE, shallow hyperreflective subretinal fluid, and small PED on the edge of central change. (CNV: choroidal neovascularization; OCTA: optical coherence tomography angiography; PED: pigment epithelial detachment; RPE: retinal pigment epithelium)

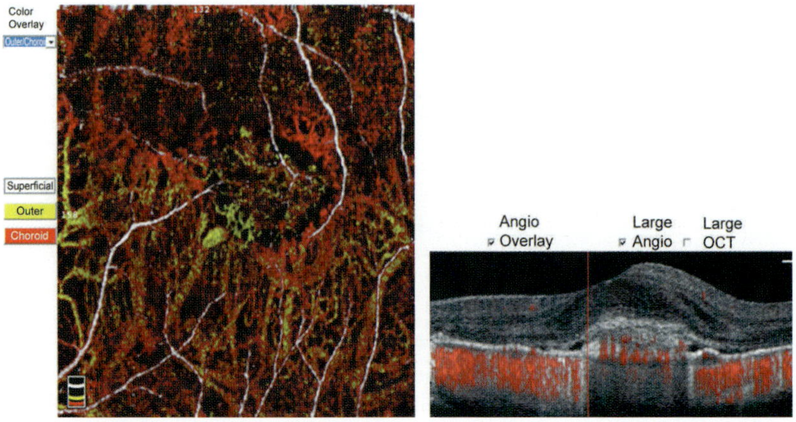

Fig. 8.7: AngioAnalytics shows a red and yellowish colored zone, which corresponds to the new neovascular membrane (CNV) in highly myopic eye. It was developed in choroid and perforated the RPE. The lower image is an OCT B-scan, which shows active and increased blood flow in the CNV. (CNV: choroidal neovascularization; OCT: optical coherence tomography; RPE: retinal pigment epithelium)

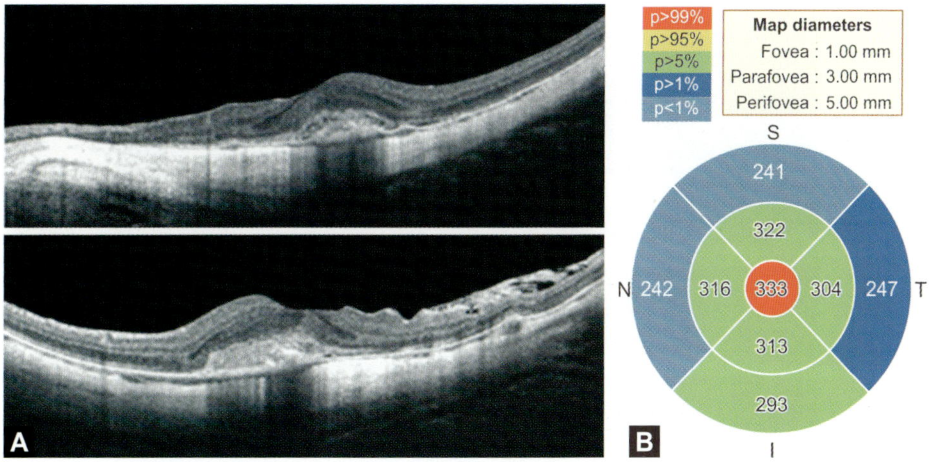

Figs. 8.8A and B: (A) An OCT B-scan of the same eye as in previous figures, a day after the application of intravitreal Eylea injection. Slightly reduced subretinal hyperreflective tissue is seen, without a serous detachment of neurosensory retina close to the CNV; and (B) Retinal thickness map shows decreased numerical values in comparison to values before the intravitreal Eylea application. (CNV: choroidal neovascularization; OCT: optical coherence tomography)

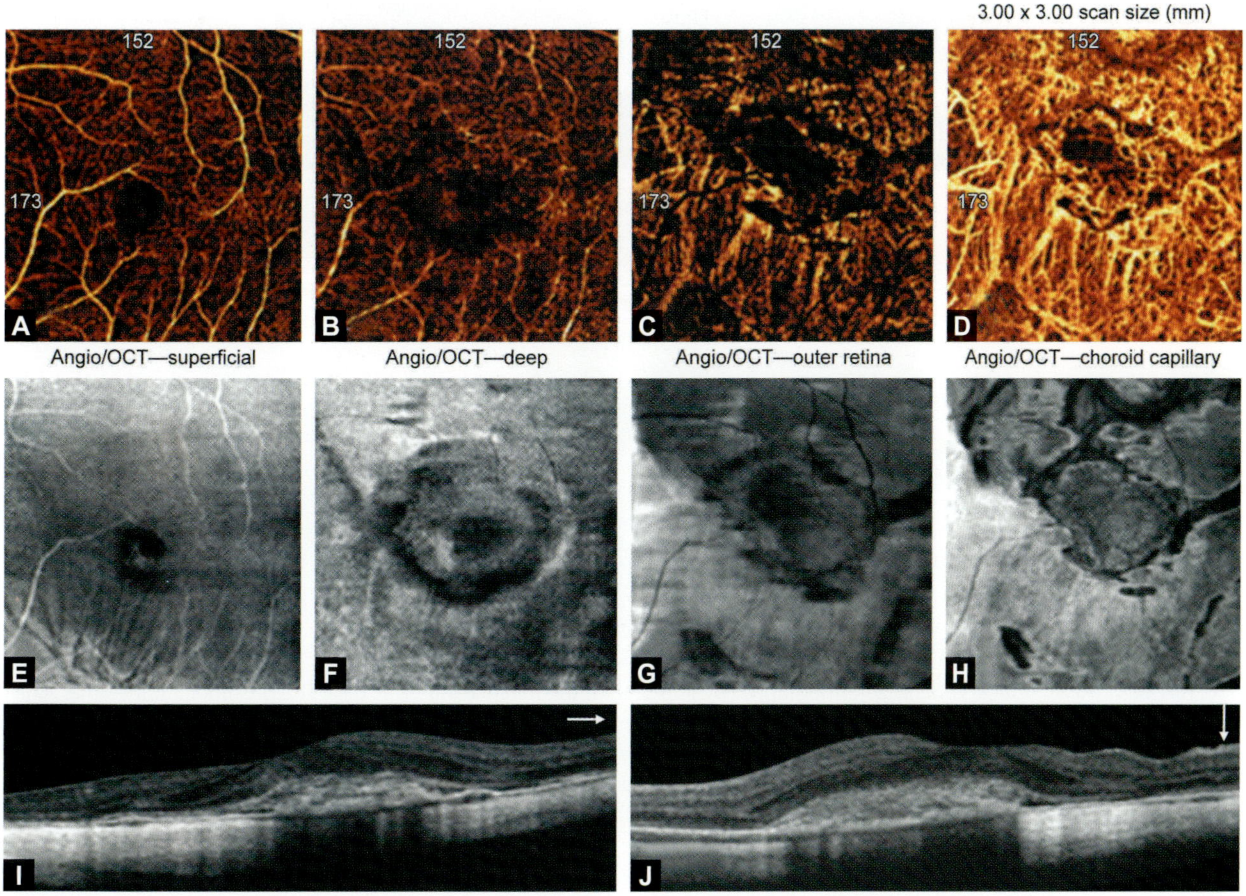

Figs. 8.9A to J: The image of superficial retinal layer shows filamentous blood vessels and fovelar avascular zone of normal size (A). In the deep vascular layer there is a large dark zone of foveolar avascular zone enlargement (B). (C and D) The CNV is equal in size, but it shows a reduced ramification and loss of small capillaries within the CNV; (E to H) En face OCT shows lower reflectivity and less pronounced retinal changes; and "B-scan shows disrupted retinal structure, the retinal pigment epithelium and Bruch membrane complex are perforated by a neovascular membrane, there is also some subretinal fluid (I and J) (CNV: choroidal neovascularization; OCTA: optical coherence tomography angiography)

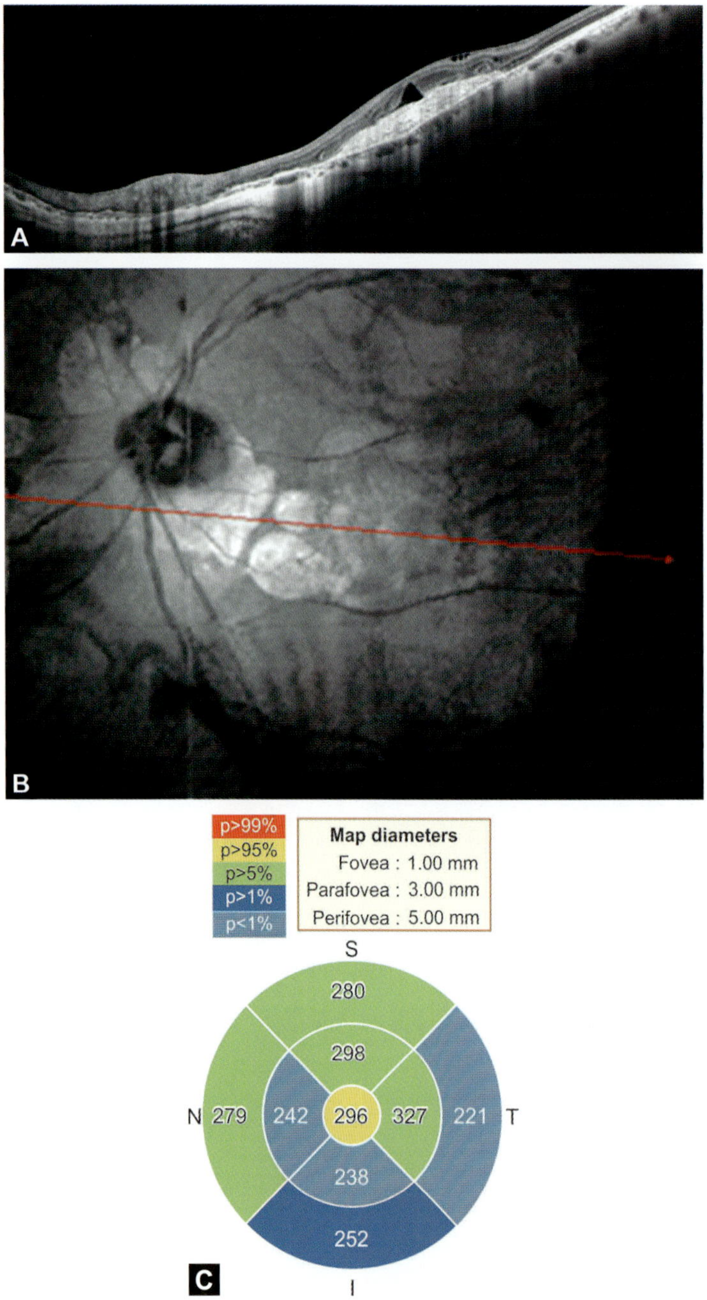

Figs. 8.10A to C: (A) An optical coherence tomography (OCT) B-scan of the macula and optic disk. The posterior staphyloma, schisis of inner and outer retinal layers, cystoid hyporeflective space in the center of macula, and subretinal hyperreflective tissue, which indicates the presence of neovascularization, can be visualized; (B) Fundus photography shows a small optic nerve head with a large myopic conus, as well as thin, straight and abnormal blood vessels, and retinal atrophy areas; and (C) Retinal thickness map shows thinning in inferior and temporal part of macula, but values in the central macula are higher than physiological ones.

very relative. Initially, 70% of patients have the visual acuity better than 20/200, while the 22% have visual acuity better than 20/40. In 5-year follow-up, 89% of patients show the deterioration of visual acuity with less than 20/200. In 10-year follow-up, the percentage of patients with significant impairment of visual acuity reaches more than 96%.

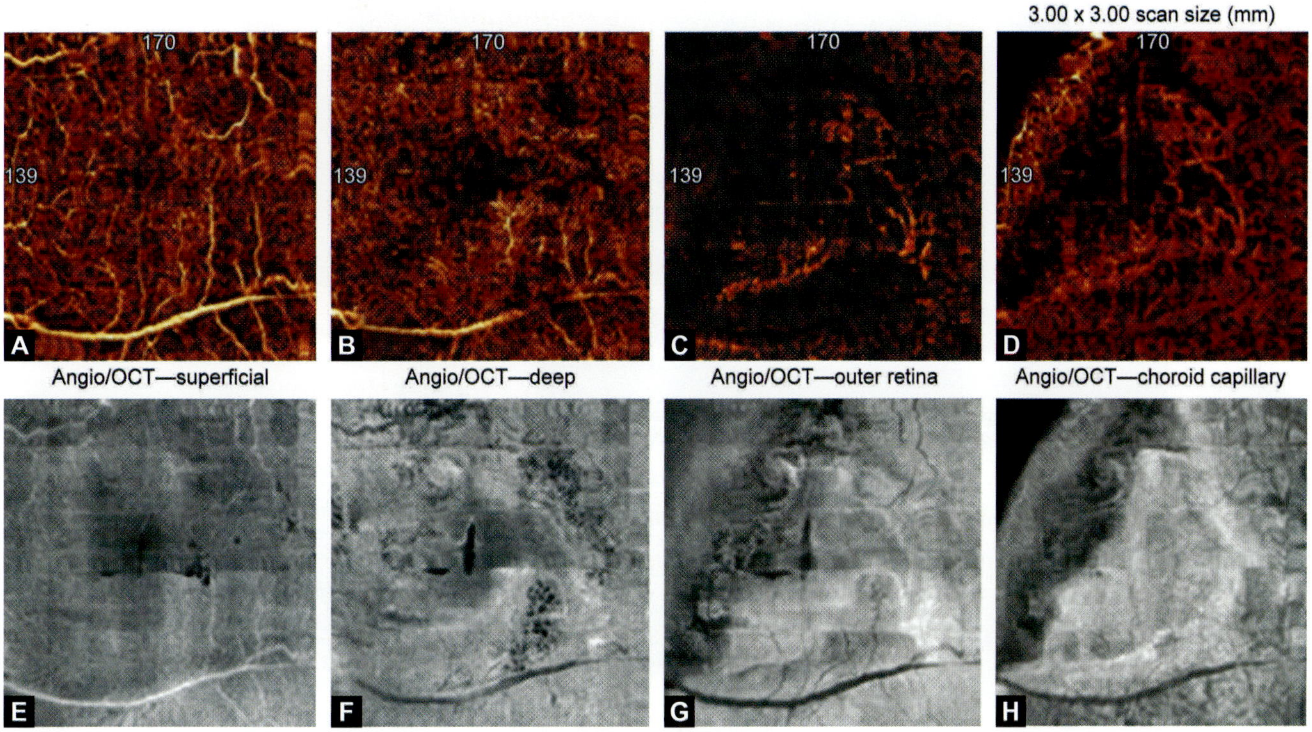

Figs. 8.11A to H: The images of retinal layers presented by the OCTA SSADA protocol and en face OCT (3 × 3 mm); the same eye as in Figures 8.10A to C. (A) OCT angiography of the superficial vascular layer shows slightly changed capillary meshwork. The FAZ is lost and small motion artifacts can be seen. This layer does not show ischemic regions; (B) The FAZ is enlarged in the deep vascular plexus and the blood flow slows down in the perimacular region. There are a lot of anastomoses and IRMA; (C) In outer retina a filamentous neovascularization with surrounding dark halo is present. Inside the new vascular network, many dark vascular dropout areas can be noted; (D) Angiogram of choriocapillaris shows a CNV of the same size and shape with dry and inactive capillaries, along with the presence of dark regions with no flow inside and around the neovascularization. The image represents the fibrotic scarification; (E) En face OCT of the same layer shows no significant changes. There are a few hyporeflective honeycomb-like spaces, which correspond to the superficial layer tear; (F) En face OCT of deep retinal layer shows grouped hyporeflective zones in the form of honeycomb pattern, which correspond to the superficial retinal tear. In the very center, a sharp stretched central zone can be seen; and (G and H) En face OCT image of the outer retina and choroid shows a central hyperreflective wide zone, which corresponds to CNV. (CNV: choroidal neovascularization; FAZ: foveal avascular zone; OCTA: optical coherence tomography angiography)

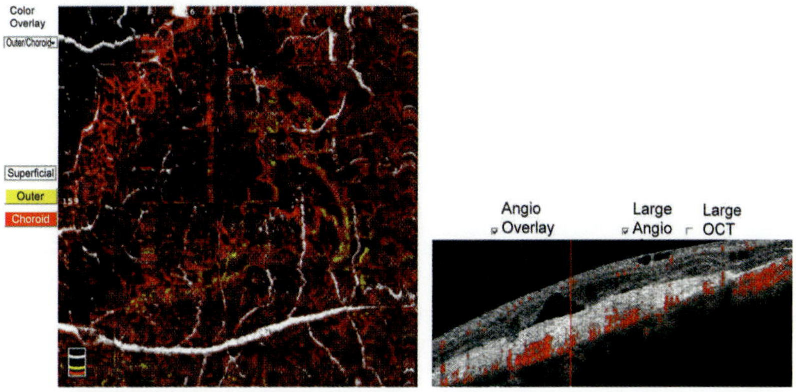

Fig. 8.12: The same CNV presented by the OCTA AngioAnalytics. A dry, rarefied, and inactive neovascular membrane inside the scar is obvious, without visible color-coded new blood vessels that would indicate an active vascularization. OCT B-scan in the lower part of the image shows the region of CNV analysis. (CNV: choroidal neovascularization; OCTA: optical coherence tomography angiography)

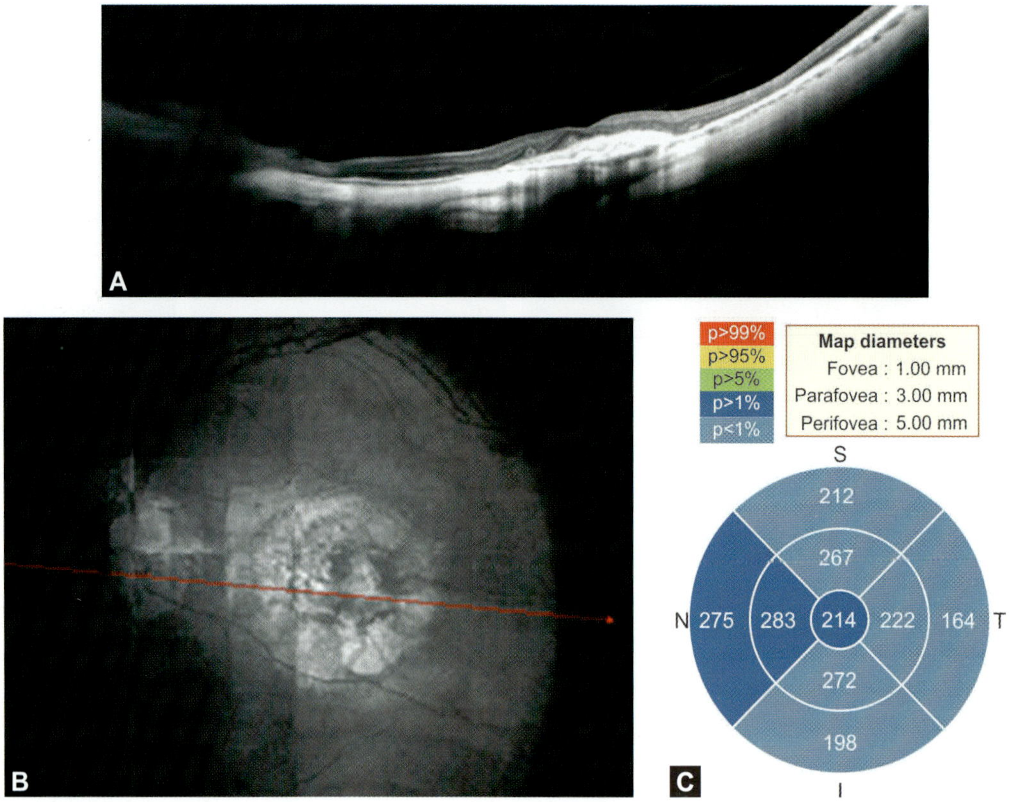

Figs. 8.13A to C: (A) An optical coherence tomography (OCT) B-scan of the macula and optic disk. Posterior staphyloma, extremely thin retina, hyperreflective subretinal tissue, and choroidal thickening are present; (B) Fundus photography reveals a small and white optic disk with myopic changes and typical myopic conus, as well as a hyperreflective macular region; and (C) Macular thickness map demonstrates the macular thinning in all segments.

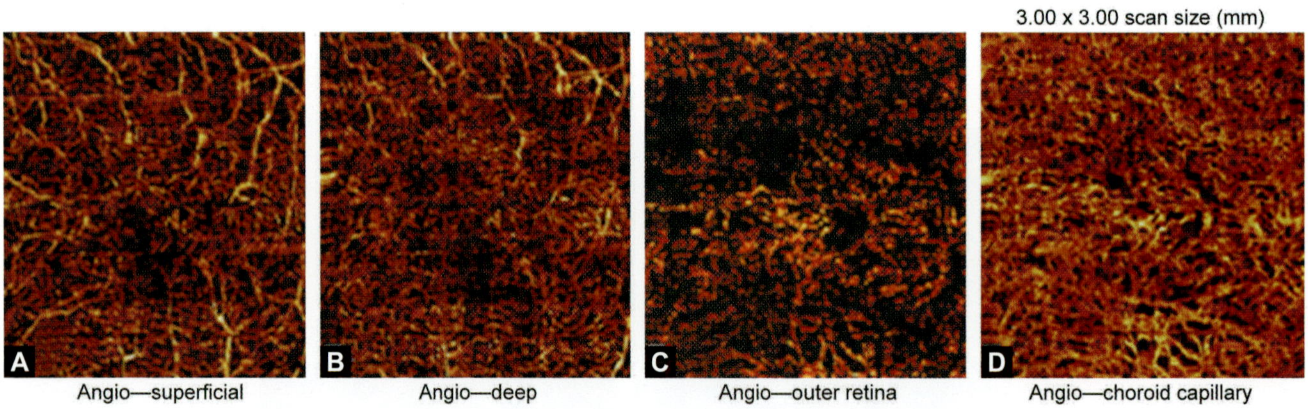

Figs. 8.14A to D: An OCTA SSADA protocol of retinal layers, the same eye as in previous figure (3 × 3 mm). (A and B) Vascular structure of superficial and deep vascular plexus is irregular and slightly changed. FAZ cannot be clearly visualized and is surrounded by a few regions of capillary dropout in the deep vascular plexus. Many anastomoses, especially in the superficial vascular plexus, can be noticed; and (C and D) In the outer retina and choriocapillaris, an irregular and ramified active neovascularization with rough appearance is visualized. A typical surrounding dark halo is missing. Neovascularization perforated the RPE (type 2 CNV). (CNV: choroidal neovascularization; FAZ: foveal avascular zone; OCTA: optical coherence tomography angiography; RPE: retinal pigment epithelium)

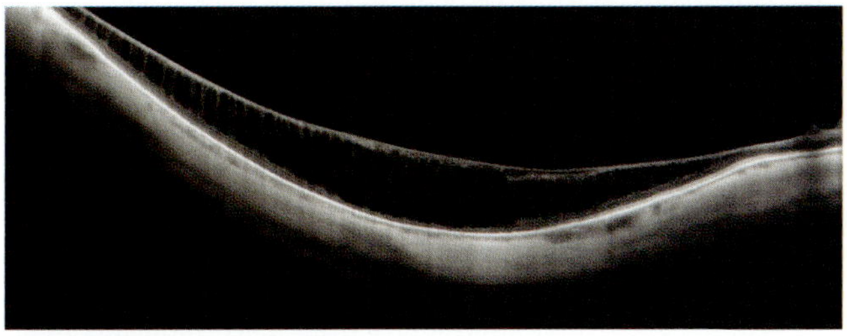

Fig. 8.15: An optical coherence tomography (OCT) B-scan presents a posterior staphyloma and complete intraretinal tear (schisis) in the inner retinal part. Many small gaps and cracks, which are separated by thin small parts of retinal tissue, are presented.

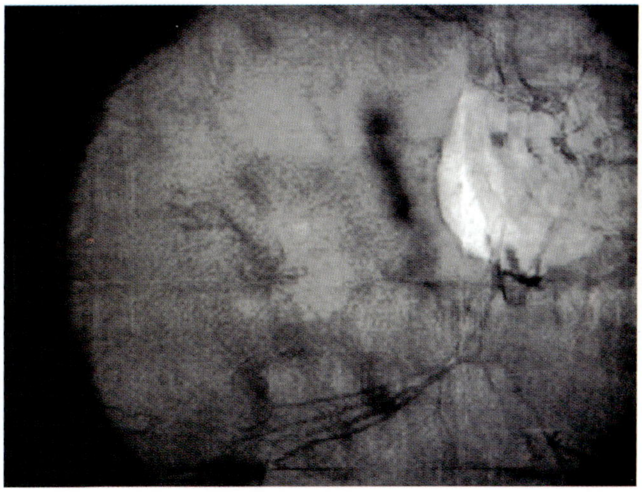

Fig. 8.16: Fundus photography of the same eye. Many floaters, that look like snowflakes in a snow globe, are seen in the vitreous and they cause shadows and blurring of the image. The optic disk is hardly seen. A huge peripapillary myopic degenerative conus and filamentous straight blood vessels are observed.

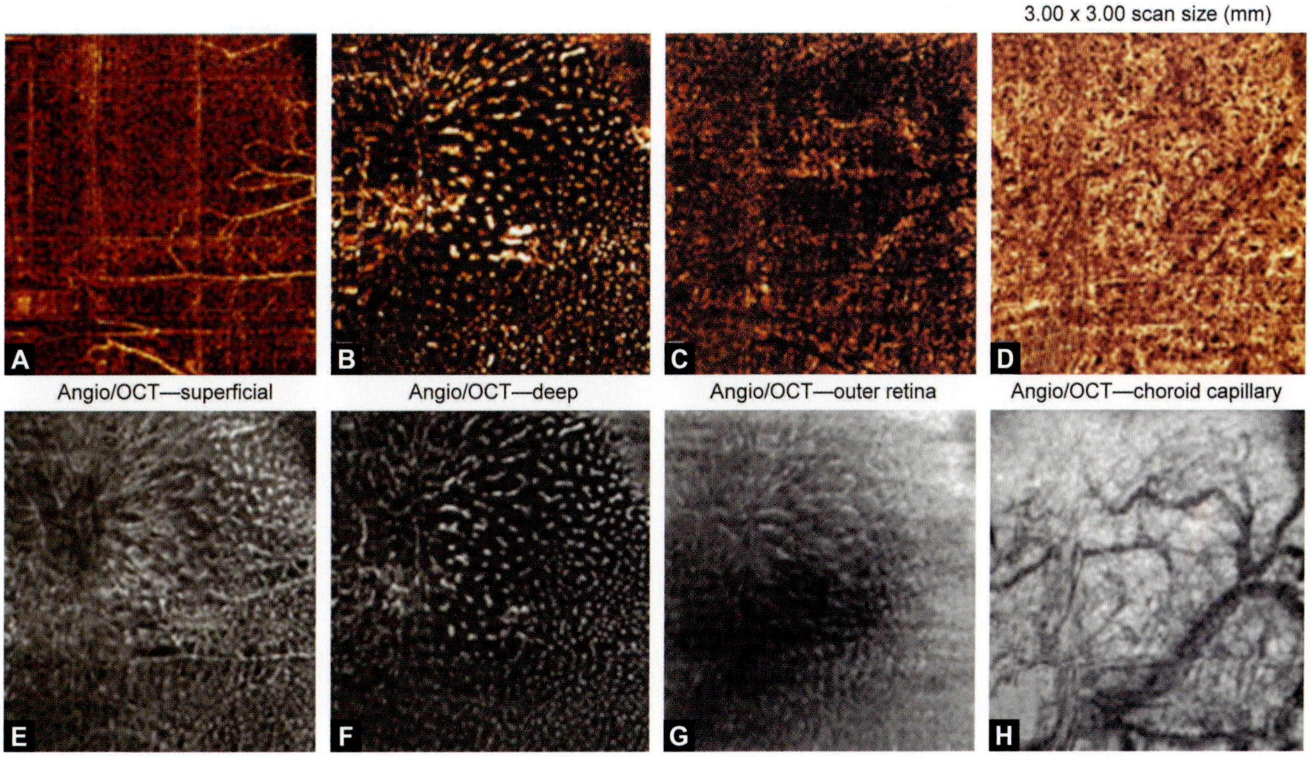

Figs. 8.17A to H: The image of OCTA and en face OCT of retinal layers of the same eye as in the Figure 8.16 (3 × 3 mm). (A) The superficial vascular plexus cannot be recognized. Nice, symmetric, and lacy structure is lost, with only a few visible irregular blood vessels. The FAZ cannot be visualized; (B) A complete loss of vascularization in deep vascular plexus is also seen. FAZ is not present, so the angiography finding resembles of the corresponding image of the en face OCT; (F) Both images show honeycomb and sponge-like structural changes, which can look like changes seen in juvenile retinoschisis; (C and D) The outer retina and choroid do not show any pathognomonic changes, and honeycomb-like spaces cannot be visualized, due to fact that the schisis occurred in inner retina. The outer retina is avascular, but the choroid shows irregular and rough lobular vascular structure; and (E to H) En face OCT imaging corresponds to angiographic changes and provides a clear visualization of retinoschisis and sponge or honeycomb-like retinal structure. (FAZ: foveal avascular zone; OCTA: optical coherence tomography angiography)

BIBLIOGRAPHY

1. Battaglia Parodi M, Iacono P, Bandello F. Correspondence of leakage on fluorescein angiography and optical coherence tomography parameters in diagnosis and monitoring of myopic choroidal neovascularization treated with bevacizumab. Retina. 2016;36(1):104-9.
2. Fischer MD, Inhoffen W, Ziemssen F. Spectral domain optical coherence tomography in the treatment of myopic choroidal neovascularization. Ophthalmologe. 2012; 109(8):758-65.
3. Hong YJ, Miura M, Makita S, et al. Noninvasive investigation of deep vascular pathologies of exudative macular diseases by high-penetration optical coherence angiography. Invest Ophthalmol Vis Sci. 2013;54(5):3621-31.
4. Hopf S, Pfeiffer N. Epidemiology of myopia. Ophthalmologe. 2017;114(1):20-3.
5. Ikuno Y, Sayanagi K, Soga K, et al. Lacquer crack formation and choroidal neovascularization in pathologic myopia. Retina. 2008;28(8):1124-31.
6. Ikuno Y, Sayanagi K, Soga K, et al. Intravitreal bevacizumab for choroidal neovascularization attributable to pathological myopia: one-year results. Am J Ophthalmol. 2009;147(1):94-100.
7. Lai TY, Cheung CM. Myopic choroidal neovascularization: diagnosis and treatment. Retina. 2016;36(9):1614-21.
8. Louzada RN, Ferrara D, Novais EA, et al. Analysis of scleral feeder vessel in myopic choroidal neovascularization using optical coherence tomography angiography. Ophthalmic Surg Lasers Imaging Retina. 2016;47(10):960-4.
9. Matsuo M, Honda S, Matsumiya W, et al. Comparison between anti-vascular endothelial growth factor therapy and photodynamic therapy for myopic choroidal neovascularization. Eur J Ophthalmol. 2012;22(2):210-5.
10. Milani P, Massacesi A, Moschini S, et al. Multimodal imaging and diagnosis of myopic choroidal neovascularization in Caucasians. Clin Ophthalmol. 2016;10:1749-57.
11. Milani P, Massacesi A, Setaccioli M, et al. Sensitivity of fluorescein angiography alone or with SD-OCT for the diagnosis of myopic choroidal neovascularization. Graefes Arch Clin Exp Ophthalmol. 2013;251(8):1891-900.
12. Moghadas Sharif N, Shoeibi N, Ehsaei A, et al. Optical coherence tomography and biometry in high myopia with tilted disc. Optom Vis Sci. 2016;93(11):1380-6.
13. Munk MR, Rückert R, Zinkernagel M, et al. The role of anti-VEGF agents in myopic choroidal neovascularization: Current standards and future outlook. Expert Opin Biol Ther. 2016;16(4):477-87.
14. Ng WY, Ting DS, Agrawal R, et al. Choroidal structural changes in myopic choroidal neovascularization after treatment with antivascular endothelial growth factor over 1 year. Invest Ophthalmol Vis Sci. 2016;57(11):4933-9.
15. Querques G, Corvi F, Querques L, et al. Optical coherence tomography angiography of choroidal neovascularization secondary to pathologic myopia. Dev Ophthalmol. 2016;56:101-6.
16. Tideman JW, Snabel MC, Tedja MS, et al. Association of axial length with risk of uncorrectable visual impairment for Europeans with myopia. JAMA Ophthalmol. 2016;134(12):1355-63.
17. Yoshida T, Ohno-Matsui K, Ohtake Y, et al. Long-term visual prognosis of choroidal neovascularization in high myopia: a comparison between age groups. Ophthalmology. 2002;109(4):712-9.
18. Yoshida T, Ohno-Matsui K, Yasuzumi K, et al. Myopic choroidal neovascularization: a 10-year follow-up. Ophthalmology. 2003;110(7):1297-305.

CHAPTER 9

Retinal Artery Occlusion

INTRODUCTION

Retinal artery occlusion is a disease characterized by ischemic infarctions of the entire retina or just a certain part of it. Anatomically, it can be classified into the central retinal artery occlusion (CRAO), branch retinal artery occlusion (BRAO), and ciliary retinal artery occlusion.

EPIDEMIOLOGY AND ETIOLOGY

Etiologically, all arterial occlusive diseases can be divided into nonartery and artery. Nonartery retinal artery occlusions are frequent and affect patients between the ages of 60 years and 65 years. Artery occlusions generally affect people above the age of 70 years, so along with vision loss, some extraocular symptoms may occur. The main etiopathologic mechanism of CRAO is thrombosis in area of lamina cribrosa (LC). Most frequently, it is related to atherosclerosis. In 25% of these cases, the embolus is the cause of occlusion. Conditions that carry a high risk for the development of artery occlusion include disorders of coagulation factors, traumas, optical nerve drusen, active eye infections, migraines, and congenital malformations of the central retinal artery. Men are affected more frequently than women. BRAO is more frequent on the right eye and is related to emboli appearance and formation (in 75% of cases). Usually the embolus is seen on the artery bifurcation, while the location of the embolus origin may be at any place between the heart and the ophthalmic artery. Risk factors are hypertension, hypercholesterolemia, diabetes, smoking, and a positive family history.

SYMPTOMS AND SIGNS

Symptoms of CRAO are sudden and unpainful. The patient has decreased visual acuity, a narrowed field of vision in all quadrants, and the presence of a relative afferent pupillary defect. In the case of BRAO, there is sudden and unpainful vision loss in certain sectors, while central visual acuity is preserved unless the macula is affected. Ciliary retinal artery occlusion causes significant decrease of central vision acuity. Patients often complain of transitory vision loss that precedes occlusion (*amaurosis fugax*). Fundoscopic examination reveals pallid retina as a consequence of the sudden ischemia. On some occasions, it is possible to see a well-described phenomenon referred to as a cherry-like stain (*cherry red spot*) in the central macula. The sign is present due to retinal ischemia which changes the regular choroid color in all parts except the macular area where the nerve fibers are extremely thin. Other associated signs and conditions include embolus visualization in 25% of patients, changes and plaques in the carotid artery in 33% of patients, 5% of patients with giant cell arteritis, and 18% of patients with iris neovascularization and visible arterial collaterals on the optical disk.

DIAGNOSTICS

Fundus photography shows the cherry color stain standing out from the surrounding ischemic pale colored retina. In chronic cases, optical coherence tomography (OCT) can depict retinal flatness along with the loss of the inner layers of the retina in regions of previous ischemia. In acute cases, the OCT can show swelling and edema in the ischemic region. Fluorescence angiography (FAG) shows prolonged arterial filling, often with accentuated colored edges in regions with obstructed arterioles. FAG can emphasize the presence of an embolus. OCT angiography (OCTA) may help in BRAO diagnostics where there are changes in the superficial and deep vascular network. The number and quality of collateral capillaries is lost, especially in the deep vascular network. This layer shows an increase in the number and area of the intercapillary spaces (capillary *dropout*) (Figs. 9.1 to 9.3).

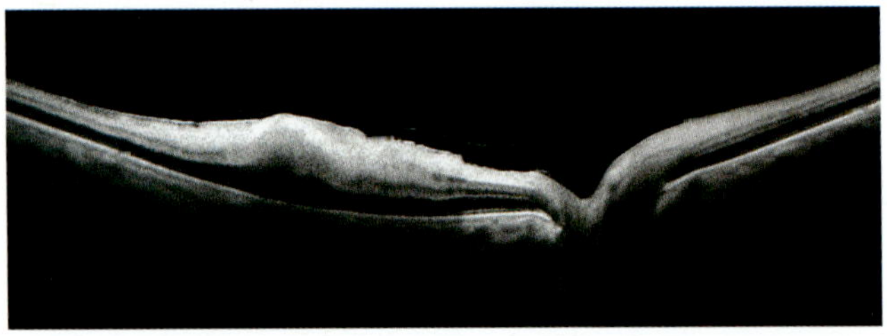

Fig. 9.1: An OCT B-scan in an 82-year-old female patient, 4 days after complete vision loss. An abnormal retinal profile can be visualized with the loss of normal foveal depression. The inner retina is thickened and highly reflective. The outer retina is hyporeflective and seems as if it is swelling, due to the acute central retinal artery occlusion. The external limiting membrane and RPE are intact. The posterior hyaloid membrane can also be visualized. (OCT: optical coherence tomography; RPE: retinal pigment epithelium)

TREATMENT

There is no clearly proved therapy for CRAO. Irreversible damage to the retina occurs within 90–100 minutes from the moment of occlusion, and therapeutic procedures are performed if the patient seeks medical attention within 24 hours of the onset of the first symptoms. Basic treatment includes lowering the intraocular pressure by massaging the eyeball, paracentesis, the use of hyperosmotic drugs to reduce eye pressure, and medication that induces peripheral vasodilatation. If the occlusion is secondary, due to giant cell arteritis, high doses of corticosteroids should be given to prevent the other eye from being affected. Unfortunately, most retinal obstructions end with permanent and severe loss of visual acuity. A third of the patients experience a certain degree of visual acuity recovery. Patients must also be treated by an internist to prevent the onset of a heart attack. In patients who develop neovascularization of the retina, optical disk, or iris, with the consequence of neovascular glaucoma, complications are treated with panretinal photocoagulation.

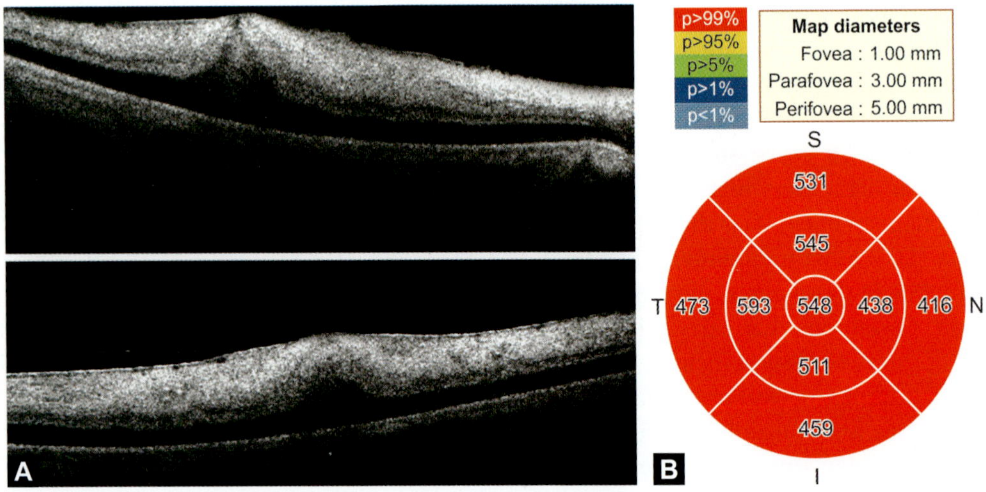

Figs. 9.2A and B: (A) An optical coherence tomography (OCT) B-scan of the same eye as in the previous image, scanned with a bigger magnification. The epiretinal membrane is hyperreflective and is starting to separate from the retinal surface. The whole inner retina is thickened and hyperreflective; and (B) The retinal thickness map shows increased values of macular thickness in all parts, even up to 548 microns.

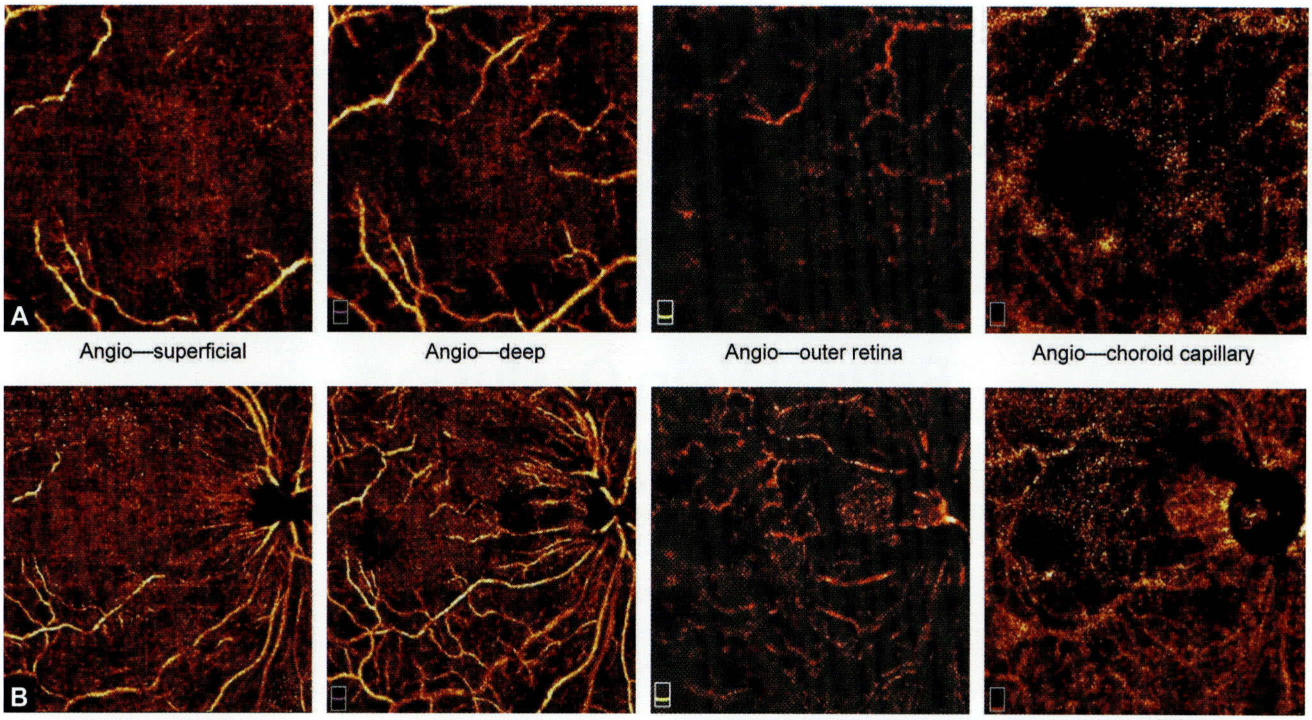

Figs. 9.3A and B: Angiography images of the same eye with the CRAO. Angiograms, scanned with a bigger magnification, 3 × 3 mm. These scans can emphasize the foveal avascular zone (FAZ) and macular area, along with associated vascular structures. In these images, the superficial and deep vascular plexus show a completely lost and dried area, without small and gentle capillaries. Regular capillary networks cannot be seen. There are only a few straight, dry, and bigger blood vessels, with segmented flow. FAZ cannot be visualized and measured. The outer retina is avascular but a reflection from big choroidal vessels can be seen. The fine lobular vascular structure of the choroid is lost; (B) Presents the images scanned in a smaller magnification (6 × 6 mm). It allows a physician a better insight into the exact size of the affected area. The superficial vascular plexus shows a big nonflow area, which can also be seen in the deep vascular plexus. The outer retina is avascular, and the choroid shows a harsh irregular, dry vascular structure.

BIBLIOGRAPHY

1. Baumal CR. Optical coherence tomography angiography of retinal artery occlusion. Dev Ophthalmol. 2016;56:122-31.
2. Bhanushali DR, Yadav NK, Dabir S, et al. Spectral domain optical coherence tomography angiography features in a patient of central retinal arterial occlusion before and after paracentesis. Retina. 2016;36(5):e36-8.
3. Bonini Filho MA, Adhi M, de Carlo TE, et al. Optical coherence tomography angiography in retinal artery occlusion. Retina. 2015;35(11):2339-46.
4. Dattilo M, Biousse V, Newman NJ. Update on the management of central retinal artery occlusion. Neurol Clin. 2017;35(1):83-100.
5. de Castro-Abeger AH, de Carlo TE, Duker JS, et al. Optical coherence tomography angiography compared to fluorescein angiography in branch retinal artery occlusion. Ophthalmic Surg Lasers Imaging Retina. 2015;46(10):1052-4.
6. Varma DD, Cugati S, Lee AW, et al. A review of central retinal artery occlusion: clinical presentation and management. Eye (Lond). 2013;27(6):688-97.
7. Wang R, Qian L, Wang Y, et al. Evaluation of ophthalmic artery branch retrograde intervention in the treatment of central retinal artery occlusion (CRAO). Med Sci Monit. 2017;23:114-20.

CHAPTER 10

Retinal Vein Occlusion

INTRODUCTION

Retinal vein occlusion (RVO) is a condition characterized by hemorrhagic infarctions of the entire retina or its part, and is manifested by a sudden painless loss of vision, numerous retinal bleedings, an appearance of soft retinal exudates, and a macular edema. Anatomical localization divides the condition into the central retinal vein occlusion (CRVO), the primary occlusion of the superior or inferior retinal vein [hemi-retinal vein occlusion (HRVO)], and occlusion of the more distal branches of the central retinal vein [branch retinal vein occlusion (BRVO)]. Due to the perfusion status, which is determined by the fluorescein angiography (FAG), RVO can be divided into a nonischemic, milder form, and ischemic, more severe form. This division determines the clinical course, prognosis, and development of complications.

EPIDEMIOLOGY AND ETIOLOGY

Retinal vein occlusion is one of the most common retinal vascular diseases. Both sexes are equally affected, and it is particularly common in the elderly population over 65 years of age. The condition is usually unilateral, although in 6–14% of the cases it can be bilateral. BRVO appears three times more often than CRVO. RVO essentially presents with a blockage of the venous blood flow, resulting in the increased intracapillary pressure and consequent leakage of fluid and blood. If the leakage is near the macula, a macular edema may occur. Macular ischemia occurs due to capillary damage and retinal capillary nonperfusion. It leads to the retinal damage, growth of abnormal blood vessels, and neovascularization, which can cause secondary complications such as neovascular glaucoma, vitreous hemorrhage, or retinal detachment. The most common cause of CRVO is the obstruction of venous blood vessels with a thrombus, while the BRVO is most commonly caused by compression of the atherosclerotically modified arterious blood vessel on the vein, resulting in turbulent venous blood flow, endothelial damage, and consequent thrombosis. The most known risk factors for RVO are older age, diabetes, arterial hypertension, obesity, smoking, hypercoagulable states, and glaucoma. The risk factors for BRVO are hypertension, hyperlipidemia, disorders of coagulation factors, systemic inflammatory conditions, and glaucoma. CRVO is always linked with hypertension and diabetes. In younger patients, RVO is usually a secondary change due to hypercoagulable states or general inflammatory diseases.

SYMPTOMS AND SIGNS

The main symptom is a quick, painless loss of the vision on one eye. The visual acuity can vary from 20/20 to the point of appreciating hand movements in front of the face.

The patient can also complain about blurred vision. The percentage of visual acuity depends on the severity of retinal ischemia and of the size of the present macular edema. Fundoscopic examination may reveal flame-shaped intraretinal hemorrhages, if they occur in the superficial parts of the retina, and dot or blot-shaped intraretinal hemorrhages, if they occur deeper in the retina and are arranged along the occluded vein following a curving stream of the dilated blood vessels. Occasionally, fundoscopic examination may reveal the edema of a part or the entire optic disk area, along with cotton-wool patches and a macular edema. Fundoscopical changes usually appear serious and dramatic, and most of them occur suddenly (this appearance is described as a *blood and thunder* fundus).

DIFFERENTIAL DIAGNOSIS

- Branch retinal vein occlusion
- Occlusion of the superior or inferior retinal vein (HRVO)
- Ocular ischemic syndrome (OIS)
- Preproliferative and proliferative diabetic retinopathy
- Hypertensive retinopathy.

It should not be forgotten that similar clinical findings may also occur in cases of radiation retinopathy, optic disk vasculitis (papillophlebitis), papillary edema, and in all papillary inflammatory conditions with a secondary appearance of vein occlusion.

DIAGNOSTICS

Fundus examination can reveal the previously described signs of the disease. Fundus photography can show the presence of large retinal bleeding in one part or the entire half of the retina. Those hemorrhages can sometimes be seen throughout the entire retinal surface. They may be very different in shape, depending on the depth of their appearance. Usually, fundus photography can show a flame-like shape of the hemorrhage, and a dot or blot-like shape. Along with the described bleedings, physicians can also sometimes see soft exudates, macular edema, areas of the ischemic retina, and neovascularizations. Optical coherence tomography (OCT) is a useful diagnostic tool, which can clearly reveal macular edema. On the OCT B-scan, the macula appears significantly thickened and many intraretinal cysts of various sizes can be seen. Subretinal fluid may also be present. In the late stage of the chronic form of the disease, the macular area can be thinned due to prolonged retinal ischemia. FAG also indicates the presence of cystoid macular edema. FAG helps to distinguish the ischemic from the nonischemic form of RVO. The ischemic form of CRVO shows very large regions without any capillary flow. The risk of secondary neovascularization directly depends on the ischemia severity. FAG helps in detecting the active areas with neovascularization.

Optical coherence tomography angiography (OCTA) is the latest diagnostic tool that contributes to the effective and early detection of RVO. Vascular changes can be seen on angiograms both in the superficial and in the deep vascular plexus.

Optical coherence tomography angiography changes in the superficial vascular plexus that occur in cases of macular ischemia due to the RVO. The regions without flow and those with preserved flow can be clearly determined and are easily distinguishable. The distinction between these areas can be even better seen and more clearly demarcated in the deep vascular plexus. Along with the described areas, numerous anastomoses, vascular loops, and dilated, tortuous blood vessels can be shown. Also, blood vessels do not have a regular, proper course in their entire length, but show focal deviations. Wall thickness is irregular and a focal segmentation along with the narrowing of the lumen can occur. Abruptions of the vascular vessels can often be seen as well as terminal dilations around the foveal avascular zone (FAZ). The FAZ is wider and irregular, usually oval in shape, and compared to the FAZ of a healthy eye. Many microvascular abnormalities can also be seen in the superficial vascular network by the OCTA. Areas without capillary blood flow (capillary dropouts) are shown as areas with rare, scattered, and completely irregular capillaries. On the OCTA, the region with a retinal edema is recognized as an area of widely separated, irregular, curvy, and enlarged blood vessels, which have very unclear edges (Figs. 10.1 to 10.5).

The deep vascular plexus, in cases of RVO, shows even more significant changes, mainly in the regions of ischemia. The capillary arrangement is asymmetrical and irregular, especially in regions without flow. In the angiograms, dilated capillaries with an enlarged caliber alternate with capillaries with a reduced caliber and/or with capillaries that are seemingly occluded. Capillaries in the deep vascular network appear to be enlarged, attenuated in formation, and the entire network seems to be sparse and blurry. The walls of the blood vessels are thicker in pathological zones and there are numerous irregular shunts, especially

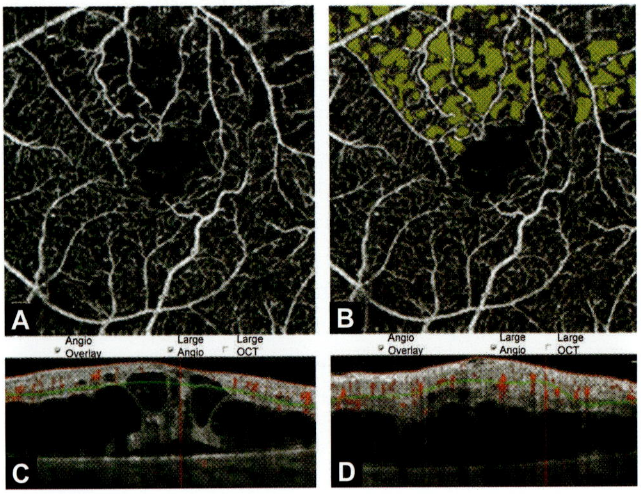

Figs. 10.1A to D: (A) An en face angiogram of the superficial vascular plexus; and (B) The Angio Analysis of areas without vascular flow (capillary dropout) in the same layer. (A) The angiography of the superficial vascular plexus shows the vascular dropouts as larger darker regions without any capillaries that are situated mainly above the FAZ. Similar changes will be seen in the deep vascular plexus; (B) Figure shows Angio Analysis and pinpointed regions without flow, which are colored in yellow. The area above the FAZ is full of vascular dropouts different in shape and size; and (C and D) OCT B-scans, where the thin horizontal red and green lines mark the thickness of the layers that are analyzed. Central macular edema along with the accumulation of the subretinal fluid is presented on these scans. (FAZ: foveal avascular zone; OCT: optical coherence tomography)

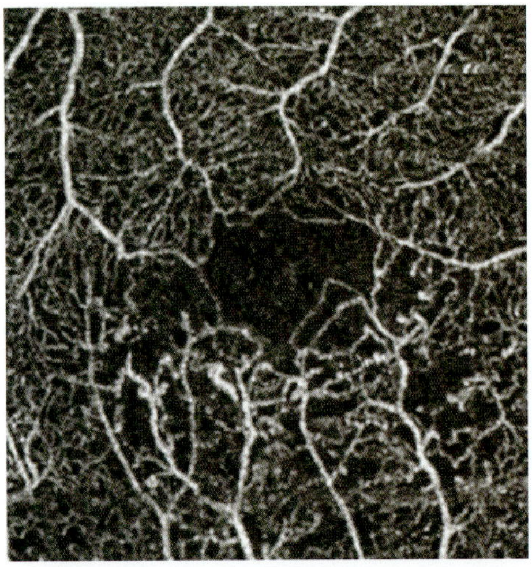

Fig. 10.3: An OCTA of the superficial vascular plexus. There is a harsh vascular network with a few arteriovenous anastomoses and many vascular loops. Vascular dropouts are mainly located inferiorly. FAZ is enlarged and irregular in shape. These changes cannot be visualized by the FAG due to the fluid leakage. Inside the affected area, capillaries look damaged and truncated, and have harsh cuts. (FAG: fluorescein angiography; FAZ: foveal avascular zone; OCTA: optical coherence tomography angiography)

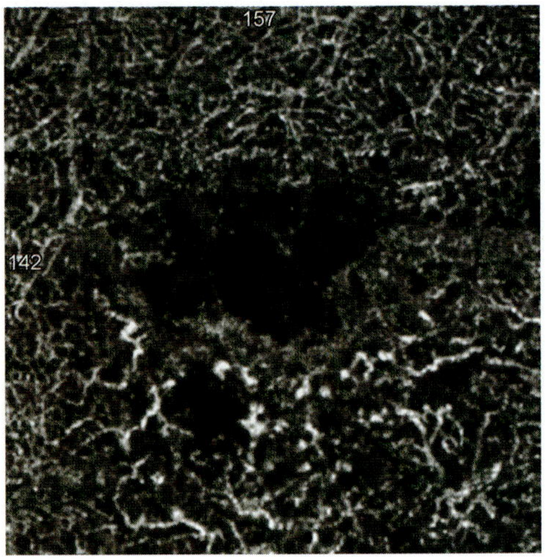

Fig. 10.2: An en face angiogram of the deep vascular plexus with a well represented vascular congestion. Vascular congestion is always the best visualized in this vascular plexus. Capillaries are irregular and different in thickness. Some of them are of greater caliber and seem to be dilated, while the others are narrowed or occluded. The vascular network seems to be rough at the places with dilated, sparsed capillaries. The whole affected region looks grayish and blurred, and the edges of the capillary walls are very unclear.

in the borders between regular and pathological parts of the retina. Vascular congestion is also the most visible in the deep vascular plexus, especially in that borderline region. The deep vascular network also shows changes in the size of blood vessels, local dilatations, aneurysms, and microaneurysms that vary in size and arrangement (Figs. 10.6 to 10.11).

THERAPY

Macular edema can be treated with intravitreal antivascular endothelial growth factor (anti-VEGF) injections, intravitreal corticosteroid injections, and/or with a laser. Patients with BRVO, macular edema, and visual acuity below 20/40 are recommended to do grid laser photocoagulation. Grid, focal photocoagulation is used in the treatment of leaking microaneurysms or regions that show leakage or ischemia in FAG. The laser should be avoided for the treatment of the FAZ. A yellow laser is recommended for its treatment, as it leaves no scars. If an argon green laser (514 nm) is used for the treatment, a recommended spot size should be between 50 μm and 100 μm with an exposure of 20–100 ms, and a power of 50–100 mW, titrated to a light gray spot color after the application. Newer studies, such

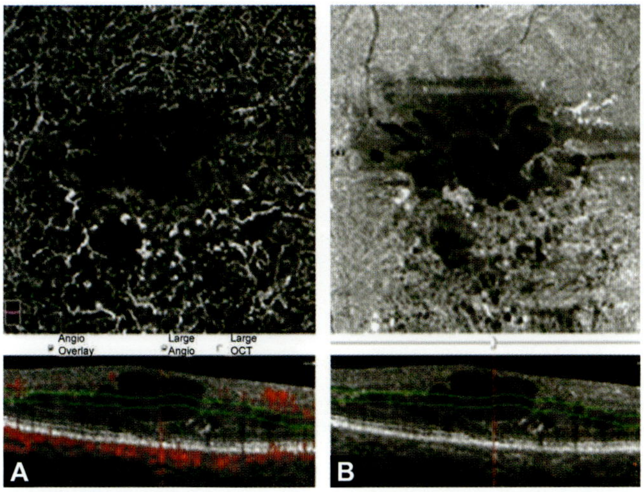

Figs. 10.4A and B: An optical coherence tomography angiography (OCTA) and en face OCT of the deep vascular plexus, the same eye as in Figure 10.3. (A) An OCTA shows many areas without flow, which are different in size and shape, and the whole capillary network has a deformed structure. Dark areas without flow match the cysts and macular edema, which is best shown on the corresponding B-scans. Venous congestion is well presented in this layer and many dilated, as well as narrowed capillaries can be seen, especially in the borderline between the "normal" and affected retina. Many anastomoses can be visualized along with numerous hyperreflective microaneurysms and aneurysms. On the corresponding OCT B-scan, cystoid macular edema is visible. The zone between two thin horizontal lines shows the localization and the depth of the analyzed layer; and (B) The corresponding en face OCT image shows many irregular, larger, and smaller, hyporeflective areas, which are sharply divided from each other by the hyperreflective retinal tissue. Those rounded areas match the macular cysts, due to the macular edema in the deep layer of the inner retina.

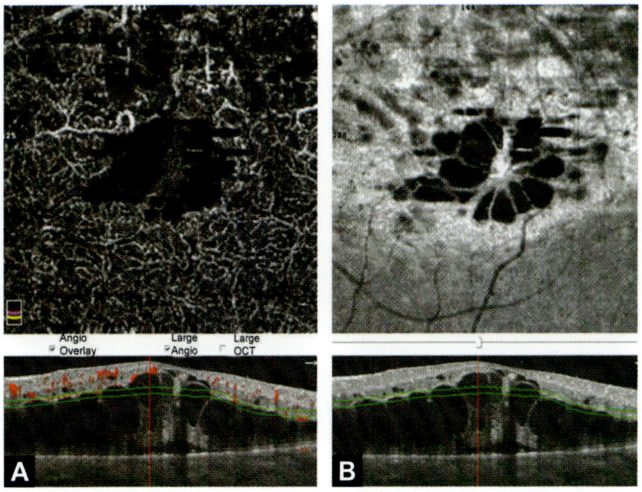

Figs. 10.5A and B: An OCTA and en face OCT of the deep vascular plexus along with the corresponding B-scans. (A) The angiography of the deep vascular plexus in the eye with CRVO. Many capillary dropouts, a vascular congestion, dilated capillaries with blurred edges, vascular loops, and anastomoses can be seen. In the FAZ, in the very center, there is one larger part of the retinal tissue. From that part there are a few thinner, smaller rays of tissue that separate the edema into a few cystic spaces. The OCT B-scan, presented in the inferior part of the image, shows the central edematous change, which is divided by the rays into cysts that are different in size and shape. Shallow accumulation of the subretinal fluid is also seen; and (B) En face OCT very clearly shows the frontal appearance of the macular edema. The cysts form a kind of shape that resembles a flower with bigger and smaller petals. When analyzing the OCT angiography finding, the comparison and parallel analysis of all the protocols is highly recommended. (CRVO: central retinal vein occlusion; FAZ: foveal avascular zone; OCTA: optical coherence tomography angiography)

as the BRAVO study, recommend treatment with intravitreal ranibizumab injections in patients with BRVO and macular edema. The study showed significant recovery of visual acuity in 6 months to 1 year after the application. A CRUISE study shows a similar effect of ranibizumab injection in cases of macular edema due to the CRVO. Newer medications, such is aflibercept, have shown efficacy in the treatment of macular edema due to the CRVO but are not allowed as a treatment option for the cases of the macular edema due to the BRVO (Galileo, Copernicus). Corticosteroids can also be used as a treatment option in cases of the macular edema caused by RVO, but nowadays they are medications of the second or third choice, after the anti-VEGF therapy and laser treatment, due to their side effects (higher risk of cataract development, as well as glaucoma). According to the results of the CVOS study (Central Vein Occlusion study), patients with the CRVO have no benefit from grid laser photocoagulation.

Panretinal photocoagulation (PRP) is recommended for patients who have neovascularization on the retina, optic nerve, or on the iris. The development of the neovascularization is more common in the patients with a CRVO, due to the presence of the larger regions of retinal ischemia. If the affected region is larger than the five papillary diameters, in patients with a BRVO, the risk of developing neovascularization is extremely high. Laser

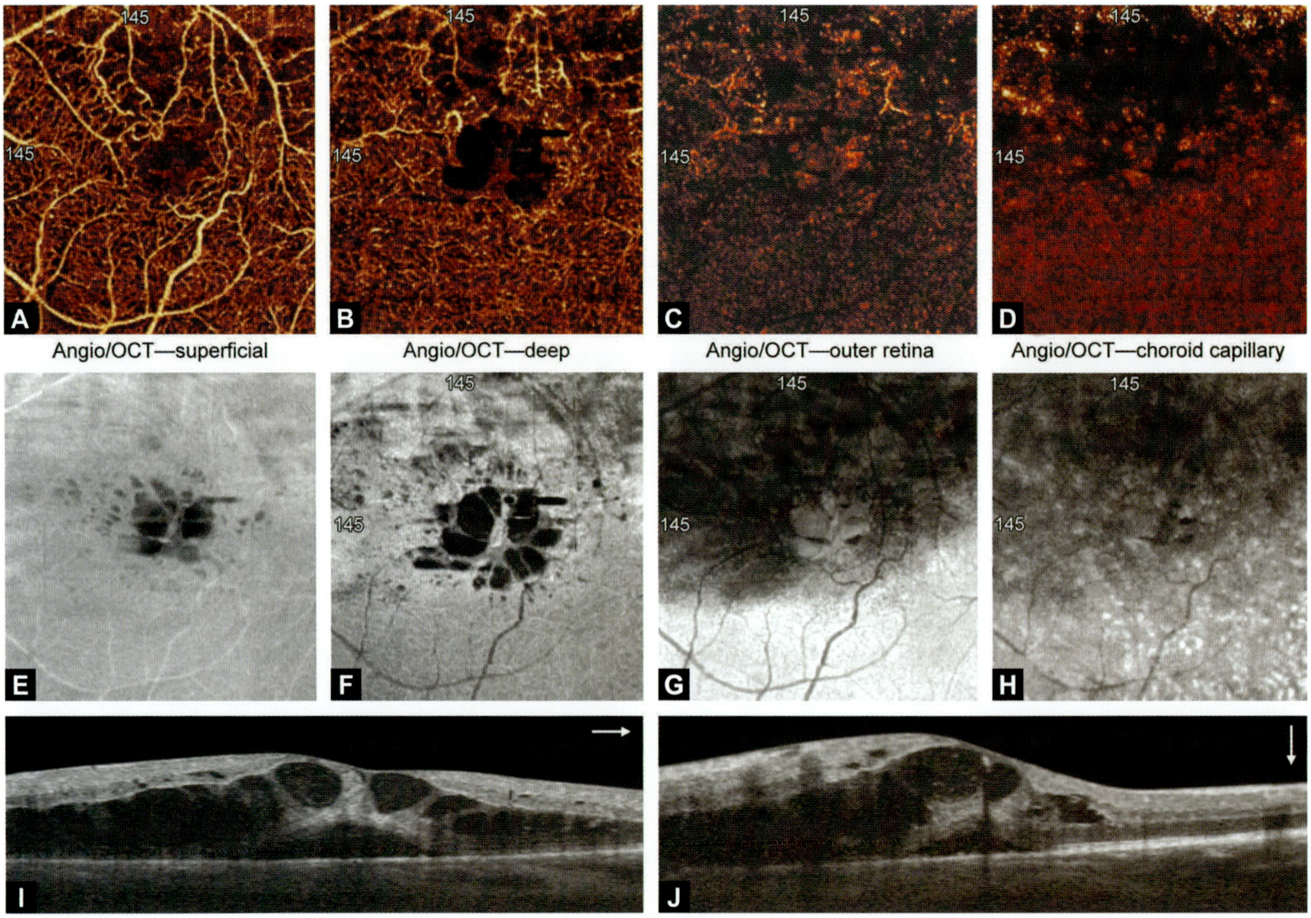

Figs. 10.6A to J: An OCTA SSADA protocol and en face OCT of the corresponding retinal layers, along with the matching OCT B-scan in a 55-year-old patient with RVO (3 × 3 mm). (A and B) Both the superficial and deep vascular plexus show obvious changes of the vascular network, which indicate RVO. Very clear separation of the normal and affected retina can be seen in both vascular networks. The superficial vascular network shows many capillary dropouts, many anastomoses, vascular loops, and microaneurysms. Affected capillaries are very tortuous and segmentally dilated. The deep vascular plexus shows signs of venous congestion, clearly bounded capillary dropouts, and many microaneurysms. FAZ forms a flower-like shape, due to the cysts that are separated between each other, and due to the macular edema; (C and D) The outer retina and choroidal layer show a big dark region above the center, which matches the location of the edema; (E to H) An en face OCT of the corresponding retinal layers, where the edema and cysts can be best seen in the deep layer of inner retina. The classic appearance with oval, petal-like cysts in the center indicates the existence of macular edema. In the outer retina and choroid, the hyporeflective area can be seen above the very center. This area corresponds to the accumulated subretinal fluid; and (I and J) OCT B-scans show the central macular edema, which is divided into smaller cysts by the residual retinal tissue. There is also a shallow sensory retinal detachment. (FAZ: foveal avascular zone; OCTA: optical coherence tomography angiography; RVO: retinal vein occlusion)

photocoagulation causes the regression of the neovascularization and reduces the risk of the vitreal hemorrhage to the 50%. The PRP is done by the argon green laser, with spots being 200–500 μm in size, exposure of 100–200 ms, and a power of 200 mW which causes light, gentle white spots to appear on the retina after the application. PRP complications include decreasement or loss of peripheral vision, night vision problems, loss of accommodation, ischemia of the anterior part of the eye (rarely), and random foveal spots (burns).

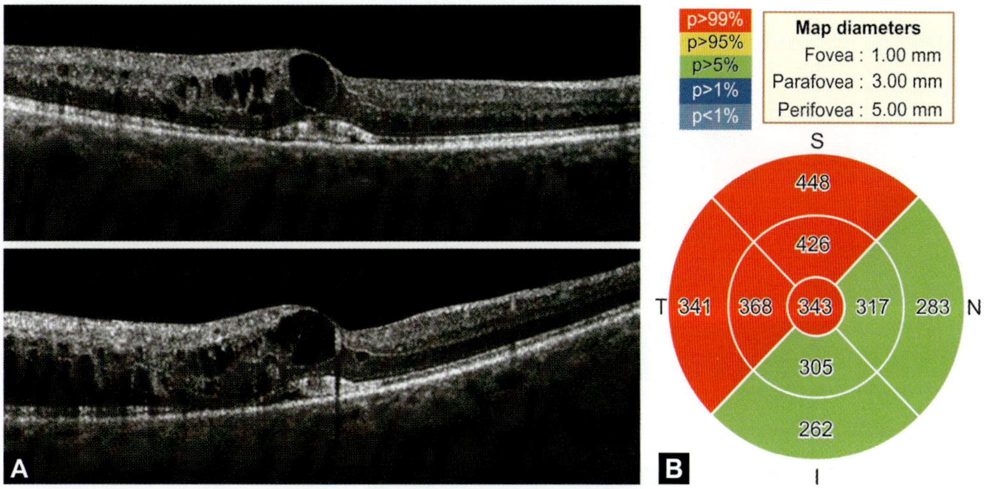

Figs. 10.7A and B: An OCT B-scan and the retinal thickness map in a 65-year-old patient with RVO. (A) The whole temporal part of the retina and macular area show the edema with the cysts, which are different in size and shape. There is also hyperreflective subretinal fluid shown, and the RPE seems to be perforated and irregular in places. The nasal part of the retina shows no pathological changes. This could implicate that this patient was affected with hemi-retinal vein occlusion; and (B) The retinal thickness map shows increased values of the foveal area both in the superior and temporal perifoveal zones. This map shows the exact division of the two halves of the retina, the normal one, and the affected one. (OCT: optical coherence tomography; RPE: retinal pigment epithelium; RVO: retinal vein occlusion)

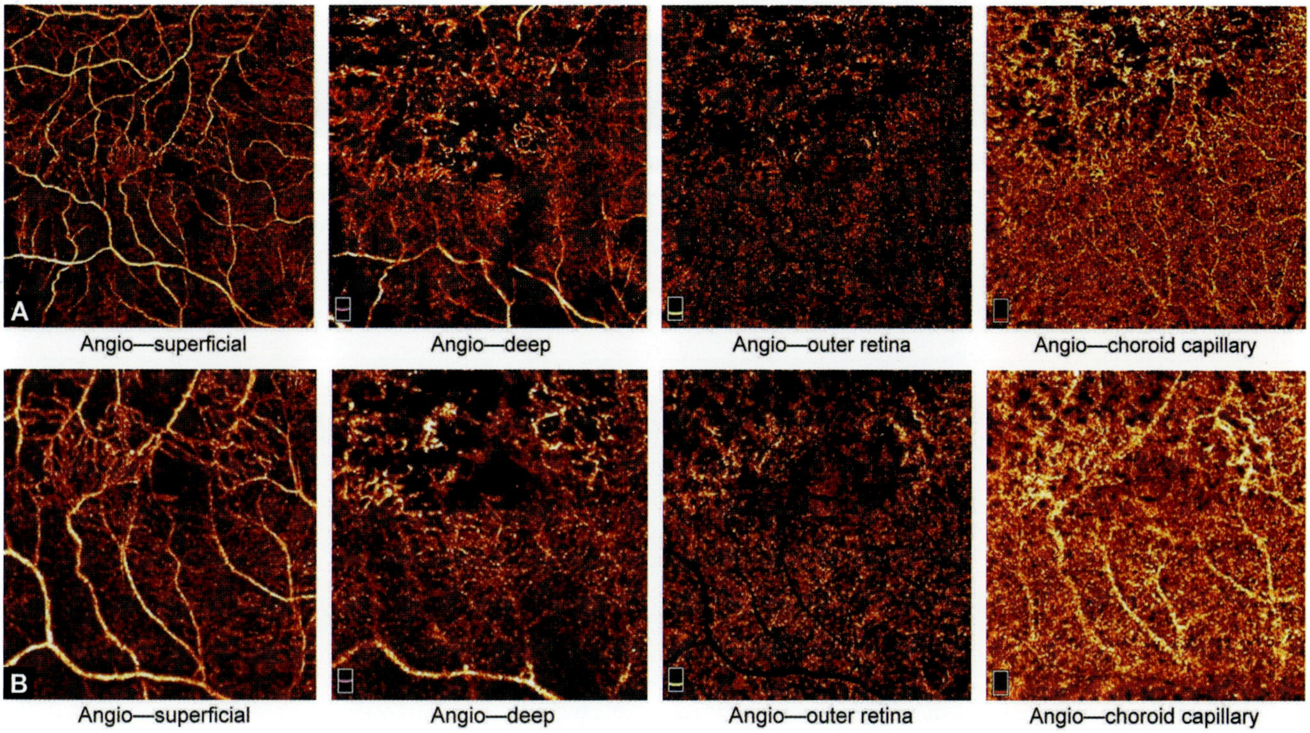

Figs. 10.8A and B: The figures show the optical coherence tomography (OCT) angiography of the retinal vascular layers, which are scanned in different magnifications. (A) The upper four images are scanned with a smaller magnification (6 × 6 mm) and they give a very good insight into the size of the affected region. Pathologically changed retina extends to the entire upper and temporal side on the angiograms; and (B) The bigger magnification (3 × 3 mm) gives a very exact insight into the vascular changes and the appearance of the capillaries. There are many vascular dropouts in the superficial vascular network. The deep vascular network shows vascular congestion and many microaneurysms.

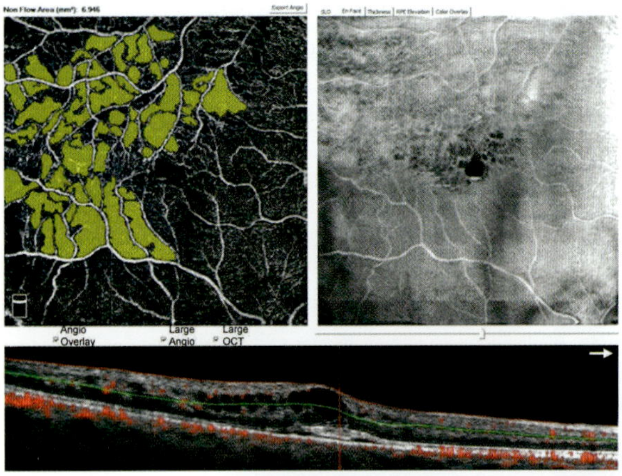

Fig. 10.9: Optical coherence tomography angiography (OCTA) Angio Analysis of the nonflow area in the superficial vascular plexus (6 × 6 mm). The yellow-colored areas are the areas without any capillary flow, and this nonflow area measures 6.946 mm^2. Most of those areas are located in the superior and temporal part of the retina. On the right side of the image, the en face OCT of the superficial part of the inner retina is shown. There are a few small cysts around the central zone. On the lower part of the image, the corresponding OCT B-scan is presented. The horizontal red and green line bound the analyzed superficial layer.

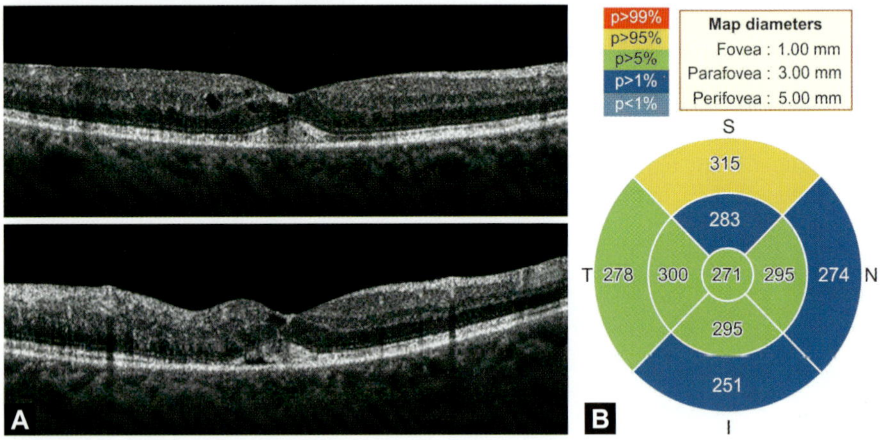

Figs. 10.10A and B: An optical coherence tomography (OCT) B-scan and a retinal thickness map of the same eye as in the previous images, 3 days after the intravitreal ranibizumab application. (A) The B-scan shows a significantly thinner retina with the decreased number of the edematous cysts. However, the retina in some places still presents with the accumulation of intraretinal fluid. The whole retinal profile seems to be irregular and still slightly edematous, but the finding is much better in comparison to the one before therapy; and (B) The retinal map showing regular values of the macular thickness after the ranibizumab application, but in places still slightly increased (in the superior part).

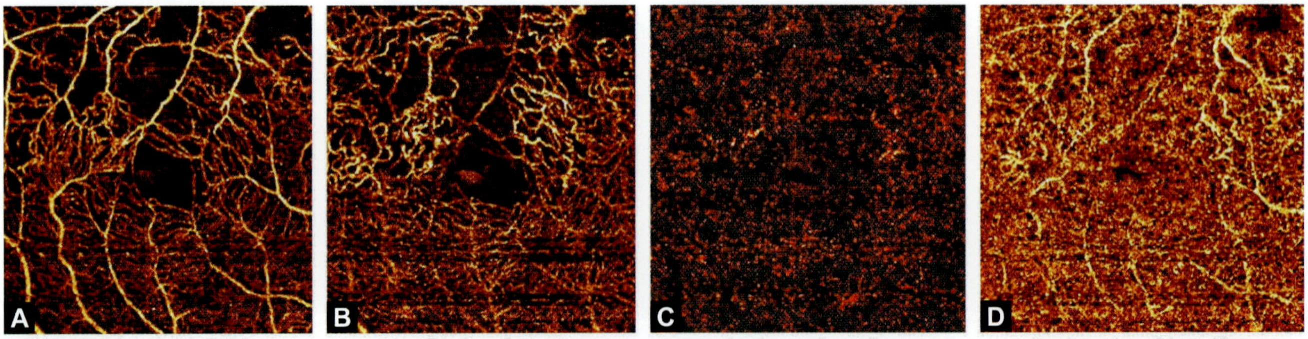

Angio—superficial | Angio—deep | Angio—outer retina | Angio—choroid capillary

Figs. 10.11A to D: An OCT angiography of the superficial and deep vascular plexus, outer retina, and choriocapillaris (3 × 3 mm) of the same eye as in previous figures, 3 days after the anti-VEGF therapy (ranibizumab). The superficial and deep vascular network still shows the classical vascular changes that are significant for the RVO. Many capillary dropouts, vascular shunts, loops, and microaneurysms can be seen in both of the vascular networks. However, there is no such expressed vascular congestion in the deep vascular plexus anymore. Capillaries do not have unclear edges, like they used to have before the therapy, and many of them can be clearly visualized. The outer retina shows no pathological changes, and the vascular structure of the choriocapillaris seems to be a bit rough. (OCT: optical coherence tomography; RVO: retinal vein occlusion; VEGF: vascular endothelial growth factor)

BIBLIOGRAPHY

1. Adhi M, Filho MA, Louzada RN, et al. Retinal capillary network and foveal avascular zone in eyes with vein occlusion and fellow eyes analyzed with optical coherence tomography angiography. Invest Ophthalmol Vis Sci. 2016;57(9):486-94.
2. Bertelmann T, Feltgen N, Scheffler M, et al. Vision-related quality of life in patients receiving intravitreal ranibizumab injections in routine clinical practice: baseline data from the German OCEAN study. Health Qual Life Outcomes. 2016;14(1):132.
3. Campochiaro PA, Aiello LP, Rosenfeld PJ. Anti-vascular endothelial growth factor agents in the treatment of retinal disease: from bench to bedside. Ophthalmology. 2016;123(10S):S78-88.
4. Casselholmde Salles M, Kvanta A, Amrén U, et al. Optical coherence tomography angiography in central retinal vein occlusion: correlation between the foveal avascular zone and visual acuity. Invest Ophthalmol Vis Sci. 2016;57(9):242-6.
5. Chhablani J, Stewart M, Paulose R, et al. Clinical characteristics and treatment outcomes of recurrent central retinal vein occlusions. Semin Ophthalmol. 2016:1-7.
6. Coscas F, Glacet-Bernard A, Miere A, et al. Optical coherence tomography angiography in retinal vein occlusion: evaluation of superficial and deep capillary plexa. Am J Ophthalmol. 2016;161:160-71.e1-2.
7. Fujihara-Mino A, Mitamura Y, Inomoto N, et al. Optical coherence tomography parameters predictive of visual outcome after anti-VEGF therapy for retinal vein occlusion. Clin Ophthalmol. 2016;10:1305-13.
8. Ghasemi Falavarjani K, Iafe NA, Hubschman JP, et al. Optical coherence tomography angiography analysis of the foveal avascular zone and macular vessel density after anti-VEGF therapy in eyes with diabetic macular edema and retinal vein occlusion. Invest Ophthalmol Vis Sci. 2017;58(1):30-4.
9. Kartasasmita AS, Takarai S, Switania A, et al. Efficacy of single bevacizumab injection as adjuvant therapy to laser photocoagulation in macular edema secondary to branch retinal vein occlusion. Clin Ophthalmol. 2016;10:2135-40.
10. Lam FC, Chia SN, Lee RM. Macular grid laser photocoagulation for branch retinal vein occlusion. Cochrane Database Syst Rev. 2015;(5):CD008732.
11. Nagasato D, Mitamura Y, Semba K, et al. Correlation between optic nerve head circulation and visual function before and after anti-VEGF therapy for central retinal vein occlusion: prospective, interventional case series. BMC Ophthalmol. 2016;16:36.
12. Panakanti TK, Chhablani J. Clinical trials in branch retinal vein occlusion. Middle East Afr J Ophthalmol. 2016; 23(1):38-43.
13. Patel A, Nguyen C, Lu S. Central retinal vein occlusion: a review of current evidence-based treatment options. Middle East Afr J Ophthalmol. 2016;23(1):44-8.
14. Sawada O, Ohji M. Retinal vein occlusion. Dev Ophthalmol. 2016;55:147-53.
15. Setta M, Ozaki S, Tabuchi A. Long-term outcomes in eyes receiving of bevacizumab early in the course of branch retinal vein occlusion. Nippon Ganka Gakkai Zasshi. 2016; 120(5):396-402.
16. Singer MA, Jansen ME, Tyler L, et al. Long-term results of combination therapy using anti-VEGF agents and dexamethasone intravitreal implant for retinal vein occlusion: an investigational case series. Clin Ophthalmol. 2016;11: 31-8.
17. Sun Y, Liang Y, Zhou P, et al. Anti-VEGF treatment is the key strategy for neovascular glaucoma management in the short term. BMC Ophthalmol. 2016;16(1):150.
18. Suzuki N, Hirano Y, Tomiyasu T, et al. Retinal hemodynamics seen on optical coherence tomography angiography before and after treatment of retinal vein occlusion. Invest Ophthalmol Vis Sci. 2016;57(13):5681-7.
19. Wylęgała A, Teper S, Dobrowolski D, et al. Optical coherence angiography: A review. Medicine (Baltimore). 2016; 95(41):e4907.
20. Yang CS, Liu JH, Chung YC, et al. Combination therapy with intravitreal bevacizumab and macular grid and scatter laser photocoagulation in patients with macular edema secondary to branch retinal vein occlusion. J Ocul Pharmacol Ther. 2015;31(3):179-85.

CHAPTER 11

Synchysis Scintillans (Cholesterolosis)

INTRODUCTION

Synchysis scintillans is a degenerative condition of the eye, characterized by the appearance of yellow-whitish glowing crystals in vitreous, which are composed of cholesterol. They float in the anterior chamber of the eye and in the liquefied vitreous.

EPIDEMIOLOGY AND ETIOLOGY

The condition appears quite rarely. Mostly, it occurs secondarily in eyes with previous episodes of inflammation, chronic, or repetitive vitreous hemorrhage and in posttraumatic ocular conditions. It can also appear in patients who had repeated surgical interventions of the posterior ocular segment. Cholesterol crystals originate due to the disintegration of erythrocytes or plasma cells. These characteristic deposits usually appear after the recovery of vitreous hemorrhage. This condition occurs rarely than the asteroid hyalosis (AH).

SYMPTOMS AND SIGNS

Patients complain of motley floaters in their visual field, while the ophthalmologist notes them in the anterior and posterior segment of the eye. The condition is usually bilateral. The key thing which differentiates cholesterolosis from AH is that the deposits are present both in anterior and posterior, vitreal eye segment in this condition. These deposits freely float and move slowly, and are not connected to other structures of the eye. AH refers to a condition where deposits are always fixated and their movements may always be foreseen. An anamnesis of prior surgical intervention in the affected eye always helps in diagnosis. It is important to differentiate other similar entities, such as bubbles or droplets of the silicon oil, which are often shown in the superior portion of anterior chamber. Perfluorocarbon droplets are transparent, larger, and located inferiorly in the anterior chamber.

DIFFERENTIAL DIAGNOSIS

- Asteroid hyalosis
- Emulsification of silicone oil
- Stagnation of perfluorocarbon.

DIAGNOSTICS

Diagnosis is proved by the slit-lamp examination and ocular ultrasound. Fluorescein angiography (FAG) is not recommended and cannot assist in a diagnosis. Optical coherence tomography (OCT) B-scans can visualize hyperreflective dots in the vitreous (Figs. 11.1 to 11.3).

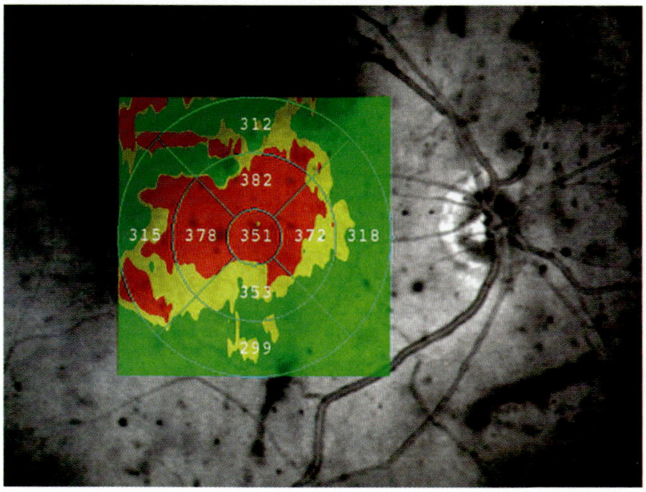

Fig. 11.1: Fundus photography. Numerous dark dots, which are different in size, can be seen all over the image. In some places they consolidate and cover underlying structures. Centrally is a superposed map of the macular, with thickening in its central portion.

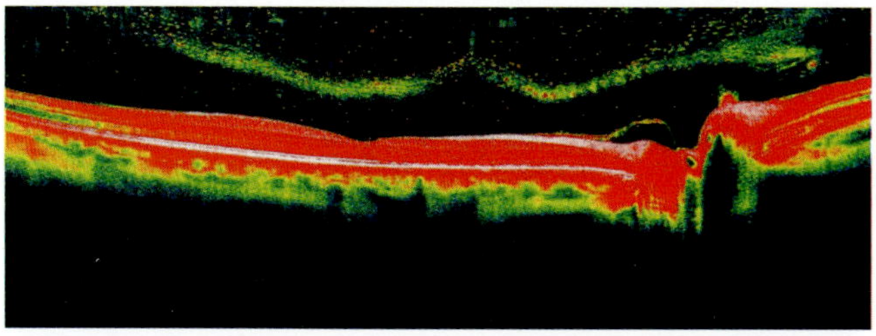

Fig. 11.3: An optical coherence tomography (OCT) B-scan of the macula and optic nerve in a 45-year-old male patient. In the vitreous, numerous small, dotted deposits are evident. Posterior hyaloid membrane, which raises from the edge of papilla and extends toward the macula, can be seen.

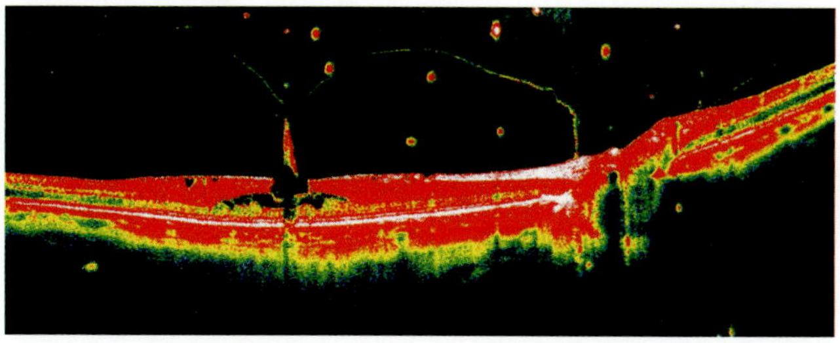

Fig. 11.2: An optical coherence tomography (OCT) B-scan of macular area and optic nerve in the same eye as in the first Figure 11.1. Sagittal cross-section shows significant changes in central macula. Vitreomacular traction, epiretinal membrane, and detached operculum with posterior hyaloid membrane can be seen. The retinal tissue is edematous and schisis can be seen, which was formed due to the force of dragging. In the vitreous, many hyperreflective dots, which are different in size, are visible. They represent cholesterol deposits.

TREATMENT

Treatment is advised only if the density of cholesterol deposits causes a significant decrease in visual acuity or if the pain and headache is present. Surgical treatment implies pars plana vitrectomy.

BIBLIOGRAPHY

1. Banc A, Stan C. Anterior Chamber Synchysis Scintillans: A Case Report. Rom J Ophthalmol. 2015;59(3):164-6.
2. Brodsky MC. Synchysis Scintillans in a Child. JAMA Ophthalmol. 2015;133(7):e150793.
3. Grigorian AP, Grigorian F. Observational study about biometry in patients with cataract and synchisis scintillans. Oftalmologia. 2005;49(1):46-9.
4. Kumar V, Goel N, Piplani B, et al. Spontaneous posterior dislocation of nucleus with synchysis scintillans. Cont Lens Anterior Eye. 2011;34(3):144-6.

CHAPTER 12

Posterior Vitreous Detachment

INTRODUCTION

A posterior vitreous detachment (PVD) is defined as a separation of posterior vitreous cortex from the inner retinal membrane.

EPIDEMIOLOGY AND ETIOLOGY

Posterior vitreous detachment presents the physiological condition in elderly. However, it can appear in patients with high myopia, due to increased axial length of the eye, as well as postoperatively or after traumatic injuries and inflammations of eyes. PVD occurs due to the aging, liquefaction, and syneresis of the vitreous, which results with pathological changes in area of vitreoretinal junction. In the late phase of PVD development, separation progresses to the optic disk and causes the formation of a Weiss ring and accompanying symptoms. Vitreous separation, in some cases, occurs suddenly (acute PVD) and can be pathophysiological, due to the fact that it can peel off areas of adhesion to the neurosensory retina. Vitreomacular tractions, macular holes, or peripheral retinal tear/detachment can occur.

SYMPTOMS AND SIGNS

Patients complain on appearance of floating objects in their vision field (floaters) and transitory flashes (photopsias), which are more noticeable in dimly lit environments. They can also be described as flies, or a cobweb distracting their central or peripheral vision.

According to the PVD range, it can be a "complete" PVD, in cases where entire posterior vitreous is separated from the retina, or "partial", when the vitreous gel is still attached at the macula or optic nerve head.

According to the time of appearance, it can be acute (it develops suddenly and often turns into the complete PVD shortly after the appearance) or chronic (it develops slowly and becomes complete after several weeks or months).

In young patients and those without vitreoretinal separation, vitreous is tightly connected to the optic nerve and macula. As PVD develops, it firstly separates in the macular area, while remains still attached to the optic nerve. In later stages, detachment becomes complete and the vitreous separates from the optic nerve as well. This becomes visible as a Weiss ring on examination. The ring presents pathognomonic clinical sign for the acute PVD. Usually, the ophthalmologist can see many vitreous opacities instead of typical Weiss ring.

DIFFERENTIAL DIAGNOSIS

- Retinal detachment
- Retinal holes
- Ocular migraine
- Intraocular inflammations (uveitis).

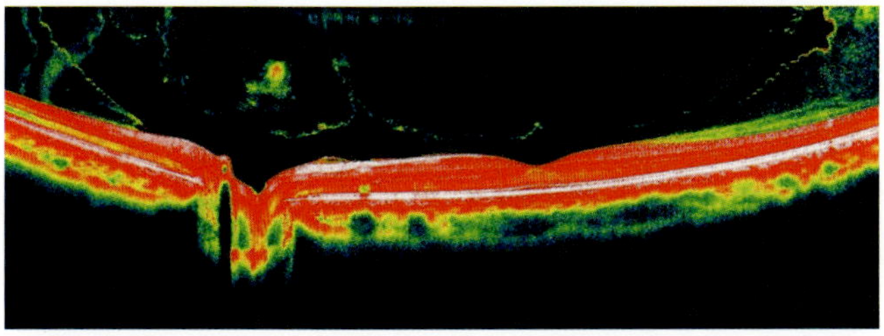

Fig. 12.1: An optical coherence tomography (OCT) B-scan shows a partial detachment of posterior hyaloid membrane, with many hyperreflective dots and opacities in the vitreous. Posterior hyaloid membrane is still attached to the macula and optic nerve.

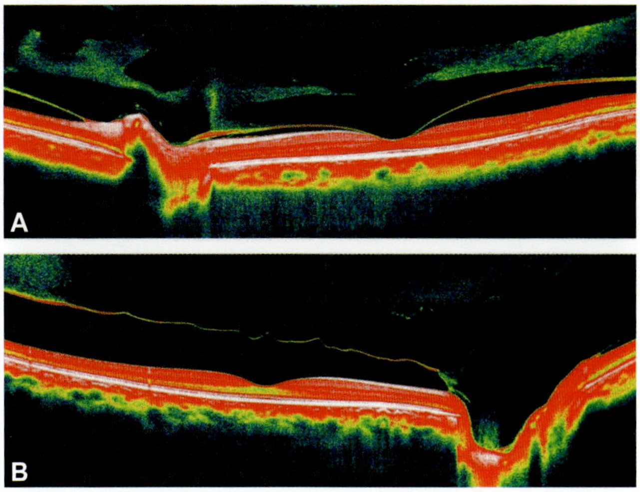

Figs. 12.2A and B: (A) An OCT B-scan shows a partial detachment of posterior hyaloid membrane, which can be clearly seen separating itself from the retinal surface. It is still attached at the macular area and optic nerve. Parts of the vitreous start to condense, creating opacities; and (B) OCT of the retina in a patient who had complete separation of the vitreous from the fovea center. Posterior hyaloid membrane is seen as a wavy hyperreflective line above the retina. However, the vitreous is still attached at the optic nerve, indicating only a partial PVD has occurred. (OCT: optical coherence tomography; PVD: posterior vitreous detachment)

DIAGNOSTICS

Along with the clinical examination, ocular ultrasound and optical coherence tomography (OCT) are used for diagnosing the condition. Fluorescein angiography (FAG) cannot be used for diagnosing posterior vitreous detachment, but it can be used to detect its complications (cystoid macular edema). OCT can clearly present the separation of posterior hyaloid membrane as a hyperreflective wavy membrane above the retina. OCT can also be useful in detection and presentation of retinal pathological complications, such are epiretinal membrane, macular microruptures, vitreofoveal tractions, etc. (Figs. 12.1 and 12.2).

TREATMENT

If PVD without complications occurs, treatment is not advised. Regular ophthalmology control examinations are enough. There is no recommended therapy for PVD. In many cases most of symptoms withdraw spontaneously by the time. The crucial thing is a detailed examination, with the aim to detect possible retinal detachments and/or other complications. Patients should be educated by the ophthalmologist to detect changes in their vision, and which symptoms they should pay attention to.

BIBLIOGRAPHY

1. Carrero JL. Incomplete posterior vitreous detachment: Prevalence and clinical relevance. Am J Ophthalmol. 2012;153(3):497-503.
2. Gella L, Raman R, Kulothungan V, et al. Prevalence of posterior vitreous detachment in the population with type II diabetes mellitus and its effect on diabetic retinopathy: Sankaranethralaya diabetic retinopathy epidemiology and molecular genetic study SN-DREAMS report no. 23. Jpn J Ophthalmol. 2012;56(3):262-7.
3. Hikichi T, Hirokawa H, Kado M, et al. Comparison of the prevalence of posterior vitreous detachment in whites and Japanese. Ophthalmic Surg. 1995;26(1):39-43.
4. Johnson MW. Posterior vitreous detachment: Evolution and complications of its early stages. Am J Ophthalmol. 2010;149(1):371-82.
5. Kim YC, Harasawa M, Siringo FS, et al. Assessment of posterior vitreous detachment on enhanced high density line optical coherence tomography. Int J Ophthalmol. 2017;10(1):165-7.
6. Shen B, MacIntosh PW. Posterior vitreous detachment associated with non-arteritic ischaemic optic neuropathy. Neuroophthalmology. 2016;40(5):234-23.
7. Shen Z, Duan X, Wang F, et al. Prevalence and risk factors of posterior vitreous detachment in a Chinese adult population: the Handan eye study. BMC Ophthalmol. 2013;13(1):33.
8. Ştefănescu-Dima AŞ, Corîci CA, Mănescu MR, et al. Posterior vitreous detachment and macular anatomical changes: A tomographic-electroretinographic study. Rom J Morphol Embryol. 2016;57(2):751-8.

CHAPTER 13

Epiretinal Membrane, Cellophane Maculopathy, and Macular Pucker

INTRODUCTION

Epiretinal membrane (ERM) in the macula (epiretinal gliosis, epimacular membrane) is an avascular fibrocellular structure made from glial cells that, like a delicate film, proliferates above or on the surface of the retina in the macular area, and due to its contractile properties may cause changes in the structure of the retina on which it formed. Depending on the clinical presentation, it can have various names: preretinal macular gliosis/fibrosis, ERM in the macula, cellophane maculopathy, and macular pucker (macular wrinkling).

EPIDEMIOLOGY AND ETIOLOGY

Most frequently, ERM is idiopathic with a 7% incidence in the general population, and in about 10% of cases it is bilateral. It occurs around the age of 65 years and prevalence increases with the patient's age. Following a surgery of the primary retinal detachment, clinically significant ERM occurs in 3–8.5% of patients. There are many causes of ERM, the most common being eye inflammations, infections, previous retinal vein occlusions, and trauma. ERM is most commonly related to changes in the posterior vitreous splitting (*vitreoschisis*). This residual vitreous is the foundation and the trigger for proliferation of inflammatory cellular elements [stemming from retina and retinal pigment epithelium (RPE)] forming the ERM. Therefore, ERM is a fibrous tissue growing and proliferating into the macula or over it, between the posterior hyaloid membrane and inner limiting membrane. Fibrous tissue contractions lead to macular distortion with symptoms typical of macular pulling.

SYMPTOMS AND SIGNS

The condition is asymptomatic in the early stage, but metamorphopsia and distortion occur in later stages as the primary symptoms that could be linked to ERM. It is important to note that the symptoms are always present even when there is no damage to visual acuity. Patients cite micropsia or monocular diplopia less frequently. Visual acuity can be between 20/20 and 20/400.

Epiretinal membrane is attached to the macula and is described as a delicate and transparent cellophane-like membrane. Due to traction and pulling of the retinal tissue, secondary changes to the fundus such as macular pseudohole, intraretinal bleeding, vascular network disorder, and less frequently, cystoid macular edema may occur.

DIFFERENTIAL DIAGNOSIS

- Vitreomacular traction
- Lamellar macular hole
- Full thickness macular hole

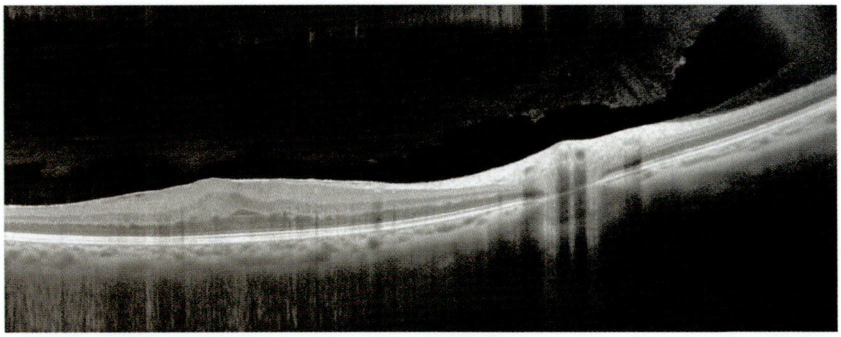

Fig. 13.1: An OCT B-scan of the macular area and optic nerve in a 45-year-old female patient. Preoperative ERM image. Clearly visible thickening of the macular area and loss of normal foveolar depression can be seen. There is an impression that the macula has a serrated shape as seen in the sagittal cross section. A thin hyperreflective ERM is visible across the macular area pulling the retinal tissue toward itself. (ERM: epiretinal membrane; OCT: optical coherence tomography)

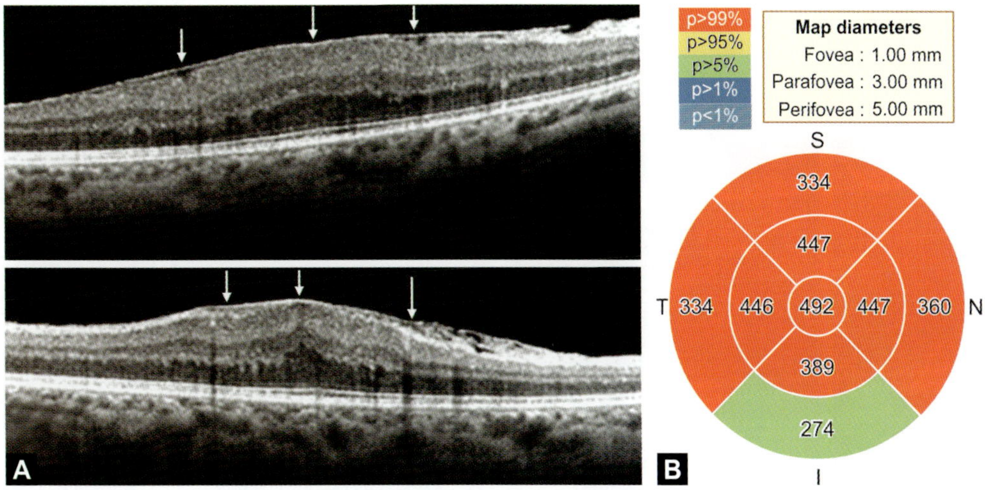

Figs. 13.2A and B: (A) An OCT B-scan of the macular area. Arrows mark the hyperreflective ERM causing thickening of the macula; and (B) The image shows the retinal thickness map with values significantly above reference values. Thickening of the entire macular area is present. (ERM: epiretinal membrane; OCT: optical coherence tomography)

- Macular schisis
- Cystoid macular edema.

DIAGNOSTICS

In addition to a clinical examination, optical coherence tomography (OCT) is an irreplaceable method for diagnosing ERM. OCT helps with the differentiation of this entity and similar conditions. Fluorescein angiography (FA) is not of great help in diagnosing ERM. An OCT image will show a hyperreflective preretinal membrane adhering across the surface of the macula. The macula will show different degrees of disorder in foveal shape and structure. The macula can sometimes appear normal but also completely changed, depending on the stage of the disease. Macular thickening is present, which is best represented by the retinal thickness map. Intraretinal cysts can sometimes be seen, as well as subretinal fluid (Figs. 13.1 to 13.4).

THERAPY

In the initial, nonprogressive stages, monitoring of the condition is recommended as well as self-monitoring using the Amsler grid test. Without the surgical procedure the condition will gradually worsen and symptoms intensify to the point when the visual acuity will change and decline. Most patients with ERM do not experience symptoms or experience only negligible symptoms. Surgical treatment is advised if the visual acuity is in decline. Following surgery, visual acuity in most patients (75%) improves by at least two lines on the Snellen chart. Recovery is slow and takes months, sometimes even a year following the surgical intervention.

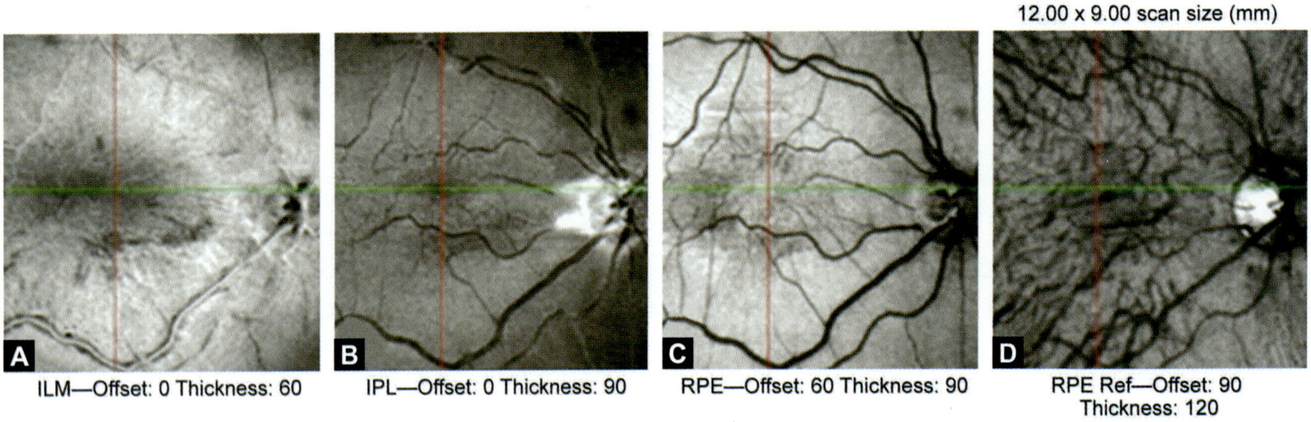

Figs. 13.3A to D: An OCT en face view from the inner to the choroidal retinal layer of the same eye (12 × 9 mm). The scan shows the macular area and regular optical nerve papilla with large blood vessels. The macula is not clearly visible and the entire area is hyporeflective with wrinkles extending in circles from the periphery toward the foveolar area. The wrinkles are consistent with the ERM fibrous tissue pulling the retinal tissue. (ERM: epiretinal membrane; OCT: optical coherence tomography)

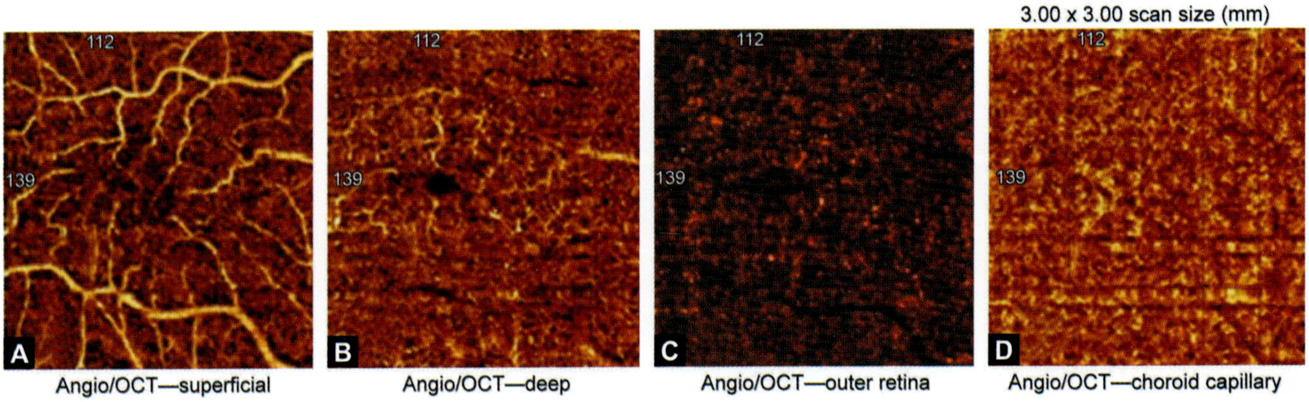

Figs. 13.4A to D: An OCTA of the macular area, showing a superficial, deep, outer, and choriocapillary layer (3 × 3 mm). The FAZ shape and configuration are completely lost in the superficial vascular plexus, while a significantly diminished FAZ is visualized in the deep plexus. There is an impression that blood vessels in both vascular plexuses are spanning across the FAZ, filling it. The avascular outer retinal layer and choriocapillary layer are without significant changes. (FAZ: foveal avascular zone; OCTA: optical coherence tomography angiography)

BIBLIOGRAPHY

1. Aydın R, Karahan E, Kaya M, et al. Evaluation of inner segment/outer segment junctions in different types of epiretinal membranes. Arq Bras Oftalmol. 2016;79(5):319-22.
2. Dell'omo R, Cifariello F, Dell'omo E, et al. Influence of retinal vessel printings on metamorphopsia and retinal architectural abnormalities in eyes with idiopathic macular epiretinal membrane. Invest Ophthalmol Vis Sci. 2013;54(12):7803-11.
3. Jeon S, Baek J, Lee WK. Gli1 Expression in Human Epiretinal Membranes. Invest Ophthalmol Vis Sci. 2017;58(1):651-9.
4. Lavinsky F, Lavinsky D. Novel perspectives on swept-source optical coherence tomography. Int J Retina Vitreous. 2016; 2:25.
5. Miguel AI, Legris A. Prognostic factors of epiretinal membranes: A systematic review. J Fr Ophthalmol. 2017;40(1): 61-79.
6. Romano MR, Cennamo G, Cesarano I, et al. Changes of tangential traction after macular peeling: Correlation between en-face analysis and macular sensitivity. Curr Eye Res. 2017;42(5):780-8.
7. Romano MR, Cennamo G, Schiemer S, et al. Deep and superficial OCT angiography changes after macular peeling: Idiopathic vs diabetic epiretinal membranes. Graefes Arch Clin Exp Ophthalmol. 2017;255(4):681-9.
8. Shahzadi B, Rizvi SF, Latif K, et al. Visual and anatomical outcomes following idiopathic macular epiretinal membrane surgery. J Coll Physicians Surg Pak. 2016;26(12): 971-4.

CHAPTER 14

Vitreomacular Traction Syndrome

INTRODUCTION

Vitreomacular traction (VMT) syndrome, or just a vitreomacular traction is a disorder of vitreoretinal connection, which is characterized by the partial posterior vitreous detachment and its strong adhesion with macula.

EPIDEMIOLOGY AND ETIOLOGY

Vitreomacular traction occurs among the elderly population. About 1.5% of general population is considered to suffer of visual impairment which is caused by VMT. The incidence is higher in patients who suffer from diabetic retinopathy and other macular diseases. Posterior vitreous detachment can lead to the incomplete separation of the posterior hyaloid membrane from the retina, and cause traction of superficial retinal layers, mainly in macula. According to the international VMT classification study (*International Vitreomacular Traction Study Classification System, Duker et al.*), in order to define a condition as VMT, posterior vitreous detachment along with anatomic and structural macular distortion is visible in optical coherence tomography (OCT). No signs of full thickness macular hole can be presented. Before the OCT, diagnosis was hard to establish. Latest nomenclature includes different VMT stages, beginning with stage 1 and ending with the impending macular hole stage.

SYMPTOMS AND SIGNS

Vitreomacular traction is frequently completely asymptomatic and the OCT finding usually does not correspond to the symptomatology. If symptoms exist, they usually include decreased visual acuity, blurry vision, photopsia, micropsia, and metamorphopsia. VMT is classified as focal, if it is smaller than 1500 µm, or broad, if it is larger than 1500 µm. Assessment is based on the OCT finding. Secondary changes occur as the result of traction and pulling by membranes, and include a schisis of inner retinal layers, macular edema, and thickening.

DIFFERENTIAL DIAGNOSIS

- Macular dystrophy
- Macular degeneration
- Full thickness macular hole
- Cystoid macular edema
- Epiretinal membrane.

DIAGNOSTICS

After a clinical examination, the OCT is usually performed. OCT B-scans can clearly show the presence of VMT, foveal distortion and posterior vitreous detachment. It reveals the absence of other macular diseases that may potentially be considered in differential diagnosis (Figs. 14.1 to 14.9).

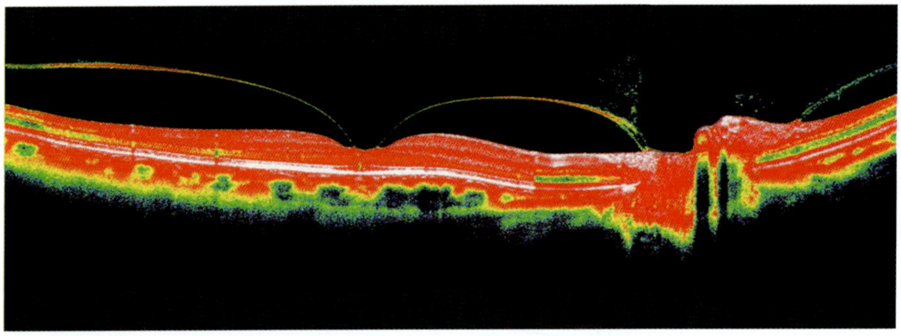

Fig. 14.1: An optical coherence tomography (OCT) B-scan of the macular area and optic nerve in 49-year old female patient. Posterior hyaloid membrane is hyperreflective and forms the "V" shape. It is still attached to the macula and edges of papilla, and it corresponds to the finding of partial posterior vitreous detachment (PVD). In the macular area, membrane slightly lifts the macular tissue and changes the appearance of standard foveal depression. Photoreceptors are interrupted in the very center.

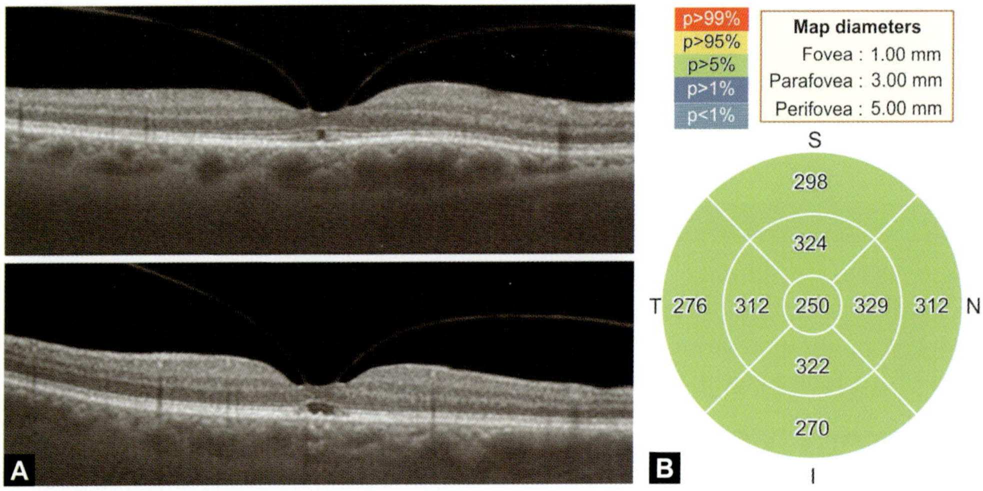

Figs. 14.2A and B: (A) The optical coherence tomography (OCT) B-scan of macular area; the same eye as in Figure 14.1. The structure of fovea can be better seen in larger magnification. The fibrous membrane, which is still attached to the macular surface, pulls out the underlying tissue and causes detachment of retina. Also, irregular wavy retinal pigment epithelium (RPE) and interruption of photoreceptors can be seen; and (B) Retinal thickness map shows regular values of macular thickness.

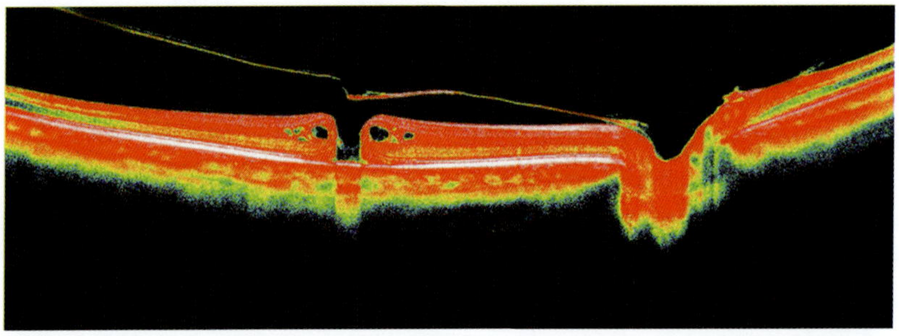

Fig. 14.3: An optical coherence tomography (OCT) B-scan of the macular area and optic nerve in 57-year-old male patient. A fully formed traction membrane is shown, along with the detachment of posterior vitreous. In the center, full thickness macular hole is visualized, which occurred due to the membrane traction. Around the central defect, retinal tissue is edematous and filled with cysts. Retinal pigment epithelium (RPE) is wavy and irregular in center.

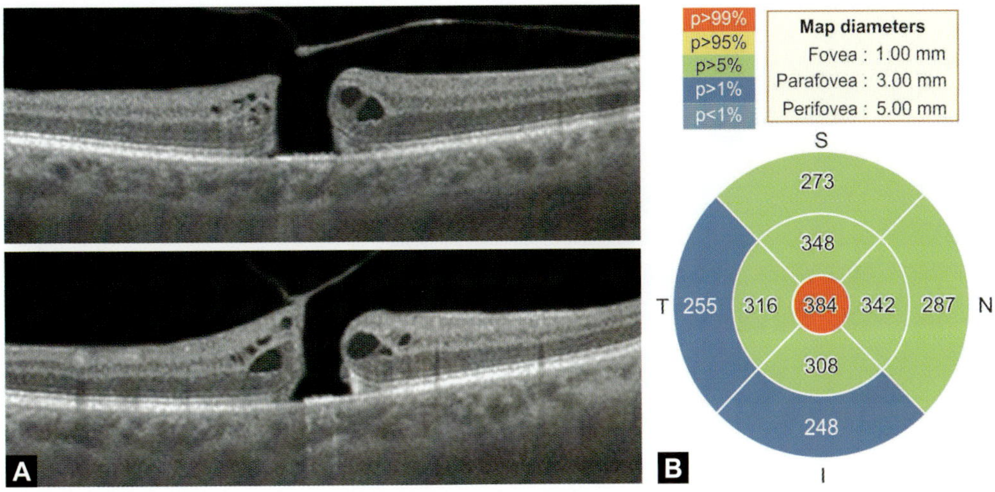

Figs. 14.4A and B: (A) An optical coherence tomography (OCT) B-scan of the macular area in the same eye as in Figure 14.3. The lower cross-section scan highlights the traction membrane, which pulls the macula and separates it from RPE. RPE appears irregular and wavy. Both cross-sections show a full-thickness macular hole reaching to the retinal pigment epithelium (RPE). On edges of the defect, retinal tissue shows visible cystoid changes and schisis of inner retinal layers; (B) Retinal thickness map shows increased central thickness (384 microns), which is caused by the elevation of macular hole edges.

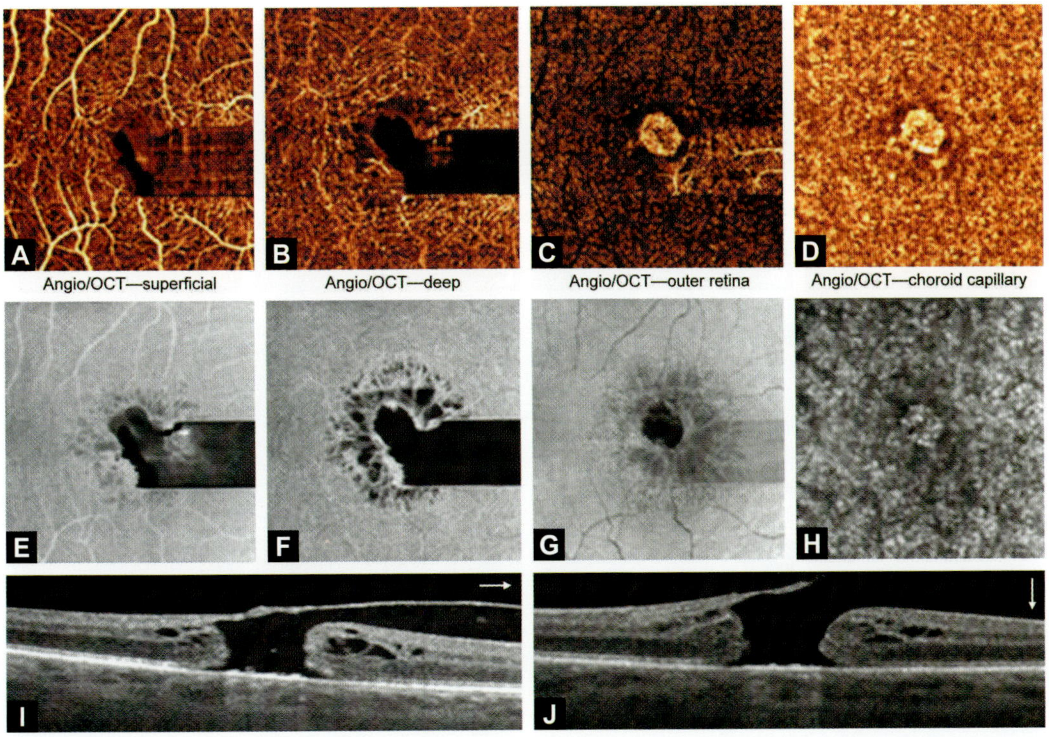

Figs. 14.5A to J: Comparative images of an optical coherence tomography angiography (OCTA) and en face optical coherence tomography (OCT) of superficial and deep vascular plexus, outer retina and choroid, the same eye as in Figure 14.4 (3 × 3 mm). Horizontal black stripes, seen in superficial and deep plexus, are artifacts that do not diminish the value of the image made through the above mentioned protocols. (A to D) Angiograms show the central defect in all retinal layers, which is consistent with the regular appearance of foveal avascular zone (FAZ) in superficial and deep vascular plexus, while in outer and choroidal layer is hyperreflective and atypical. Angiography does not show specific changes and is not aiding much in the diagnostics; (E to H) En face OCT of superficial and deep layer of inner retina shows typical honeycomb-like hyporeflective and sharply circumscribed areas around the central defect, which are consistent with the schisis of inner retinal layers. Central, dark and sharply circumscribed region matches the full thickness macular hole; and (I and J) It is clear that OCT B-scan is crucial and irreplaceable in the diagnostics of vitreomacular traction (VMT) and macular hole.

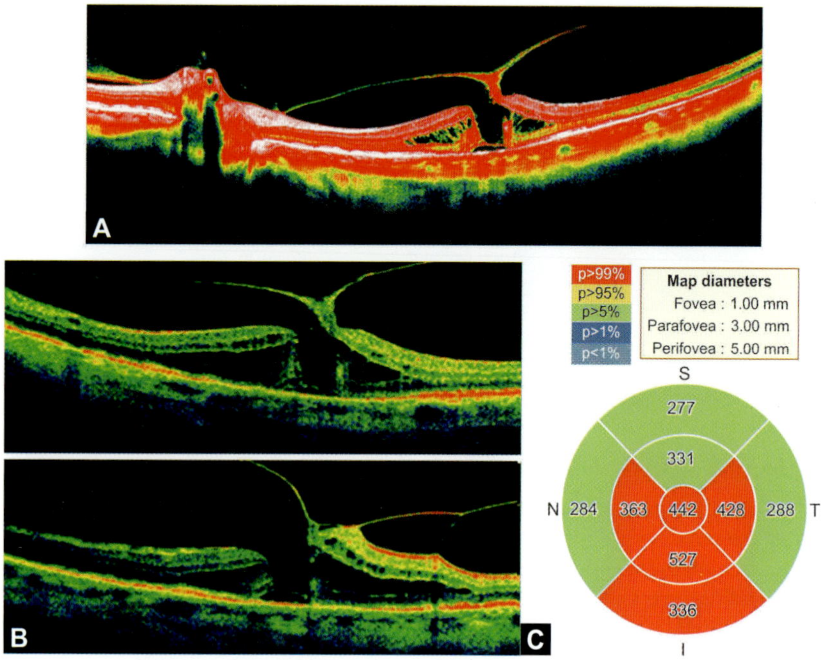

Figs. 14.6A to C: (A and B) Optical coherence tomography (OCT) B-scans of macula and optic nerve in 72-year-old female patient. "Y-shaped" fibrous membrane is shown, which lifts the entire macular region and pulls out the macula. Schisis of inner retinal layers, intraretinal edema and sensory retinal detachment can be seen; and (C) Retinal thickness map shows the increased numeric values in macular area centrally and inferiorly.

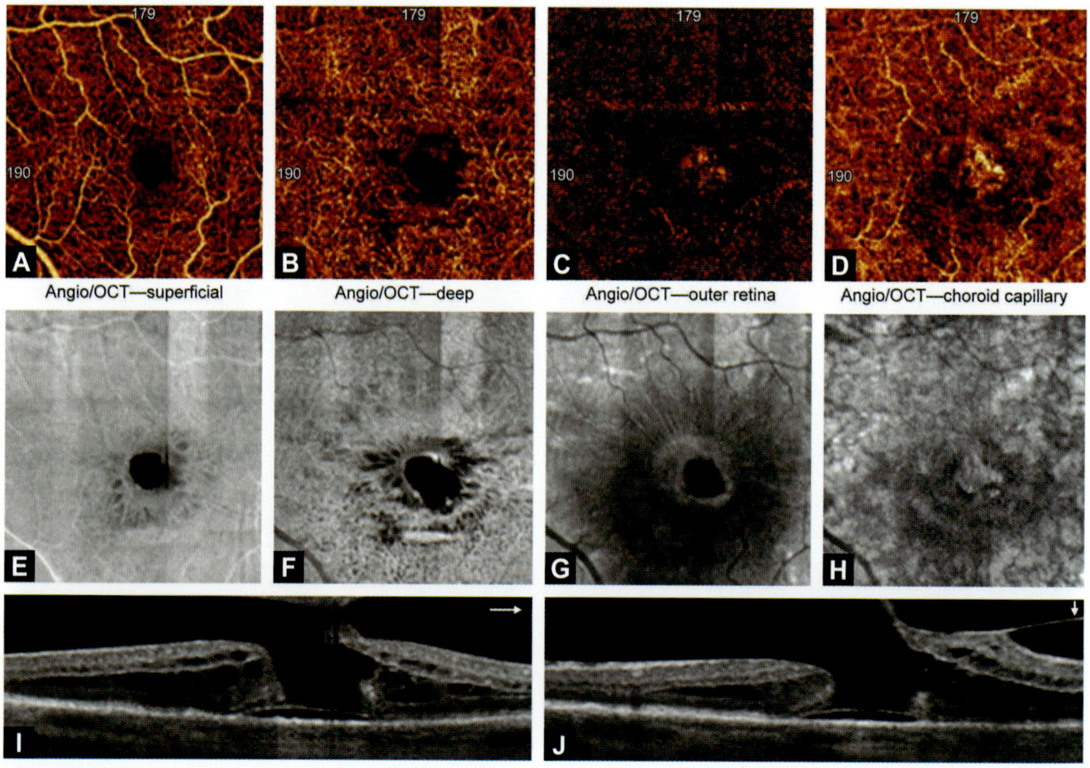

Figs. 14.7A to J: Comparative images of an optical coherence tomography angiography (OCTA) and en face optical coherence tomography (OCT) of superficial and deep vascular plexus, outer retina and choroid, the same eye as in Figure 14.6 (3 × 3 mm). (A to D) Angiograms do not provide significant information related to the diagnosis. Mild sclerotical changes in the superficial and deep vascular plexus can be noticed, while outer retina and choriocapillaris show a central, intensely colored, lumpy formation resembling of neovascularization; however this is a reflection of flow in surrounding retinal layers; (E to H) En face OCT shows a central hyporeflective, sharply limited defect in superficial and deep layer of inner retina, as well as in outer retina, which is consistent with a macular hole. Around the central defect, dark, honeycomb-like roundish cystoid spaces, which are consistent with a schisis of inner retinal layers, can be seen; and (I and J) OCT B-scan can very accurately confirm the diagnosis of vitreomacular traction (VMT), which caused the macular hole.

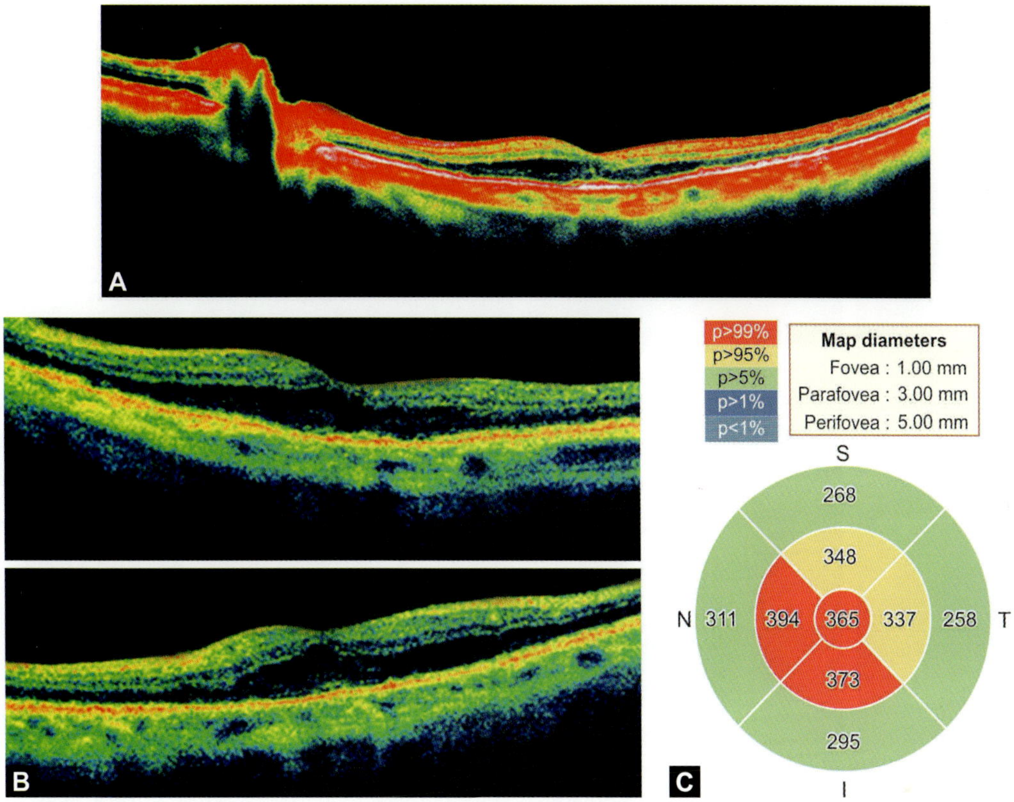

Figs. 14.8A to C: (A and B) Optical coherence tomography (OCT) B-scans of the same eye as in Figures 14.6 and 14.7, seven days after pars plana vitrectomy (PPV). Traction membranes cannot be visible on these scans. Also, schisis of inner retinal layers, as well as macular hole, are not present. Macula is regular in continuity and no more tractions and pulling can be seen. However, a diffuse macular edema and intact retinal pigment epithelium (RPE), which is wavy and grouped in places, can be seen; and (C) Retinal thickness map shows a thickening of the central zone of macular area, due to the diffuse macular edema.

TREATMENT

Treatment for VMT depends on the severity of symptoms and OCT finding. In less severe, asymptomatic cases, patients are advised to do a regular checkups. Patients are also advised about self-monitoring by using the Amsler grid test. Occasionally, these conditions can recover spontaneously and not require more aggressive therapy. If the VMT does not spontaneously heal, the process can progress, causing more dramatic symptoms. In these cases, surgical approach is recommended. Pharmacologic vitreolysis with ocriplasmin can be an effective nonsurgical treatment option for focal VMT cases. Surgical approach implies vitrectomy, peeling and removal of membranes that cause the traction. In broad and more severe VMT cases, vitrectomy is the only advised option. The prognosis is generally good. However, it depends on the severity of each case, as well as on the appearance of possible complications and adequate timing of surgery.

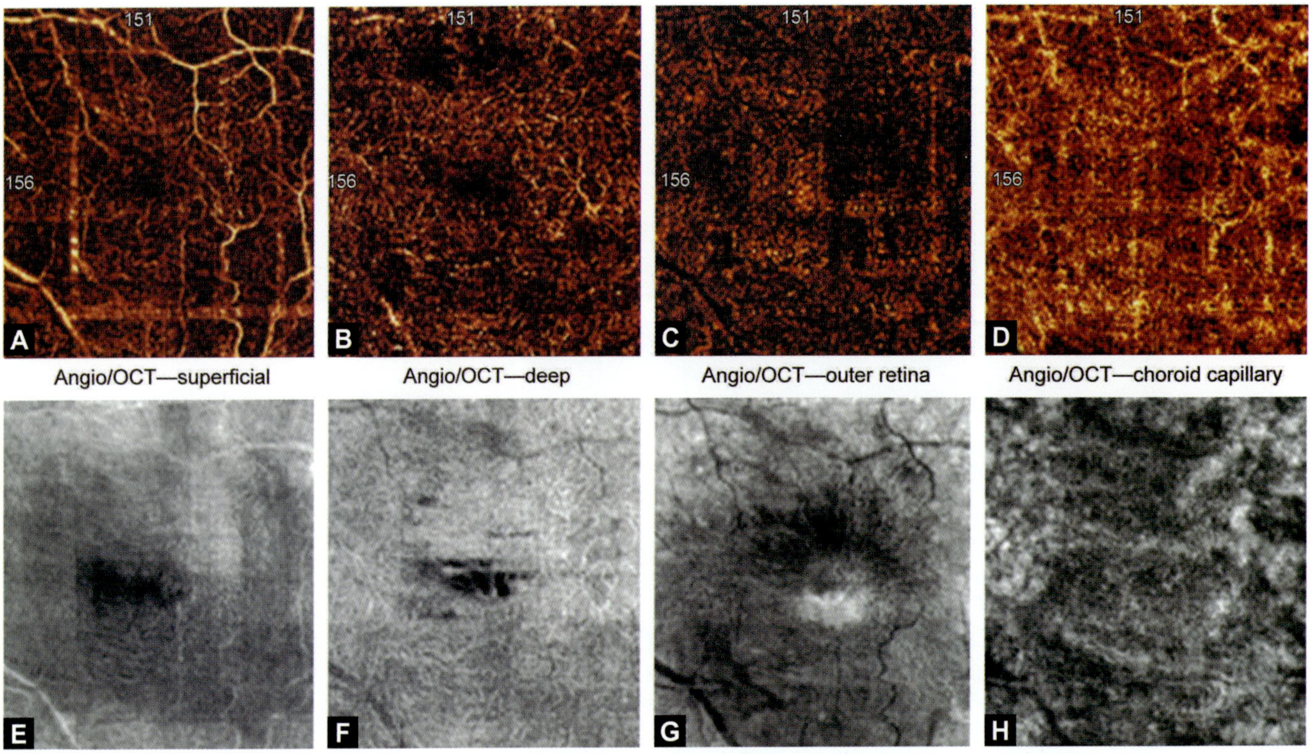

Figs. 14.9A to H: Optical coherence tomography angiography (OCTA) split-spectrum amplitude decorrelation angiography (SSADA) protocol and en face optical coherence tomography (OCT) images of corresponding retinal layers of the same eye as in Figure 14.8, seven days after pars plana vitrectomy (PPV) (3 × 3 mm). En face angiograms show no significant changes and regular appearance of all retinal layers. Symmetry of the capillary network is mildly disturbed, several prominent anastomoses and regions of decreased blood flow in the deep vascular plexus can be seen. En face OCT shows slightly irregular foveal avascular zone (FAZ). Central defect is not present and cannot be visualized after the PPV.

BIBLIOGRAPHY

1. Corvi F, Souied EH, Querques G. Resolution of vitreomacular traction and pigment epithelium detachment. Eur J Ophthalmol. 2015;26(4):0.
2. Duker JS, Kaiser PK, Binder S, et al. The International Vitreomacular Traction Study Group classification of vitreomacular adhesion, traction, and macular hole. Ophthalmology. 2013;120:2611-19.
3. Français-Maury C, Cornut PL, Mauget-Faÿsse M. Examination of vitreomacular traction syndrome. J Fr Ophtalmol. 2008;31:187-91.
4. Hale BP, Au AK, Falk NS, et al. Flat Electroretinography and Acute Visual Loss After Ocriplasmin Injection for Vitreomacular Adhesion Complicating Macular Schisis. Ophthalmic Surg Lasers Imaging Retina. 2015;46:888-92.
5. Jackson TL, Verstraeten T, Duchateau L, et al. Visual function response to ocriplasmin for the treatment of vitreomacular traction and macular hole. Acta Ophthalmol. 2017;95:e740-5.
6. Petrou P, Kontos A, Errera MH, et al. Pars Plana Vitrectomy for Vitreomacular Traction Syndrome: Analysing the Preoperative Prognostic Factors. Semin Ophthalmol. 2016;1-5.
7. Stopa M, Marciniak E, Rakowicz P, et al. Imaging and Measurement of the Preretinal Space in Vitreomacular Adhesion and Vitreomacular Traction by a New Spectral Domain Optical Coherence Tomography Analysis. Retina. 2017;37:1839-46.

CHAPTER 15

Macular Pseudohole

INTRODUCTION

Macular pseudohole (MPH) along with the epiretinal membrane represents a limited vitreomacular disorder which differs from the lamellar macular hole and full thickness macular hole. It occurs due to the centripetal contraction of the epiretinal membrane that lays right above macular tissue. Visual acuity is usually physiological, but sometimes metamorphopsia can occur.

SYMPTOMS AND SIGNS

Patients complain about blurred vision, distorted image, or even the appearance of a central scotoma on one eye. Patients do not see a break in the light beam during the biomicroscopic examination as cited in cases of full thickness macular holes (Watzke-Allen sign is negative).

DIFFERENTIAL DIAGNOSIS

- Lamellar macular hole
- Full thickness macular hole
- Vitreomacular traction syndrome
- Macular scars
- Cystoid macular edema.

DIAGNOSTICS

A macular pseudorupture is, with a clinical examination, manifested as an irregular, but clearly limited, reddish defect in the fovea. This defect is always related to the epiretinal membrane. The optical coherence tomography (OCT) confirms the diagnosis. The OCT B-scan can very nicely show the hyperreflectivity of an epiretinal membrane, as well as a clustered foveal tissue in the center. The key to understanding this condition is that there is no thinning in the center nor is there any loss in the macular tissue because of the MPH. OCT usually shows the macula with still preserved or slightly increased central thickness, but with abrupt, harsh and irregular foveal edges and a decreased diameter of the foveal area.

EXAMPLES OF EYES WITH THE MACULAR PSEUDOHOLE SHOWN BY OPTICAL COHERENCE TOMOGRAPHY ANGIOGRAPHY

In Figures 15.1 to 15.6 are demonstrated examples of eyes with macular pseudohole shown by optical coherence tomography angiography.

THERAPY

A regular ophthalmology checkup with continuous monitoring is recommended. The treatment depends on the severity of the symptoms and visual acuity. In the cases of progression or deterioration of the symptoms, and if the condition leads into the development of epiretinal

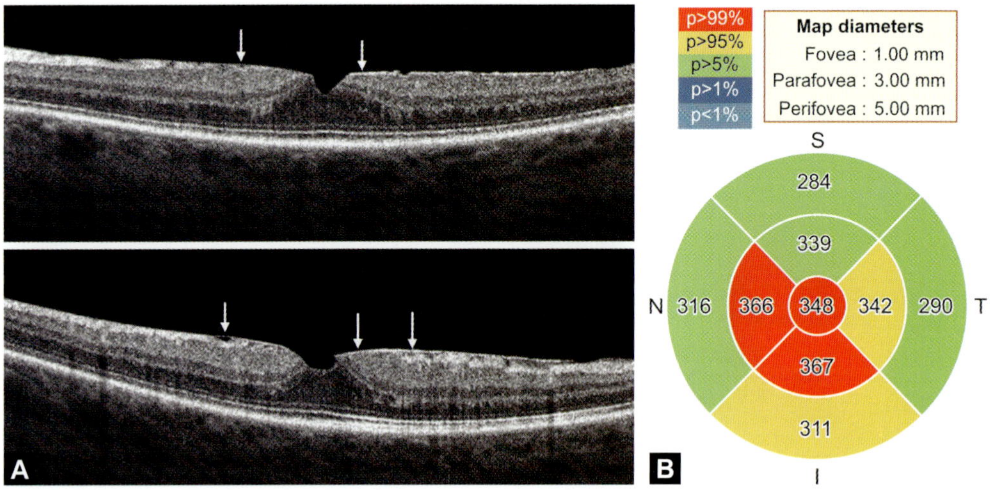

Figs. 15.1A and B: (A) An optical coherence tomography (OCT) B-scan of a macular and perimacular area of a 66-year-old female patient. Arrows exactly point out the hyperreflective epiretinal membrane which pulls out and clusters macular and foveal tissue. The macula seems like its edematous, but that is just pulled and stretched tissue due to the sclerotic fibrous epiretinal membrane (ERM). Edges of the foveolar depression are harsh and its diameter is decreased; and (B) The map of macular thickness shows increased values of central and inferior parts of the macula, with a central foveal thickness of 348 μ.

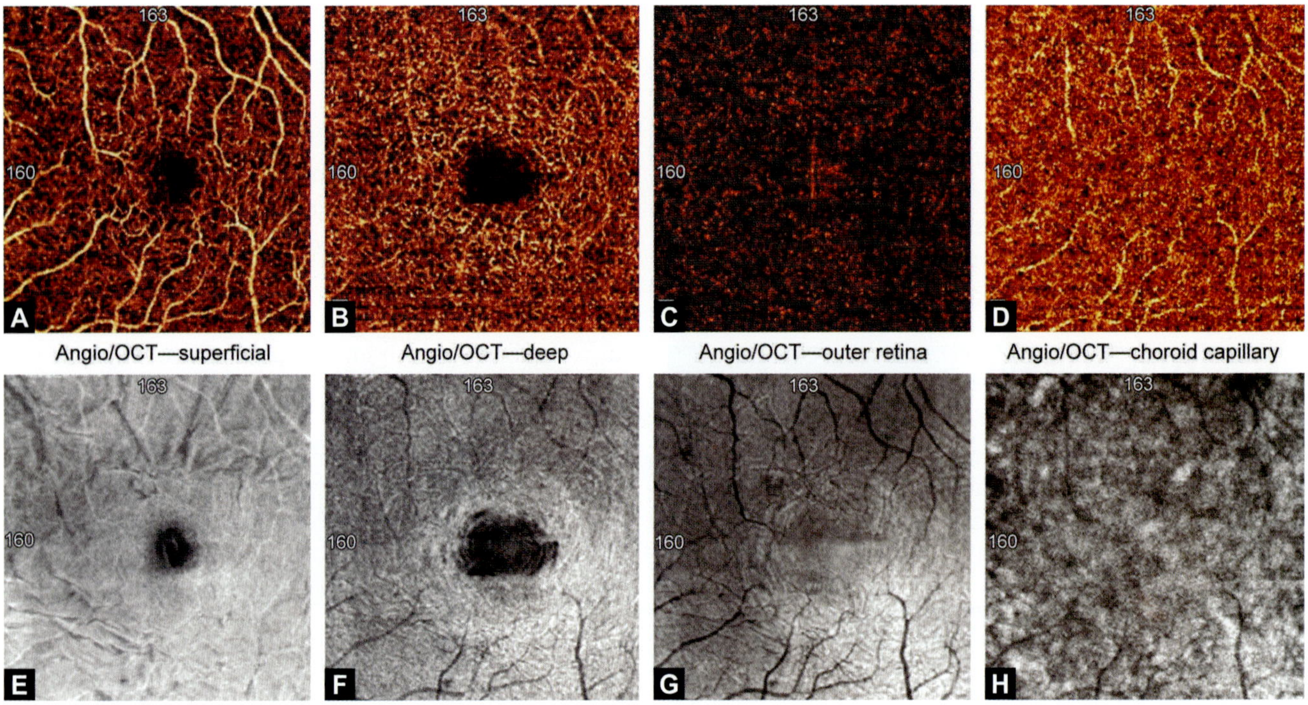

Figs. 15.2A to H: An optical coherence tomography angiography (OCTA) split-spectrum amplitude decorrelation angiography (SSADA) protocol 3 × 3 mm of superficial and deep vascular layer, outer retina and choroid, and corresponding images of enface OCT. The same eye as in Figure 15.1. (A to D) En face angiograms of the retinal layers. There are not any pathological signs nor any significant disruption in either vascular network (superficial and deep); the outer retina is regular and avascular and the choroid shows no changes. Angiography is usually not of much use in this condition and can help if there are some additional retinal diseases. (E) although shows epiretinal membrane (ERM) from the front, and in this image, irregular, harsh creases can be seen. Those creases represent a rough, sclerotic ERM which pulls the macula up. Foveal avascular zone (FAZ) seems to be slightly irregular in the deep layer of inner retina (F) while the other layers seem to be normal (G and H).

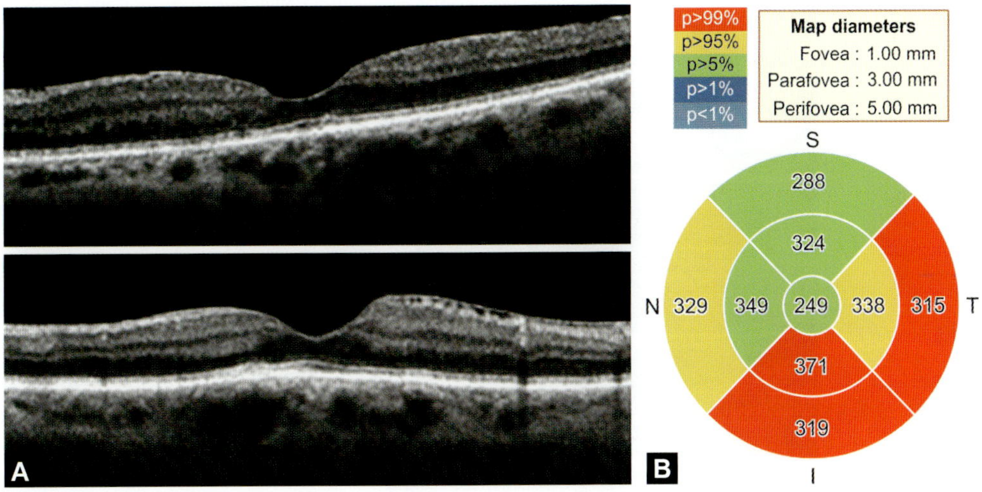

Figs. 15.3A and B: (A) An optical coherence tomography (OCT) B-scan of a macular and perimacular area of a 61-year-old female patient. On the retinal surface, a thickened, hyperreflective epiretinal membrane (ERM) is shown. Arrows exactly point out the places where it affects the macula and pulls it up. ERM causes the contracture and drawing of the macular tissue below. The macular thickness map on Figure (B) confirms the finding by showing the increased thickness values of the inferior, temporal and nasal parts of the macula. However, the central macular thickness seems to be regular.

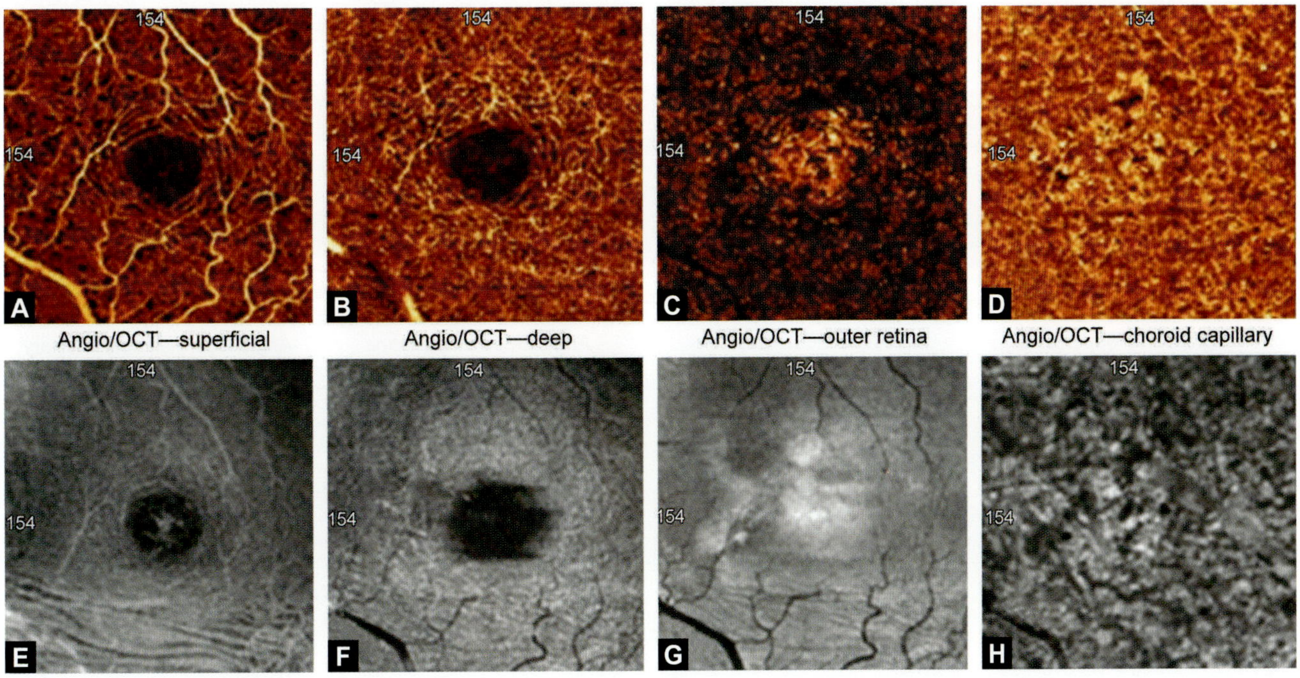

Figs. 15.4A to H: An optical coherence tomography angiography (OCTA) split-spectrum amplitude decorrelation angiography (SSADA) protocol of the retinal layers and corresponding images of enface optical coherence tomography (OCT) (3 × 3 mm), same eye as in Figure 15.3. (A to D) the regular vascularization of the inner retinal layers with the proper shape and size of the foveal avascular zone (FAZ). However, the outer retina and choroid show small granular vascular changes that are highly suspected of choroidal neovascularization (CNV). The patient probably also has an early stage of wet age-related macular degeneration (ARMD). (E to H) En face OCT scans of corresponding retinal layers. On the Figure E, in the lower part of the image, the horizontal parallel lines can be seen. Those lines are caused by the withdrawal of the epiretinal membrane. Small hyperreflective changes in the outer retina (G) and choroid (H) may adequately match the neovascular changes seen in the angiography images above.

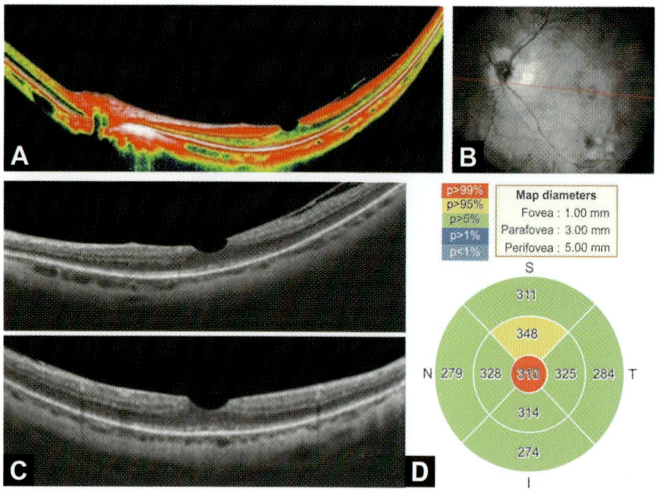

Figs. 15.5A to D: (A and C) optical coherence tomography (OCT) B-scans of the myopic eye with a macular pseudohole in a 52-year-old patient. The image shows a thickened epiretinal membrane on the very edge of the pseudorupture. It draws the retina by membrane contraction. The edges of the pseudohole are sharp and harsh and form a funnel-like shape of the macula. Figure (B) shows a fundus photograph with a small, unmatured papilla and a parapapillary degenerative cone. Blood vessels are narrow and straight, and in the retinal periphery myopic degenerative changes are seen. (D) the macular thickness map with an increased central thickness due to the pulled-out edges of the pseudohole.

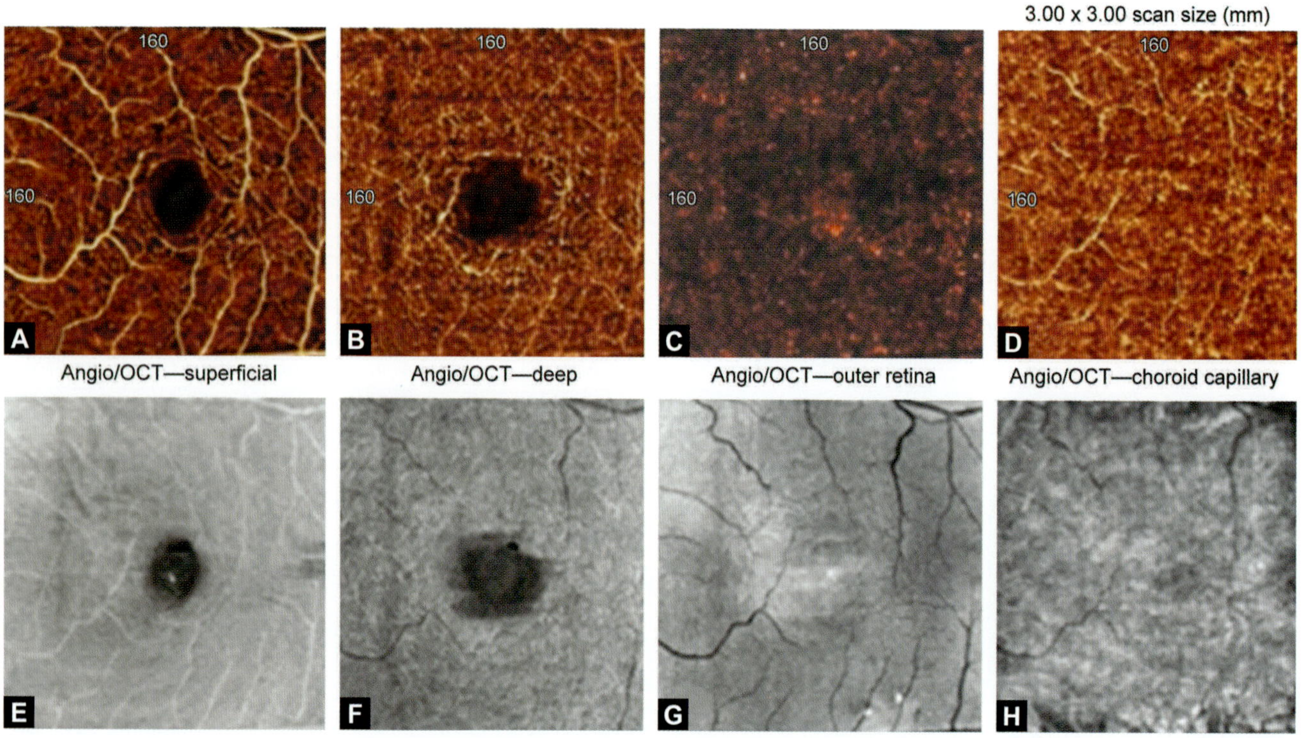

Figs. 15.6A to H: An optical coherence tomography angiography (OCTA) split-spectrum amplitude decorrelation angiography (SSADA) protocol of retinal layers and corresponding images of en face OCT (3 × 3 mm), same eye as in previous picture. (A to D) the angiography of the macular area where no significant changes in the vascularization of inner retinal layers can be seen. Slightly widened foveal avascular zone (FAZ) can be visualized in a deep vascular layer. The outer retina regularly shows no flow but has a few tiny artifacts that can imitate flow. Choriocapillaris presents with a normal, granular vascularization. (E to H) En face OCT shows a sharply edged round hyporeflective central zone that looks like a macular defect in the inner retinal layers. This zone corresponds to a sharply edged foveolar depression. Similar changes in the outer retina and in the choroidea are not detected.

membrane that significantly affects the macula, a pars plana vitrectomy along with membrane peeling is advised.

BIBLIOGRAPHY

1. Barak Y, Ihnen MA, Schaal S. Spectral domain optical coherence tomography in the diagnosis and management of vitreoretinal interface pathologies. J Ophthalmol. 2012; 2012:876472.
2. Bottoni F, Carmassi L, Cigada M, et al. Diagnosis of macular pseudoholes and lamellar macular holes: is optical coherence tomography the "gold standard"? Br J Ophthalmol. 2008;92:635-9.
3. Chen JC, Lee LR. Clinical spectrum of lamellar macular defects including pseudoholes and pseudocysts defined by optical coherence tomography. Br J Ophthalmol. 2008;92: 1342-6.
4. Compera D, Entchev E, Haritoglou C, et al. Lamellar hole-associated epiretinal proliferation in comparison to epiretinal membranes of macular pseudoholes. Am J Ophthalmol. 2015;160:373-84.
5. Haouchine B, Massin P, Tadayoni R, et al. Diagnosis of macular pseudoholes and lamellar macular holes by optical coherence tomography. Am J Ophthalmol. 2004;138:732-9.
6. Toyama T, Roggia MF, Yamaguchi T, et al. The extent of stretched lamellar cleavage and visual acuity in macular pseudoholes. Br J Ophthalmol. 2016;100:1227-31.
7. Varano M, Scassa C, Capaldo N, et al. Development of macular pseudoholes: a 36-month period of follow-up. Retina. 2002;22:435-42.

CHAPTER 16

Lamellar Macular Hole

INTRODUCTION

Lamellar macular hole is a partial defect in the retinal thickness where the inner layers of the retina are detached from the outer through traction. This is a well-circumscribed, round irregularity of the foveal area which appears bright red in a fundoscopic exam and which results from pulling and traction of the macula by the vitreous. Over time a cyst is formed on the macula that bursts in the superficial layers thus forming a lamellar macular hole or a hole in layer. The term lamellar refers to the fact that the hole encompasses a partial thickness of the macula and the change does not reach the photoreceptors and retinal pigment epithelium (RPE).

EPIDEMIOLOGY AND ETIOLOGY

Lamellar macular hole is considered to be a step in the development of a full thickness macular hole (FTMH). It is caused by the pulling forces of the vitreomacular traction. The real pathophysiological mechanism remains unknown. It is believed that epiretinal membrane through contraction or rupture of cysts from an existing central macular edema leads to the lamellar macular hole. It can also occur after acute posterior vitreous detachment (PVD).

SYMPTOMS AND SIGNS

Patients may notice blurred vision or metamorphopsia. There is a certain percentage of patients in which there is not necessarily a decline in visual acuity and the condition is asymptomatic. Lamellar macular hole usually remains stable for a longer period, but may progress into the FTMH. The importance of self-monitoring visual acuity must be explained to the patients. Varying values of visual acuity from normal to 20/40 are observed in examination.

DIFFERENTIAL DIAGNOSIS

- Macular pseudohole
- Full thickness macular hole
- Cystoid macular edema
- Pattern dystrophy
- Acute macular neuroretinopathy.

DIAGNOSTICS

Following clinical examination, an optical coherence tomography (OCT) is the method used to confirm the diagnosis. The OCT shows an irregular shape of the macula, defect in the inner foveal layers, schisis between the outer plexiform and granular layer and intact and fully preserved photoreceptors. Presence of an epiretinal membrane can frequently be seen. OCT detects macular defect and clearly indicates the depth, size and degree of damage. Absence of normal foveal depression may be noted with partial thinning of the central retinal tissue. Schisis typically occurs between the outer plexiform layer and outer granular layer of the macula. Preserved photoreceptor layer serves to differentiate the lamellar macular hole from FTMH and to assess the gravity of the condition.

Examples of an eye with lamellar macular hole shown by the optical coherence tomography angiography (Figs. 16.1 to 16.6).

THERAPY

The lamellar macular hole is most frequently a stable condition requiring constant observation and follow-ups. In certain cases where there is a presence of epiretinal membrane and in the event of severe disturbances, membrane peeling and pars plana vitrectomy are advised. Indication for surgical treatment is progressive, slow loss of vision or a documented worsening of the condition.

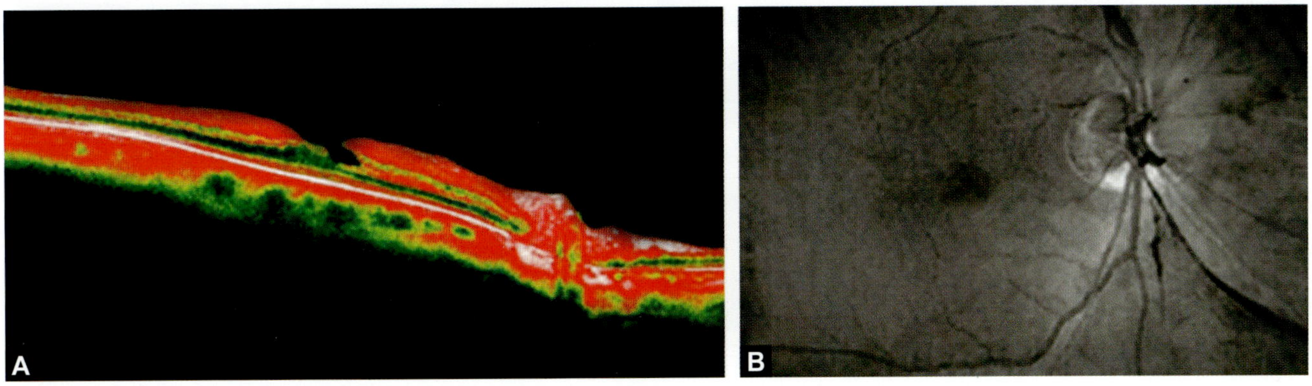

Figs. 16.1A and B: (A) An optical coherence tomography (OCT) B-scan showing the lamellar macular hole. Irregular contours and edges of the defect can be seen along with the loss of inner layers of the retina, schisis and an intact photoreceptor layer and retinal pigment epithelium (RPE). Part of retinal tissue can be seen sticking out and protruding into the central defect. A thick fibrous membrane, which is positioned vertically over the papilla can also be seen; (B) A fundus photograph shows a dark round change in the macular area consistent with retinal tissue defect.

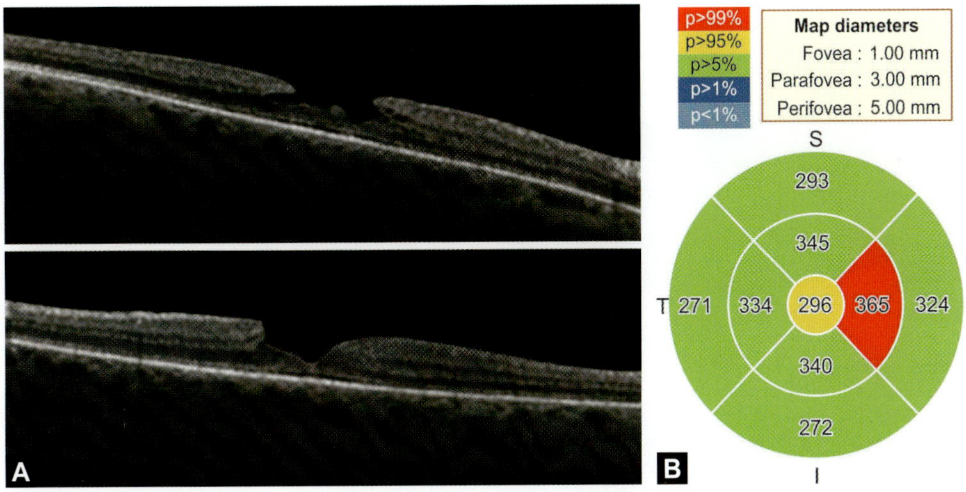

Figs. 16.2A and B: (A) An optical coherence tomography B-scan of the same eye as in Figures 16.1A and B show typical sagittal cross-sectional appearance of a lamellar macular hole. Two small cysts are visible in the retinal tissue at the edge of the defect; (B) A map of macular thickness shows thickening of the center and nasal part of the macula.

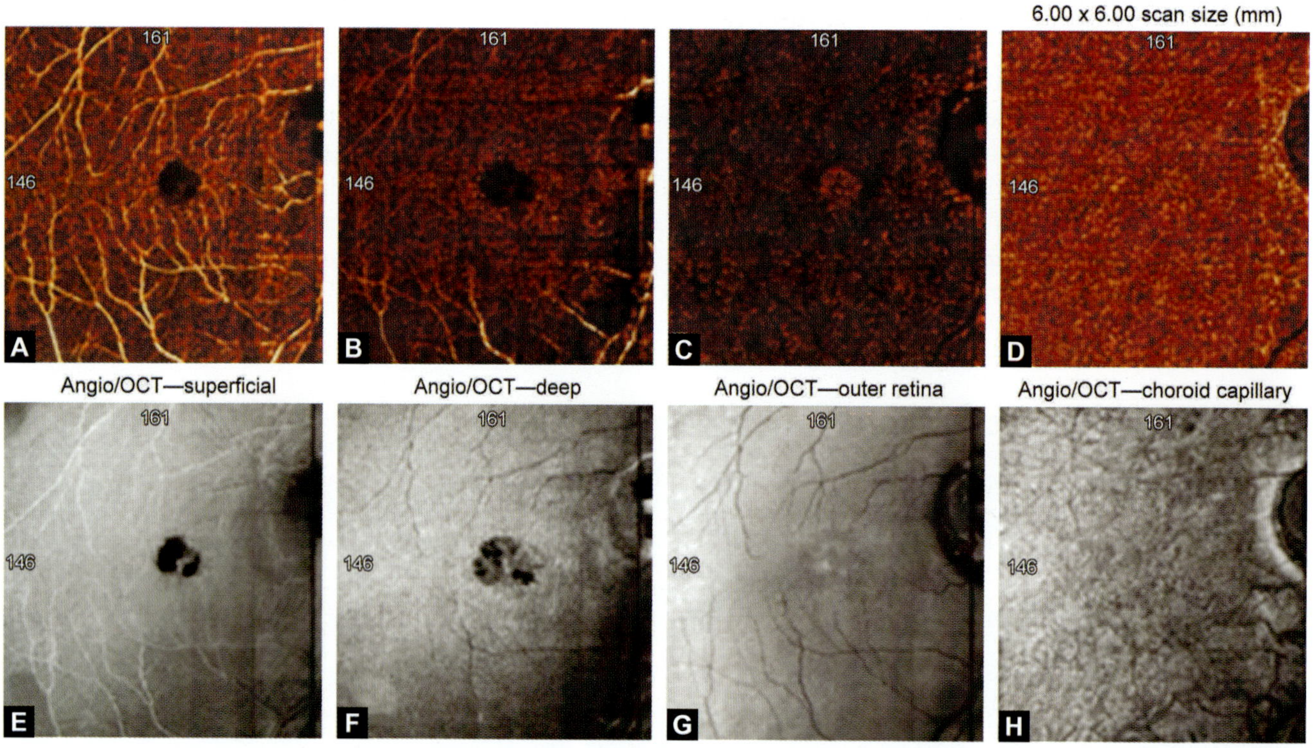

Figs. 16.3A to H: An optical coherence tomography angiography split-spectrum amplitude-decorrelation angiography (OCTA SSADA) protocol and enface OCT of corresponding retinal layers of the same eye as in the previous figures (6 × 6 mm). (A and B) An angiogram of the superficial and deep inner layer with a noticeable foveal avascular zone (FAZ) area, which has sharper and rougher edges; (C) An avascular retinal layer with a noticeable central artifact of the reflection of surrounding layers, corresponding in shape and size to the hole; (D) Regular granular and lobular structure of choriocapillaris vascularization; (E to H) En face optical coherence tomography (OCT) image of the superficial layer shows a sharply circumscribed hyporeflective round change consistent with the size of the hole. A hyperreflective trace of tissue can be seen within the dark zone overlaying the defect. The same change can be seen in the deep inner layer. The outer retina and choroidal layer present with normal structures.

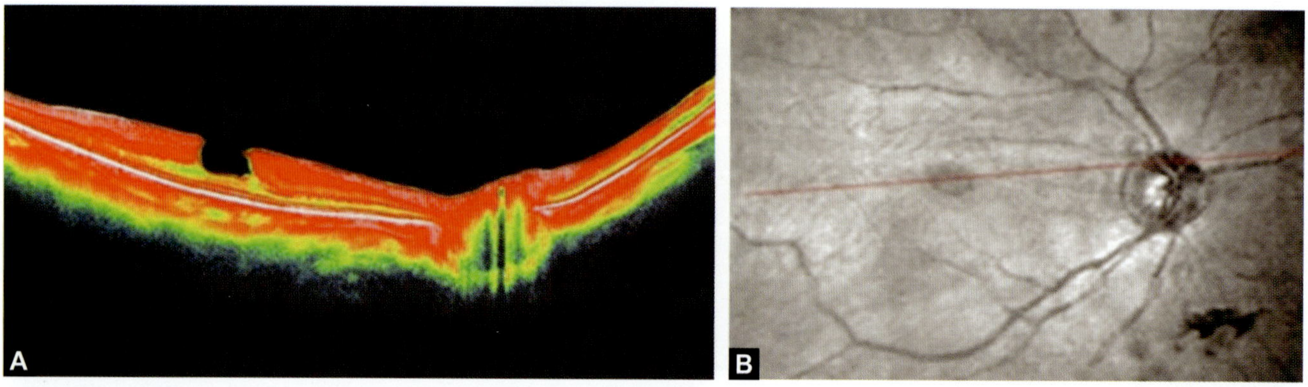

Figs. 16.4A and B: (A) An optical coherence tomography B-scan of the macula and optic nerve papilla in patient with lamellar macular hole. Irregular edges of the defect and the loss of inner retinal layers can be seen. The macular defect is deeper than the macular defect of the eye in the first example; (B) A fundus photo with a hyporeflective dark zone showing the localization of the lamellar hole.

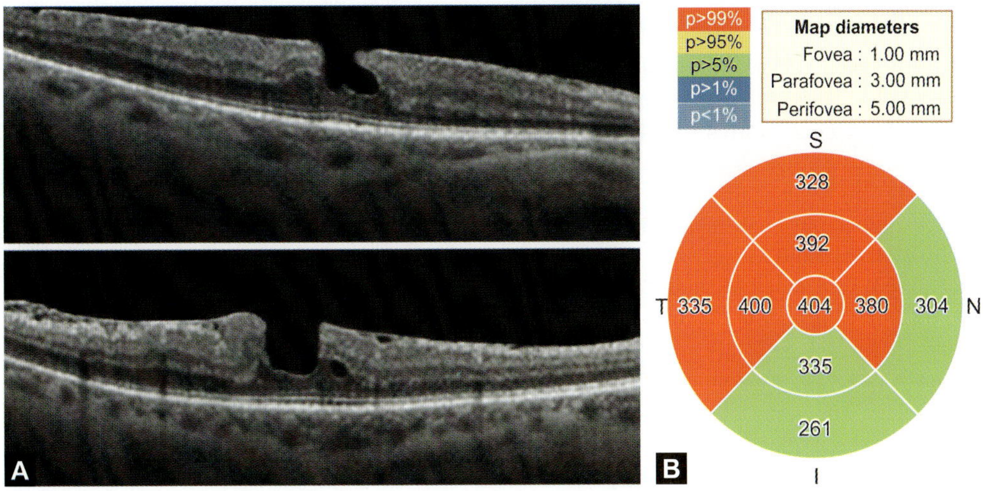

Figs. 16.5A and B: (A) An optical coherence tomography B-scan of the same eye as in Figures 16A and B showing the defect of inner retinal layers. A small accumulation of intraretinal fluid can be seen on the peripheral tissue of the defect. A fibrous hyperreflective epiretinal membrane is seen on the surface of the retina; (B) The macular thickness map shows thickening of the superior, temporal and central part of the macula and paramacular area.

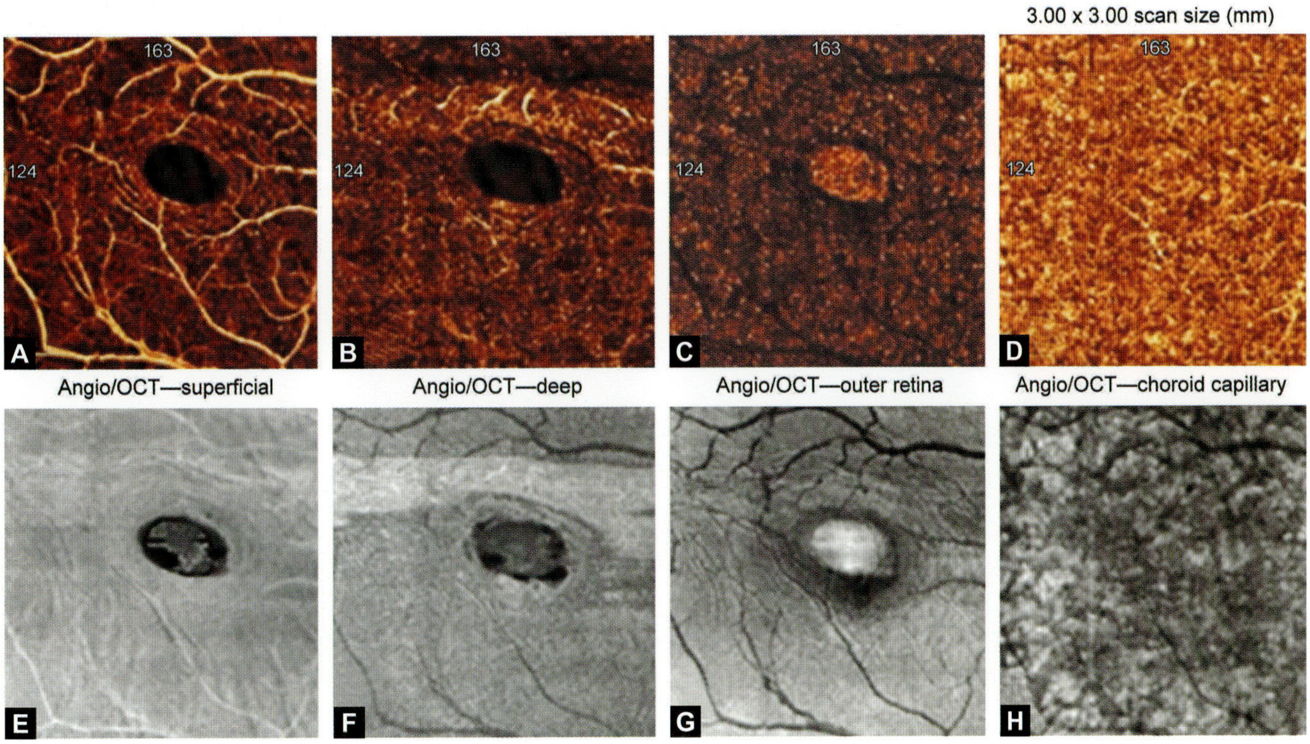

Figs. 16.6A to H: The optical coherence tomography angiography split-spectrum amplitude-decorrelation angiography (OCTA SSADA) protocol and enface OCT of the same eye as in the Figures 16.5 (3 × 3 mm). (A to C) Tissue defect stretching through the superficial and deep inner retinal layer and reaching the outer retina. Foveal avascular zone (FAZ) has a mildly ellipsoidal shape and is consistent with the defect. Distribution of blood vessels in both vascular networks is normal and the normal structure of choriocapillaris is shown (D). (E to H) En face OCT with hyporeflective, sharply circumscribed dark zone consistent with the defect of inner layers of the retina and ending in the outer part of the retina.

BIBLIOGRAPHY

1. Bottoni F, Deiro AP, Giani A, et al. The natural history of lamellar macular holes: a spectral domain optical coherence tomography study. Graefes Arch Clin Exp Ophthalmol. 2013;251(2):467-75.
2. Clamp MF, Wilkes G, Leis LS, et al. En face spectral domain optical coherence tomography analysis of lamellar macular holes. Retina. 2014;34(7):1360-6.
3. Govetto A, Dacquay Y, Farajzadeh M, et al. Lamellar macular hole: Two distinct clinical entities? Am J Ophthalmol. 2016;164:99-109.
4. Holland L, Chen JC, Lee LR. Anatomical and functional outcomes of pars plana vitrectomy for lamellar macular defects. Asia Pac J Ophthalmol (Phila). 2015;4(3):134-9.
5. Lai TT, Chen SN, Yang CM. Epiretinal proliferation in lamellar macular holes and full-thickness macular holes: Clinical and surgical findings. Graefes Arch Clin Exp Ophthalmol. 2016;254(4):629-38.
6. Parravano M, Oddone F, Boccassini B, et al. Functional and structural assessment of lamellar macular holes. Br J Ophthalmol. 2013;97(3):291-6.
7. Reibaldi M, Parravano M, Varano M, et al. Foveal microstructure and functional parameters in lamellar macular hole. Am J Ophthalmol. 2012;154(6):974-80.
8. Sanisoglu H, Elbay A, Sevim S, et al. Surgical therapy versus observation for lamellar macular hole: a Retrospective Comparison Study. Clin Ophthalmol. 2013;7:1843-8.
9. Witkin AJ, Castro LC, Reichel E, et al. Anatomic and visual outcomes of vitrectomy for lamellar macular holes. Ophthalmic Surg Lasers Imaging. 2010;41(4):418-24.
10. Witkin AJ, Ko TH, Fujimoto JG, et al. Redefining lamellar holes and the vitreomacular interface: an ultra high resolution optical coherence tomography study. Ophthalmology. 2006;113(3):388-97.

CHAPTER 17

Full Thickness Macular Hole, Stage 4

INTRODUCTION

Full thickness macular hole (FTMH) is a defect of the entire thickness of the neurosensory retina in the area of the macular center.

EPIDEMIOLOGY AND ETIOLOGY

Women in the ages between 50 and 70 are most frequently affected. FTMH can occur after an eye trauma, but it is considered to be idiopathic in over 80% of the cases. FTMH is the result of a progressive pathological perifoveolar vitreal separation with foveal adherence. The clinical presentation of the disease progression varies and includes a premacular hole (stage 0) which is in fact a vitreomacular adhesion, impending macular hole (stages 1A and 1B or vitreomacular traction) and FTMH stages from 2 to 4. Based on the size of the defect in the macula, FTMH may be described as small, medium or large FTMH. The size of the hole can be measured using the optical coherence tomography (OCT). Stages 2 and 3 of the macular hole simultaneously exhibit vitreomacular traction (VMT), while complete rupture or stage 4 does not have VMT. Impending macular holes regress spontaneously in most patients. It is important to clinically diagnose FTMH as soon as possible because the changes that occur require surgical treatment.

SYMPTOMS AND SIGNS

Patients cite abrupt decrease in visual acuity of the affected eye. Visual acuity in examination usually varies from 20/40 cases when a patient counts fingers directly in the front of their face. A complete defect of the central part is detected in macular examination. The defect is round and located in the central fovea, so deeper structures such as retinal pigment epithelium (RPE) can be visualized. Sizes of FTMH can be smaller or sometimes even larger than 500 μm. During slit-lamp examination, when the beam of light is directed straight ahead and cuts through the fovea and macula, patients report a central scotoma or hole in the center (positive Watzke-Allen sign). Attention should be given to the presence of vitreomacular traction and membrane which is a guide for the choice of therapy. A complete defect of the central part of the macula is found in examination.

DIFFERENTIAL DIAGNOSIS

- Lamellar macular hole
- Cystoid macular edema
- Pseudohole with epiretinal membrane
- Vitreomacular traction syndrome
- Central macular scar.

DIAGNOSTICS

The first step towards proper diagnosis is an examination of the fundus showing a roundish defect in the central part of the macula. Optical coherence tomography (OCT) is the best diagnostic method to confirm the presence of FTMH. Considering its invasiveness, FAG is not useful for detecting a macular hole, so preference is given to the OCT.

A detailed examination of the other eye is recommended given that bilateral macular rupture occurs in about 30% of patients. OCT will show a full thickness macular defect in the center and frequently a small operculum attached to the posterior hyaloid membrane in the vitreous. OCT is the gold standard when it comes to confirming FTMH diagnosis. It also helps in monitoring the disease following a surgical intervention-vitrectomy.

Image of an eye with full thickness macular hole (Figs. 17.1 to 17.6).

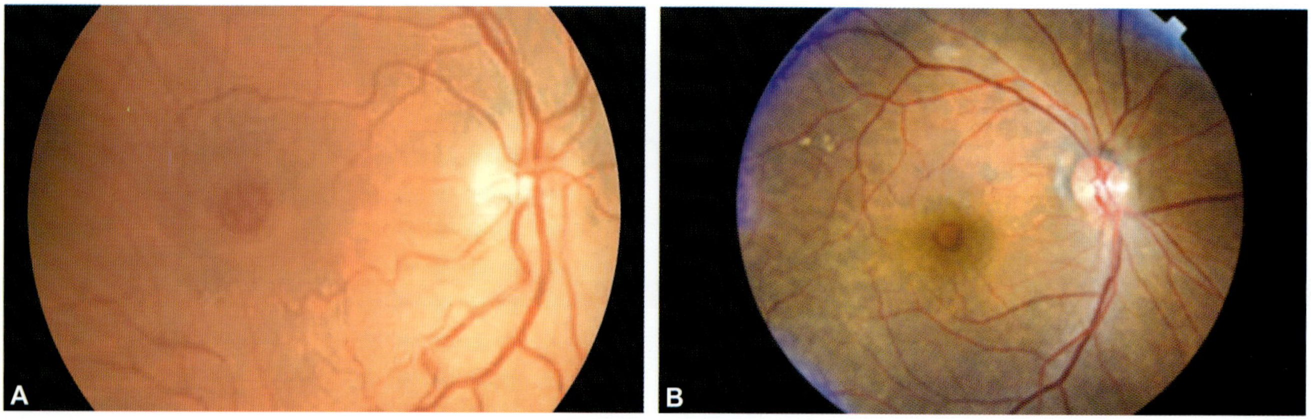

Figs. 17.1A and B: (A) Fundus photograph of a fresh full thickness macular hole. A red round change is visible, sharply circumscribed, but is not pigmented. (B) fundus photograph of a chronic full thickness macular hole with sharply circumscribed reddish hole and dark surrounding ring of the visible retinal pigment epithelium (RPE). *Taken from: http://www.palmettoretina.com/macular-hole*

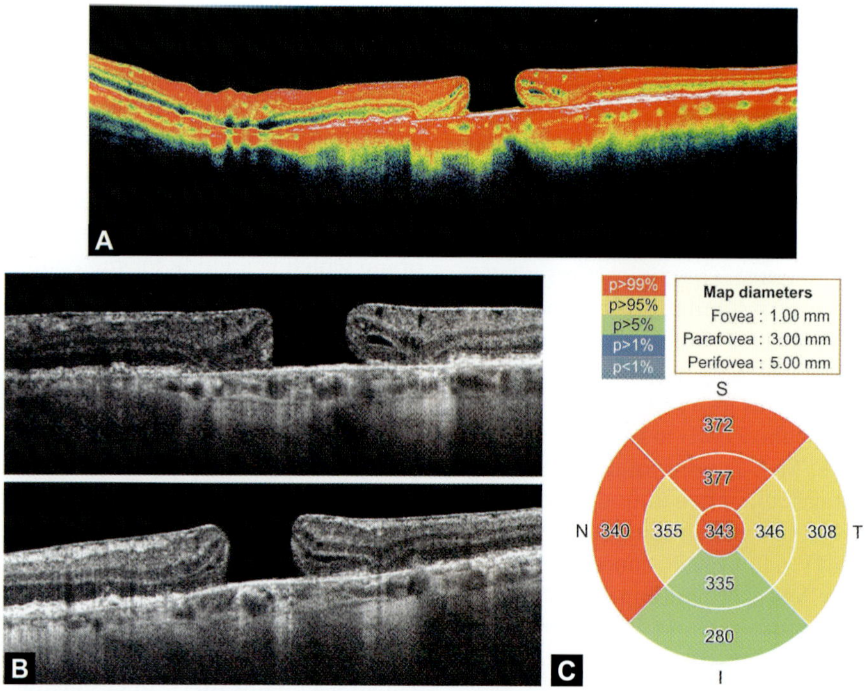

Figs. 17.2A to C: (A and B) An optical coherence tomography (OCT) B-scan of the macular area and optic nerve papilla in a 65-year-old female patient. The image of the sagittal cross-section of the macular area shows a complete defect of all retinal layers reaching to the retinal pigment epithelium (RPE). RPE is fully preserved, but wavy and irregularly grouped in places. Retinal tissue on the edges of the FTMH shows small cystoid changes filled with intraretinal fluid. (C) Retinal thickness map. An edema can be observed as well as macular area thickening of all parts except the inferior.

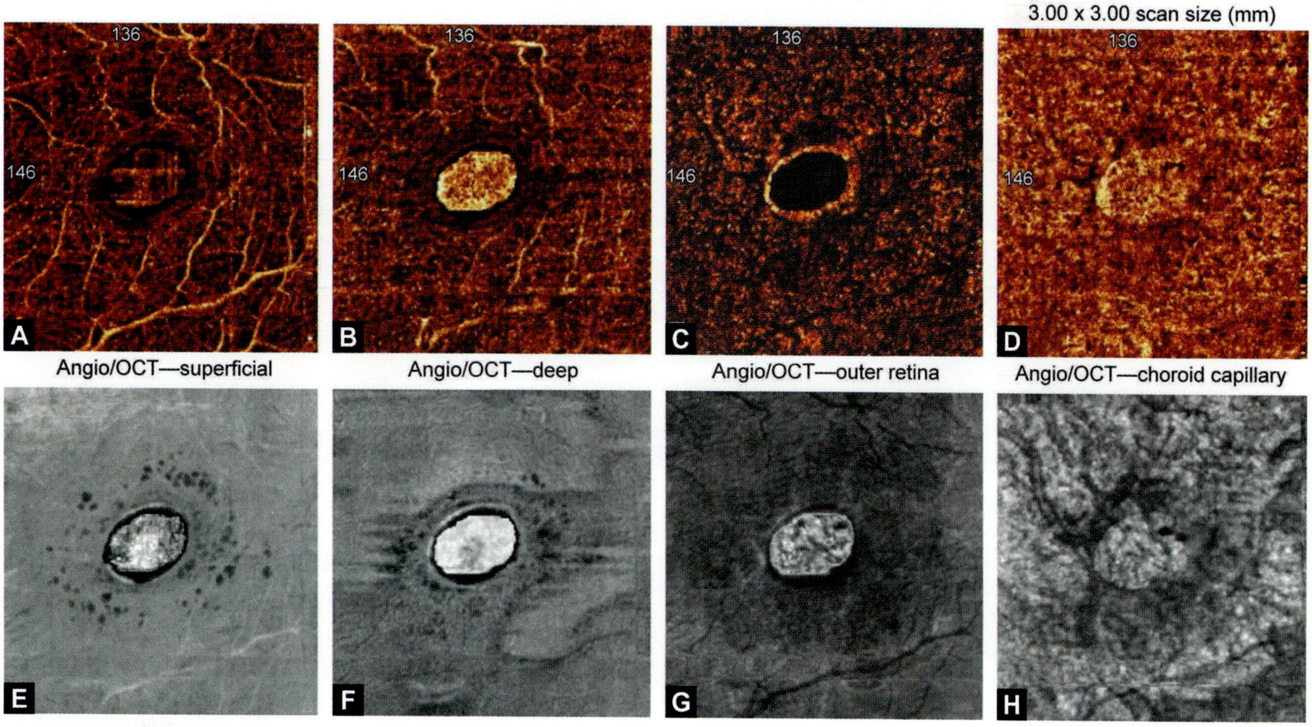

Figs. 17.3A to H: (A to H) An optical coherence tomography angiography split-spectrum amplitude-decorrelation angiography (OCTA SSADA) protocol and OCT en face of vertically corresponding layers of the same eye (3 × 3 mm); (A to D) Angiogram of an eye with full thickness macular hole (FTMH). Central defect is visible in all retinal layers (up to choroidal, which shows the reflection of the shape of the defect). It is sharply circumscribed from the surrounding vascularized tissue; (E to H) OCT en face images of the corresponding retinal layers showing a whitish defect. Along edges of the defect there are numerous small honeycomb-like changes consistent with cystoid changes of the retinal tissue around the FTMH.

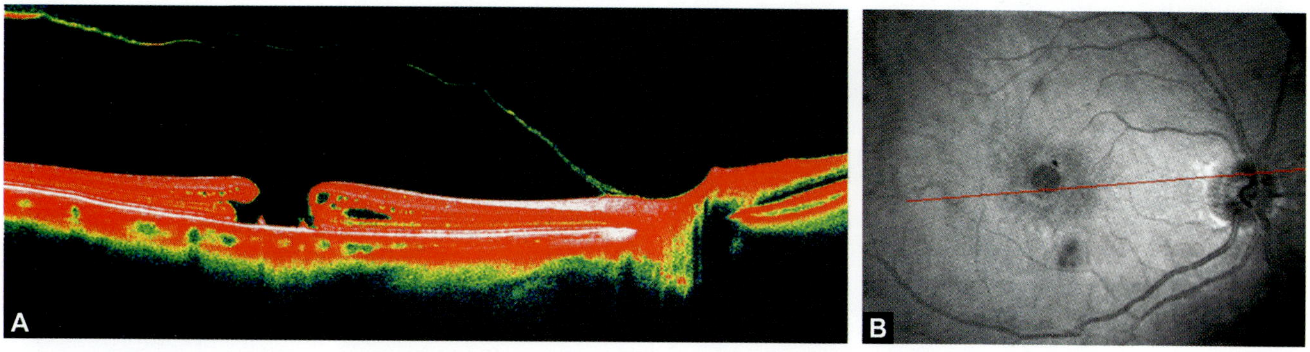

Figs. 17.4A and B: (A) An optical coherence tomography (OCT) B-scan of the macular area and optic nerve papilla in a 70-year-old female patient. Sagittal cross-section of the retina shows defect of the macular area reaching up to the retinal pigment epithelium. There is a mild wrinkling and grouping of the RPE. Edges of the FTMH are irregular and showing cystoid changes in the surrounding retinal tissue. Hyperreflective posterior hyaloid membrane is also shown; (B) A fundus photograph of the same eye. Sharply circumscribed darker area is seen which is consistent with the macular hole, as well as the surrounding tissue edema.

THERAPY

Pars plana vitrectomy is the only choice in treating full thickness macular hole. The procedure removes inner limiting membrane (ILM) around the edges of the macular hole (epiretinal membrane *peeling*) and removes the cause of posterior vitreous separation by way of gas tamponade using sulfur hexafluoride (SF6) or perfluoropropane (C3F8). Postoperatively, for the first week,

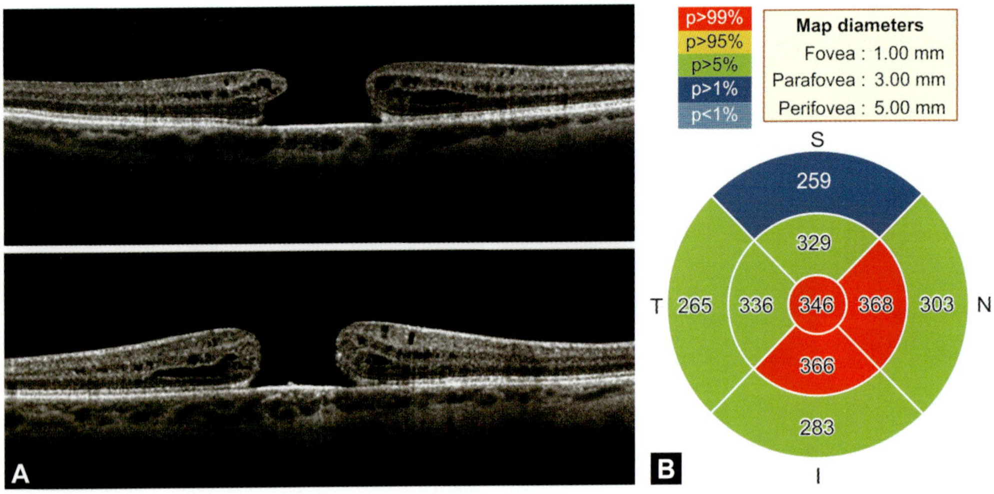

Figs. 17.5A and B: (A) An optical coherence tomography B-scan of the same eye as in Figures 17.4A and B. Sagittal cross-section of the macular area with a clearly shown defect stretching through the entire thickness of the tissue. Retinal schisis is visible as well as the accumulation of intraretinal fluid in the tissue adjacent to FTMH. (B) The retinal thickness map shows central thickening of the macular area consistent with the occurrence of edema in the retinal tissue around the FTMH.

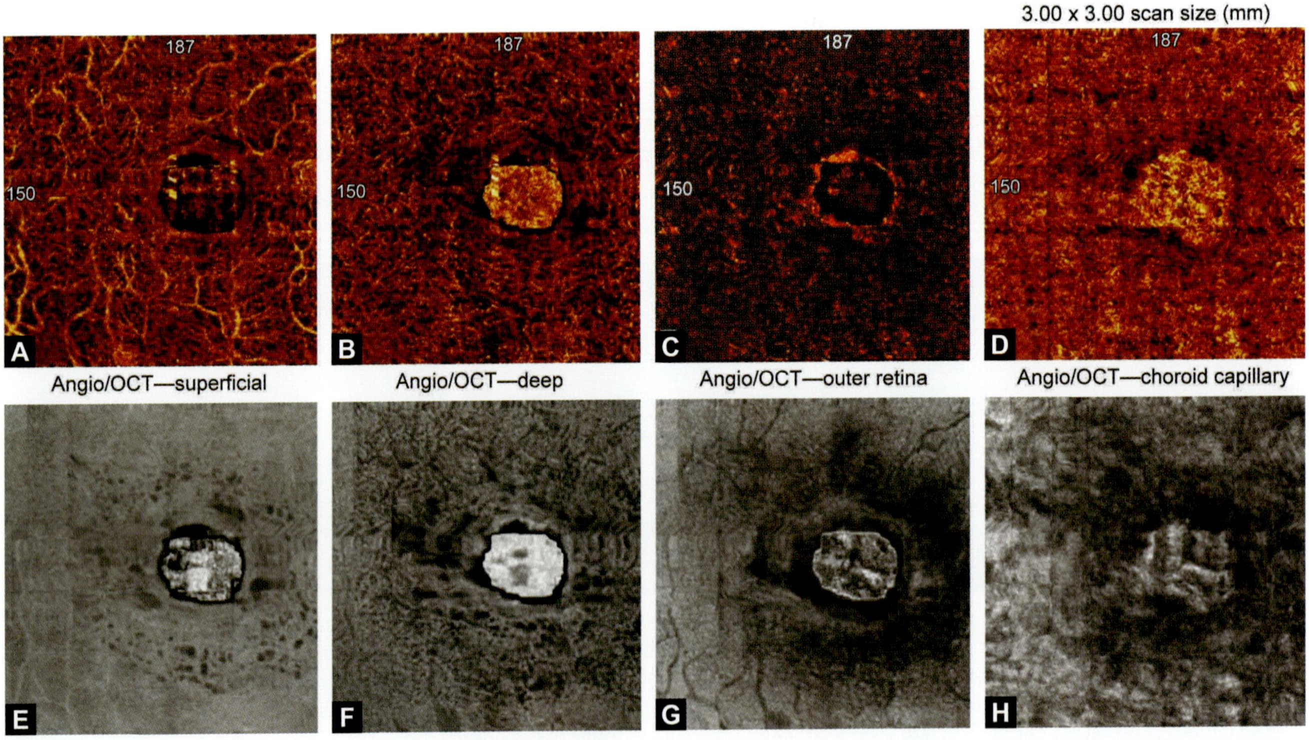

Figs. 17.6A to H: An optical coherence tomography angiography split-spectrum amplitude-decorrelation angiography protocol and OCT *en face* of the vertically corresponding layers of the same eye as in the Figures 17.5A and B (3 × 3 mm). Sharply circumscribed hole is detected through all the retinal layers without changes in the surrounding vascularization and capillary networks. En face optical coherence tomography (OCT) images show the macular hole in all retinal layers as the hyperreflective round central area with clearly pronounced rim. In the surrounding area, on the edges of the defect, small honeycomb-like hyporeflective round spaces, which are consistent with accumulated intraretinal fluid can be seen.

face-down positioning is recommended for as long as possible, depending on the size of the hole. The success of surgical treatment depends on the preoperative duration of the disease and on the size of the hole. Surgically closed holes can reopen again in a period over a year following a successful surgery, and it is considered that ILM peeling performed during the primary surgery reduces this risk.

BIBLIOGRAPHY

1. Gao M, Liu K, Lin Q, et al. Management modalities for traumatic macular hole: A systematic review and single-arm meta-analysis. Curr Eye Res. 2017;42(2):287-96.
2. Hattenbach LO, Framme C, Junker B, et al. Intraoperative real-time OCT in macular surgery. Ophthalmologe. 2016;113(8):656-62.
3. Pierro L, Iuliano L, Bandello F. OCT angiography features of a case of bilateral full-thickness macular hole at different stages. Ophthalmic Surg Lasers Imaging Retina. 2016;47(4):388-9.
4. Rahimy E, McCannel CA. Impact of internal limiting membrane peeling on macular hole reopening: A systematic review and meta-analysis. Retina. 2016;36(4):679-87.
5. Rizzo S, Savastano A, Bacherini D, et al. Vascular features of full-thickness macular hole by OCT angiography. Ophthalmic Surg Lasers Imaging Retina. 2017;48(1):62-8.

CHAPTER 18

Retinal Detachment

INTRODUCTION

Retinal detachment (RD) refers to the separation of sensory retina from the underlying retinal pigment epithelium (RPE).

EPIDEMIOLOGY AND ETIOLOGY

There are two types of retinal detachment: Rhegmatogenous (rhegma: Rupture) and non-rhegmatogenous retinal detachment. Rhegmatogenous retinal detachment often appears secondarily as a consequence of a defect in the entire thickness of sensory retina. Subretinal fluid (SRF), which originates from liquefied vitreous gel, penetrates into the subretinal space. Non-rhegmatogenous RD may be tractional or exudative (serous). Traction RD occurs due to the dragging of vitreoretinal adhesions and results with sensory retinal separation from RPE. The origin of SRF in this case is not entirely definite. This type of detachment is most commonly seen in the proliferative form of diabetic retinopathy, retinopathy of prematurity, sickle cell retinopathy and penetrating injuries of the posterior ocular segment. The serous or exudative form of retinal detachment is less common. In these cases, the subretinal fluid leaks from choriocapillary layer due to the perforated RPE and fills the subretinal space. Serous RD appears secondarily and is most commonly related to ocular tumors, and sometimes to systemic diseases.

SYMPTOMS AND SIGNS

Patients complain of sudden peripheral or central vision loss. The loss of peripheral vision is the most common symptom of retinal detachment. The visual field test shows a defect located on the opposite side, compared to the locus of actual retinal detachment in posterior pole. If the macula is included, the loss of central visual acuity occurs. Additional symptoms can include photopsia with/without the appearance of floaters in visual field. Fundoscopic examination can show an elevation of the retina in periphery which extends throughout the posterior pole.

DIFFERENTIAL DIAGNOSIS

- Retinoschisis
- Retinal ruptures
- Choroidal detachment
- Posterior scleritis.

DIAGNOSTICS

A diagnosis is established after a detailed clinical fundus examination. An ocular ultrasound (B-scan) is the gold standard for diagnosis of retinal detachment especially if vitreous opacities exist. Optical coherence tomography (OCT) may assist for diagnosis of rhegmatogenous retinal detachment when shallow subretinal separation exists. It can also help in differentiation of retinoschisis and retinal

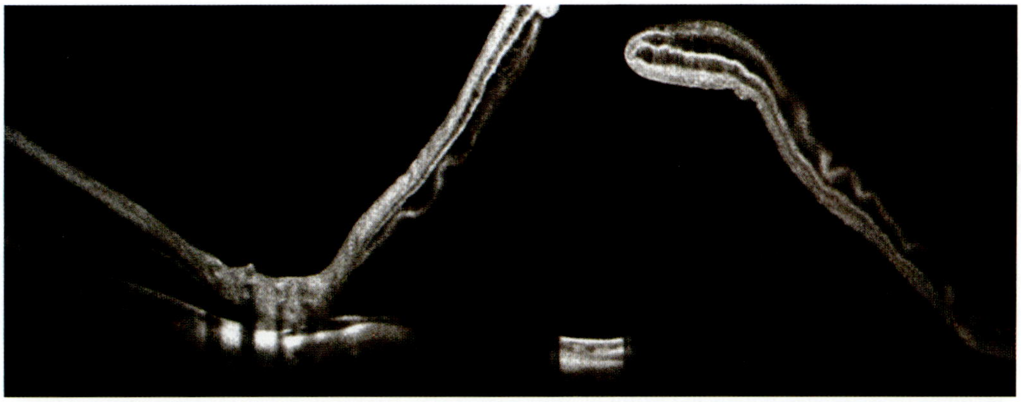

Fig. 18.1: An optical coherence tomography (OCT) B-scan of the eye with high myopia (prescription is -12 diopters) in 45 years old female patient. A complete separation of all retinal layers is presented. In this eye, a full thickness macular hole was previously operated. In separated retinal layers, edema and small cysts can be visualized.

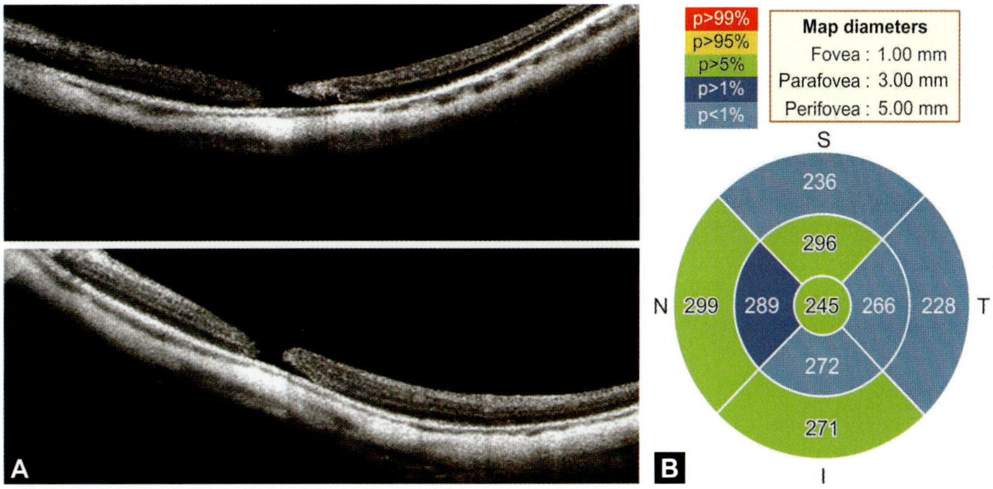

Figs. 18.2A and B: (A) An optical coherence tomography B-scan of the same eye, a month after pars plana vitrectomy. Retina adheres to the retinal pigment epithelium, but in the very center, full thickness macular hole is visible. Cysts and edema are not shown; (B) Map of retinal thickness shows referential values inferiorly and nasally, while superiorly and temporally decreased and thinned ones.

detachment, in cases when clinical differences are harder to identify (Figs. 18.1 and 18.2).

THERAPY

Rhegmatogenous retinal detachment can be treated differently varying upon the location and size of the retinal gap. Therapeutical approaches include retinopexy (only for small, asymptomatic detachments), pneumatic retinopexy, scleral buckling surgery, vitrectomy or a combined approach with vitrectomy and scleral buckling. Visualization of the retinal gap is crucial for decision about therapeutic approach. Laser retinopexy fixates the edges of retinal detachment and prevents the expanding. Other therapeutical approaches include the extraction of subretinal fluid and closure of retinal gap. Anatomical structure of the retina recovers by this approach especially the macula. If the macula is separated altogether with the periphery, postoperative visual prognosis is less certain.

BIBLIOGRAPHY

1. Chaudhary R, Dretzke J, Scott R, et al. Clinical and surgical risk factors in the development of proliferative vitreoretinopathy following retinal detachment surgery: a systematic review protocol. Syst Rev. 2016;5(1):107.

2. Daien V, Le Pape A, Heve D, et al. Incidence, risk factors and impact of age on retinal detachment after cataract surgery in France: A national population study. Ophthalmology. 2015;122(11):2179-85.
3. Georgieva V, Jochmann C, Wiedemann P. Bilateral central retinal detachment with whitish chorioretinal foci. Ophthalmologe. 2015;112(10):861-4.
4. Heimann H. Surgical technique in rhegmatogenous ablatio retinae. Ophthalmologe. 2008;105(1):5-6.
5. Ling J, Noori J, Safi F, et al. Pneumatic retinopexy for rhegmatogenous retinal Detachment in pseudophakia. Semin Ophthalmol. 2016;6:1-4.
6. Nowomiejska K, Choragiewicz T, Borowicz D, et al. Surgical management of traumatic retinal detachment with primary vitrectomy in adult patients. J Ophthalmol. 2017;2017:5084319.
7. Poulsen CD, Peto T, Grauslund J, et al. Epidemiologic characteristics of retinal detachment surgery at a specialized unit in Denmark. Acta Ophthalmol. 2016;94(6):548-55.
8. Simonett JM, Grewal DS, Fawzi AA, et al. Fundus autofluorescence patterns of submacular fluid resolution following repair of macula-involving rhegmatogenous retinal detachments. Ophthalmic Surg Lasers Imaging Retina. 2016;47(11):1020-29.
9. Tolou C, Mahieu-Durringer L, Cassagne M, et al. Treatment delay in patients with first episode of retinal detachment in the studied eye in Midi-Pyrénées. J Fr Ophtalmol. 2016;39(1):90-7.
10. Zhou J, Wei W, You Q, et al. Comparative analysis of the characteristics of bilateral rhegmatogenous retinal detachment. Zhonghua Yan Ke Za Zhi. 2016;52(5):348-53.

CHAPTER 19

Toxoplasmic Chorioretinitis

INTRODUCTION

Toxoplasmic chorioretinitis is an inflammation of the retina and choroid which is caused by the intracellular parasite *Toxoplasma gondii*.

ETIOLOGY AND EPIDEMIOLOGY

Toxoplasma gondii is the intracellular parasite and most common cause of posterior uveitis in developed Western countries. It is the second leading cause of the infective chorioretinitis in immunocompromised patients (the first cause is cytomegalovirus). The disease, in most of patients, occurs due to the acquired acute or recurrent infection by the parasite. Cases of congenital toxoplasmosis reactivation are the most frequent, although cases of primary infection can also often be diagnosed nowadays.

SYMPTOMS AND SIGNS

The most usual symptom is unilateral loss of vision. Patients complain of blurry vision and floaters, which sometimes can indicate the retinal detachment. In some cases, symptoms of the anterior segment inflammation may be present. Eye is reddish, itchy and patient complains of photophobia and epiphora. The inflammation of iris and intraocular pressure increasement can also be detected in some cases. Cornea may reveal endothelial deposits with all signs of granulomatous inflammation. Fundoscopy shows a flake-like infiltrate with unclear edges in the central macula which is a typical sign of primary toxoplasmosis. Inflammation is necrotic and it forms a lasting scar. In the cases of recurrent inflammation, a new focal inflammation is formed along pigmented edges of an old chorioretinal scar. Scarring spreads firstly through the periphery and then goes to the very center of lesion, presenting a different pigment changes. Vasculitis is not present. In immunocompromised patients, toxoplasmic retinitis can be bilateral and resemble of necrotizing retinitis.

DIFFERENTIAL DIAGNOSIS

- Macular scar,
- Cat-scratch disease,
- Ocular sarcoidosis or tuberculosis,
- Progressive ocular necrosis of the outer retinal layer caused by *aspergillus*, candida, or as a complication of syphilis.

DIAGNOSTICS

The diagnosis is based on anamnesis, clinical examination and serological tests. Colored fundus photography shows blurry posterior pole and vitreal inflammation. Blood vessels are regular and not pathologically changed. Whitish intraretinal lesion is seen near foveal area. Edges of the inflammatory lesion are unclear. Additionally, diagnosis can be proved by FAG and optical coherence tomography

(OCT). An OCT shows the exact depth of defect or retinal infiltration, as well as the effect of therapy. Usual OCT findings include macular thickening and macular edema of superior and temporal foveal part. Sagittal cross-sectional B-scan very often shows an uneven thickness of the macula (Figs. 19.1 to 19.4).

TREATMENT

Patient is treated by an infectologist. The diagnosis of toxoplasmic chorioretinitis is confirmed by the serological test with high IgM and IgG antitoxoplasmic titers. The positive IgM finding indicates the acute toxoplasmic inflammation, while the negative titer excludes toxoplasmosis as the cause of inflammation. Inflammation and infection in toxoplasmosis can pass by itself, but it must be treated in patients with affected visual acuity. Medical treatment is advised for patients with macular changes, papillary edema and/or signs of acute vitreous inflammation mainly if they are immunocompromised. Smaller lesions, which are located around the macula, should be moni-

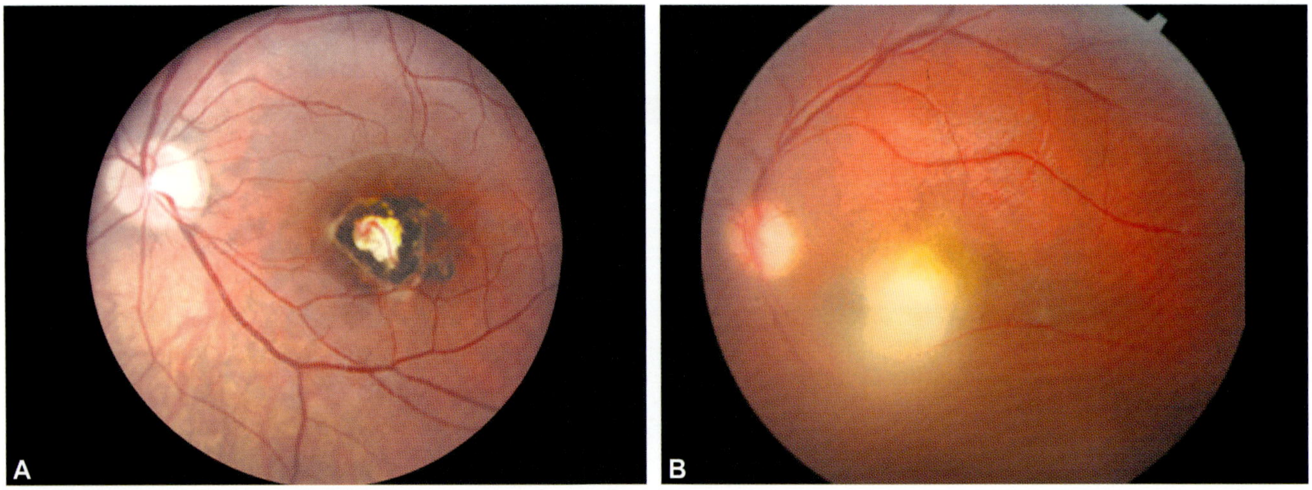

Figs. 19.1A and B: (A) A fundus photography of an old scar caused by congenital toxoplasmosis. Accumulation of pigment can be visible on the edges of lesion, indicating its oldness. A yellowish scar is seen in the center. (B) Fundus photography of an eye with the active toxoplasmosis. The change is soft, whitish and flake-like and shows no pigmented changes.
Source: https://aapos.org/

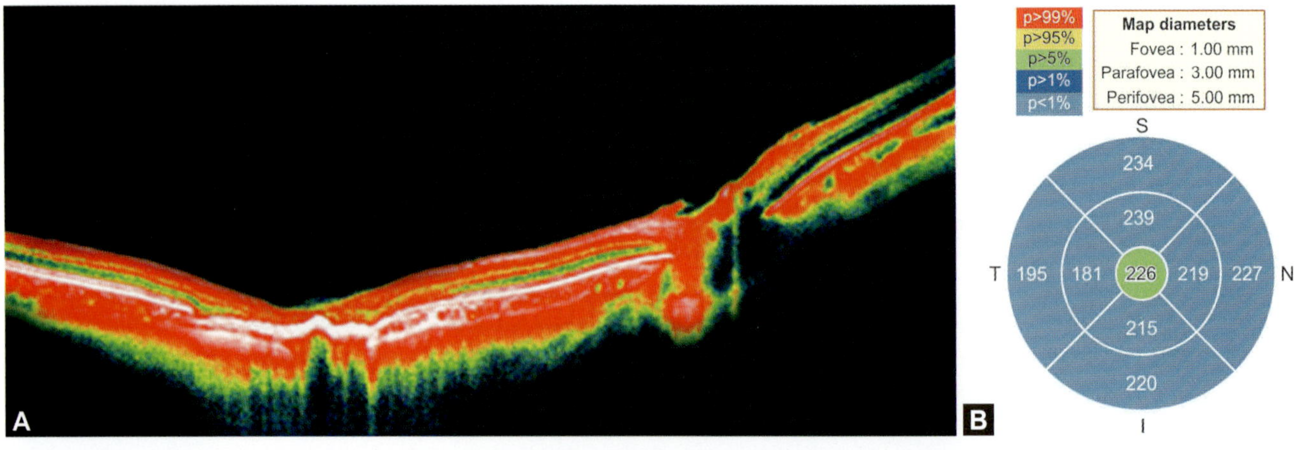

Figs. 19.2A and B: (A) Optical coherence tomography (OCT) B-scan of the macular area and optic nerve of an eye with old toxoplasmic scar. Standard foveal depression is lost, and entire retina appears thinner. However, retinal pigment epithelium (RPE) and Bruch's membrane are thickened and wavy in the macular area and choroid is very hyperreflective. (B) The retinal thickness map shows a regular thickness of macular center, due to the scar thickness, while the surrounding tissue shows decreased values.

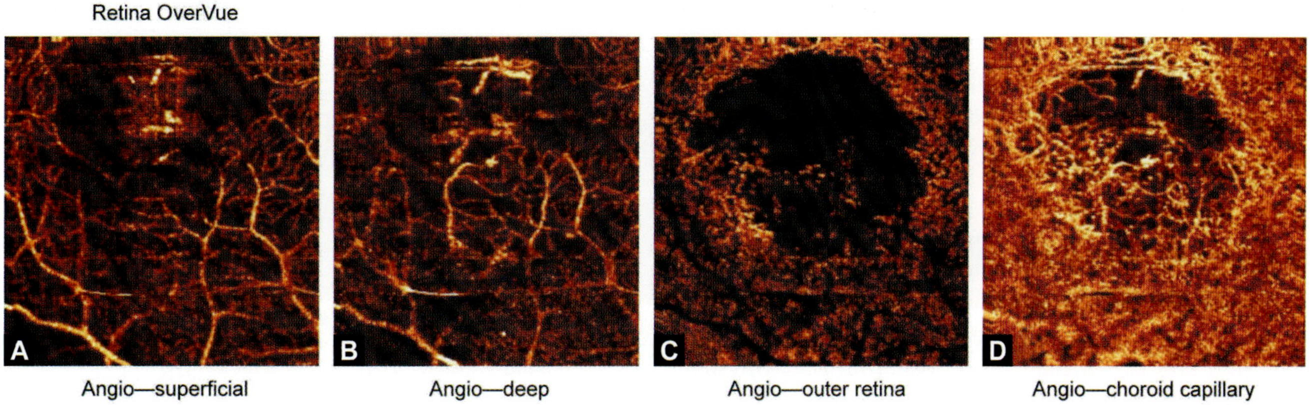

Figs. 19.3A to D: Optical coherence tomography angiography split-spectrum amplitude-decorrelation angiography (OCTA SSADA) protocol of the superficial and deep vascular plexus, outer retina and choroid, the same eye with toxoplasmosis-caused scar as in Figures 19.1 and 19.2 (3 × 3 mm). The central dark area can be seen in all retinal layers, along with dry and inactive capillaries which are surrounded by a dark halo zone (especially seen in the deep vascular plexus). A fine, dense capillary structure, usually seen in superficial and deep vascular plexus, is completely lost. A few larger dry blood capillaries with irregular flow can be visualized. Outer retina and choroid show a big dark central defect without any flow that corresponds to the sub foveloar fibrous scar. Ends of dry capillaries form vascular loops and circular connections on the periphery of the central defect.

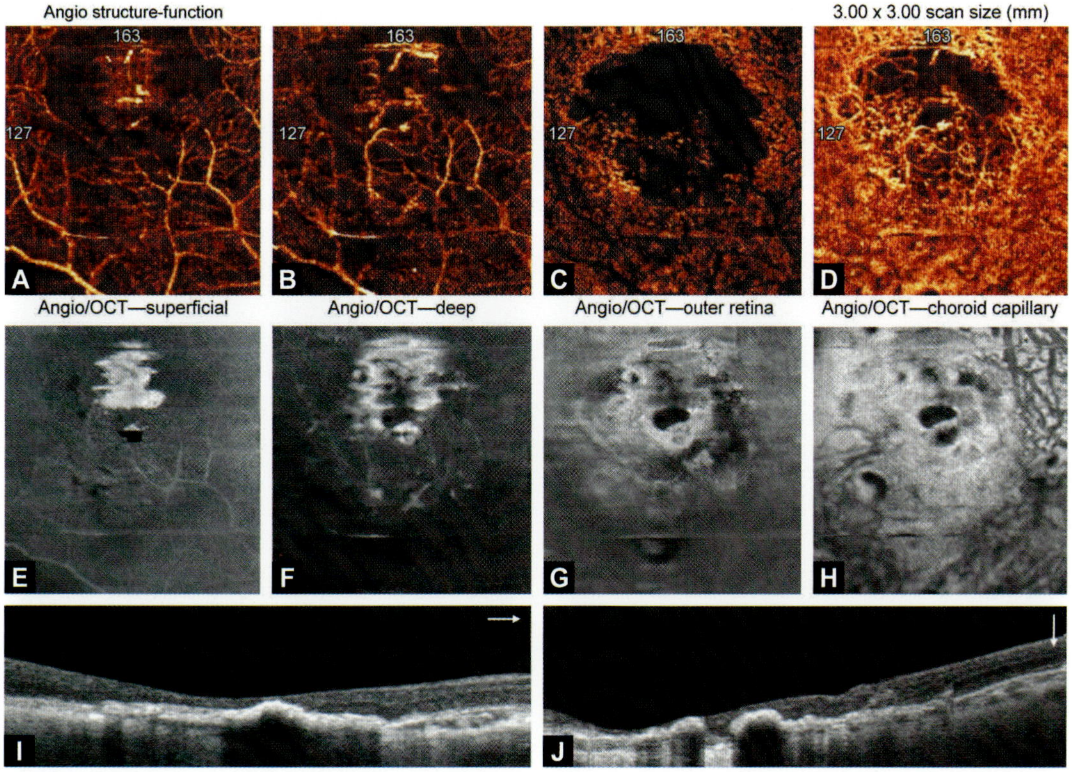

Figs. 19.4A to J: An optical coherence tomography angiography split-spectrum amplitude-decorrelation angiography protocol (3 × 3 mm), corresponding en face OCT images and B-scans of the same eye as depicted in Figures 19.1 to 19.3. Angiograms show an old, hyporeflective subfoveolar scar described in Figures 19.3A to D. (E to H) En face optical coherence tomography (OCT) images of corresponding retinal layers show the inactive retina with hyporeflective dark areas that represent defects. Hyperreflective membranous changes match the fibrous tissue without blood vessels. The choroidal region is completely dry, with several central defects and surrounding fibrous tissue. (I and J) OCT B-scan shows a matching sagittal cross-section of the hyperreflective, irregular scar which is presented as a thickness of Tela choroidea and retinal pigment epithelium (RPE).

tored. If they start to threaten the visual acuity, a long-term treatment using pyrimethamine, sulfadiazine and folic acid is advised. Intravitreal injections of clindamycin can also be administered. After the antibiotic therapy, usage of oral steroids is advised. Intravitreal application of steroids is also not excluded.

BIBLIOGRAPHY

1. Aleixo AL, Curi AL, Benchimol EI, et al. Toxoplasmic retinochoroiditis: clinical characteristics and visual outcome in a prospective study. PLoS Negl Trop Dis. 2016;10(5): e0004685.
2. Das D, Ramachandra V, Islam S, et al. Update on pathology of ocular parasitic disease. Indian J Ophthalmol. 2016;64 (11):794-802.
3. Garweg JG. Ocular toxoplasmosis: an Update. Klin Monbl Augenheilkd. 2016;233(4):534-9.
4. Hou JH, Patel SS, Farooq AV, et al. Decline in ocular toxoplasmosis over 40 years at a tertiary referral practice in the United States. Ocul Immunol Inflamm. 2016;28:1-7.
5. Khairallah M, Kahloun R, Ben Yahia S, et al. Clinical, tomographic and angiographic findings in patients with acute toxoplasmic retinochoroiditis and associated serous retinal detachment. Ocul Immunol Inflamm. 2011;19(5): 307-10.
6. Lujan BJ. Spectral domain optical coherence tomography imaging of punctate outer retinal toxoplasmosis. Saudi J Ophthalmol. 2014;28(2):152-6.
7. Nogueira AR, Leve F, Morgado-Diaz J, et al. Effect of *Toxoplasma gondii* infection on the junctional complex of retinal Pigment Epithelial Cells. Parasitology. 2016;143(5):568-75.
8. Ozgonul C, Besirli CG. Recent developments in the diagnosis and treatment of ocular toxoplasmosis. ophthalmic Res. 2017;57(1):1-12.
9. Samudio M, Acosta ME, Castillo V, et al. Clinical and epidemiological aspects of toxoplasmosis in patients with vision problems. Rev Chilena Infectol. 2015;32(6):658-63.

CHAPTER 20

Albinism

INTRODUCTION

Albinism is a genetically conditioned, heterogeneous group of diseases that are inherited in autosomal recessive pattern. Hypopigmentation of eyes and/or skin occurs due to the lack of tyrosinase, which is an enzyme needed for the conversion of tyrosine into melanin. There are two types of albinism: oculocutaneous and ocular. Oculocutaneous albinism can be tyrosinase-negative or tyrosinase-positive.

EPIDEMIOLOGY AND ETIOLOGY

Albinism affects all races, although it occurs more frequently in African Americans. It can also be part of Chédiak–Higashi syndrome and Hermansky–Pudlak syndrome. The disease is bilateral and it is characterized by the lack of pigment in retinal pigment epithelium and choroidea. Details of choroidea can be clearly seen during the fundoscopic examination. Patients usually visit the ophthalmologist in their early age, complaining of poor vision. They often don't pass basic medical examinations for the school. Nystagmus, various forms of strabismus or amblyopia can also be detected. Children complain of photophobia, they require constant use of protective sunglasses, and the darker ambience makes them feel more comfortable. Vision can vary between the regular acuity and visual acuity regarded as *legally blind*.

SYMPTOMS AND SIGNS

- *Oculocutaneous albinism* is inherited in autosomal recessive pattern.
  - *Tyrosinase-negative, type I*—Patients are not able to synthetize melanin. Usually they have light hair color and very pale skin. Both eyes show pathological changes and have a complete lack of pigmentation in eyes and skin. Slit-lamp examination reveals changes on iris (translucent and semi-transparent iris, which gives the appearance of a *red eye*). The fundoscopic examination of posterior eye segment reveals lack of regular anatomy of the macula and fovea, where retinal blood vessels cross over the expected foveolar avascular zone. The fundus periphery is without pigment and completely transparent and bright. An optical coherence tomography (OCT) shows macular hypoplasia, aplasia and/or macular schisis.
  - *Tyrosinase-positive, type II*—Patients may synthesize various melanin quantities and differ according to the skin color, which can be very light and pale, up to the almost normal color. Slit-lamp examination of the anterior eye segment can show an iris which might be very light but still pigmented, almost normal. The fundoscopic examination may reveal different hypopigmentation level.

- *Ocular albinism* is a form of disease which affects mainly eyes, with less expressed changes in skin and hair. The inheritance is sex related and rarely autosomal recessive. Female carriers are asymptomatic and have regular vision acuity. Most usual signs of disease are the existence of transparent iris parts, scattered depigmentation zones in fundus and changes in macula. Affected men show hypopigmentations in iris and fundus.

DIFFERENTIAL DIAGNOSIS

- Choroideremia,
- Thioridazine intoxication,
- Terminal phase of posterior uveitis,
- Aniridia.

DIAGNOSTICS

The first step in diagnosis is a clinical examination of anterior and posterior eye segment, where one or more signs of disease can be seen. Fundus photography is useful addition for medical documentation. An OCT can show foveal hypoplasia (absence of a regular foveal pit) in both eyes and sometimes a macular schisis. Ocular media are clear and transparent, and the optic nerve is completely regular. The complete absence of healthy, regular macula can be seen and normal foveolar depression cannot be visualized. FAG is not used as a diagnostic tool for albinism (Figs. 20.1 to 20.3).

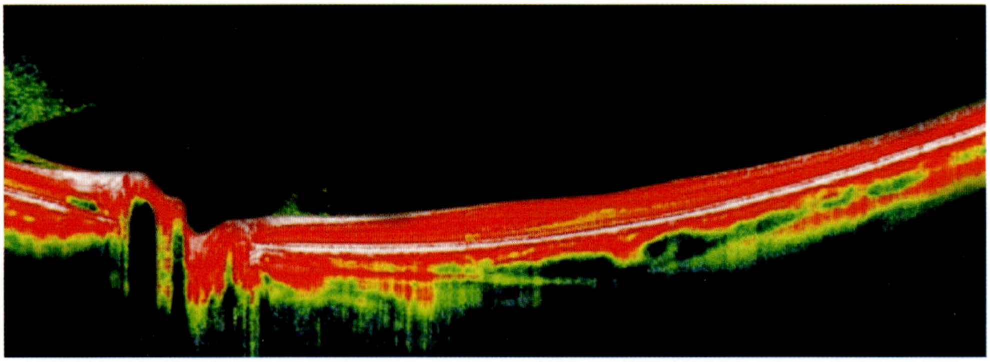

Fig. 20.1: An optical coherence tomography (OCT) B-scan with the sagittal cross-section of macular area and optic disk in 15-year old female patient. Papilla appears regular in this scan, while the expected foveolar depression cannot be visualized. Scanning must be repeated in few sections, with the aim to find macula, because it can also be a scanning error.

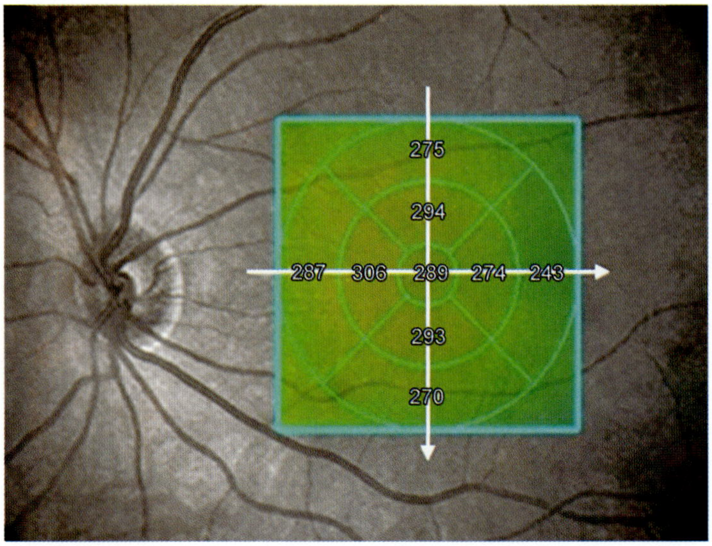

Fig. 20.2: Fundus photograph and map of macular thickness show thickness values, which are uniform and similar in size and show no foveal depression. The fovea is missing and definitely cannot be visualized.

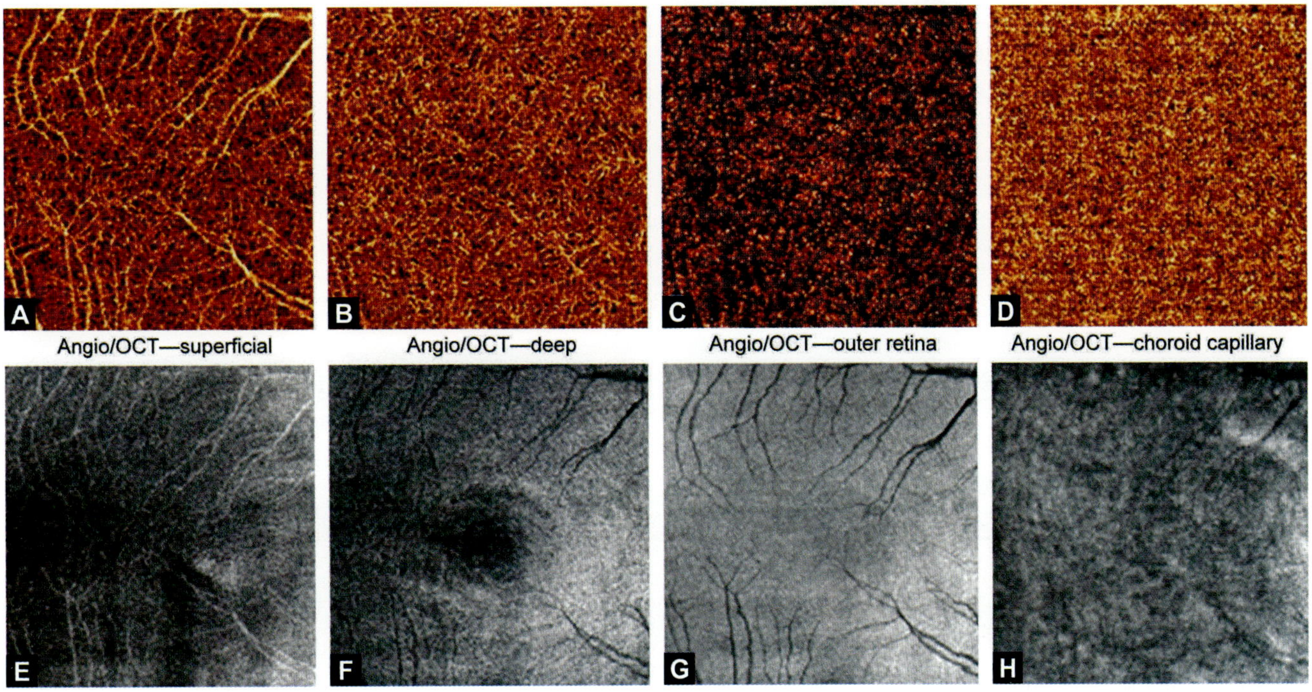

Figs. 20.3A to H: An optical coherence tomography angiography split-spectrum amplitude-decorrelation angiography (OCTA SSADA) protocol and enface optical coherence tomography (OCT) images of corresponding retinal layers in the same eye as in previous Figures (3x3 mm). Upper four images (A to D) show OCT angiography images with superficial and deep vascular plexus, where no regular roundish foveolar avascular zone (FAZ) is visualized. Capillaries seem to be crossing over the central part, where the FAZ usually appears, and form a flat uniform meshwork. Outer retina is avascular, as in normal eyes. Choriocapillary layer seems also physiological. (E to H) Enface OCT figures of matching retinal layers, which seem to be uniform, without central dark area (FAZ). A slightly darker central area can be implied in deep part of inner retina.

TREATMENT

Refractive anomalies, nystagmus, amblyopia and strabismus are treated by ophthalmologist in usual way. There is no a specific treatment for albinism, since it is hereditary condition.

BIBLIOGRAPHY

1. Bazvand F, Karkhaneh R, Roohipoor R, et al. Optical coherence tomography angiography in foveal hypoplasia. Ophthalmic Surg Lasers Imaging Retina. 2016;47(12):1127-31.
2. Benouaich X, Mahieu L, Matonti F, et al. Persistence of foveal capillary plexi in a case of fovea plana evident on OCT angiography. J Fr Ophtalmol. 2017;40(1):4-7.
3. Chong GT, Farsiu S, Freedman SF, et al. Abnormal foveal morphology in ocular albinism imaged with spectral domain optical coherence tomography. Arch Ophthalmol. 2009;127(1):37-44.
4. Costa DL, Zhuang SJ, Donsoff IM, et al. X-linked ocular albinism: Fundus of heterozygous female. Retina. 2003;23(3):410-1.
5. Dolz-Marco R, Phasukkijwatana N, Sarraf D, et al. Optical coherence tomography angiography in fovea plana. Ophthalmic Surg Lasers Imaging Retina. 2016;47(7):670-3.
6. El-Chemaly S, Young LR. Hermansky-Pudlak syndrome. Clin Chest Med. 2016;37(3):505-11.
7. Grønskov K, Jakob EK, Brondum-Nielsen K. Oculocutaneous albinism. Orphanet J Rare Dis. 2007;2:43.
8. Kamaraj B, Purohit R. Mutational analysis of oculocutaneous albinism: A compact review. Biomed Res Int. 2014;2014:905472.
9. Kaplan J, De Domenico I, Ward DM. Chediak-Higashi syndrome. Curr Opin Hematol. 2008;15(1):22-9.
10. Pakzad-Vaezi K, Keane PA, Cardoso JN, et al. Optical coherence tomography angiography of foveal hypoplasia. Br J Ophthalmol. 2016;29.
11. Summers CG. Albinism: Classification, clinical characteristics, and recent findings. Optom Vis Sci. 2009;86(6):659-62.

CHAPTER 21

X-linked Juvenile Retinoschisis

INTRODUCTION

X-linked juvenile retinoschisis (XJR) is a hereditary disease described as vitreoretinal dystrophy, which is characterized by bilateral detachment of neurosensory retina in macular area and periphery. The schisis can occur in different layers of neurosensory retina, most commonly in the nerve fiber layer, inner nuclear layer, outer nuclear layer and outer plexiform layer.

EPIDEMIOLOGY AND ETIOLOGY

X-linked juvenile retinoschisis is a rare genetic disease, with prevalence that ranges from 1 case per 5,000 to 1 case per 25,000 populations. The main cause is mutation of *XLRS1* gene, which is located on X chromosome. The gene is responsible for encoding the protein-retinoschisin, which is crucial in cellular adhesion and interactions within the inner nuclear layer as well as in synaptic connection between photoreceptors and bipolar cells. Since the disease is related to the X chromosome, females are carriers of the mutated gene and males are primarily affected.

SYMPTOMS AND SIGNS

The disease is discovered in early age, most commonly among male children at 5 years or older. Boys complain of difficulties in reading, blurry vision, and they often don't pass the vision acuity test during the basic medical examination before school. Visual acuity can vary and in some cases can be almost regular, while in other, it can range less than 20/200. Usually, children are far-sighted and the visual acuity cannot be corrected. Strabismus and nystagmus can also be associated with the condition. All patients show a maculopathy, which is characterized by the stellate-pattern cystoid changes in macula. Peripheral retinoschisis can be detected in the half of patients. Blood vessels, which are crossing over cystoid changes, are strained and can often burst and bleed, leading to the vitreous hemorrhage. XJR is, after the trauma, the most common cause of vitreous hemorrhage in boys and men of younger age. Women are asymptomatic, although sometimes they can present with mild symptoms and loss of peripheral vision.

DIFFERENTIAL DIAGNOSIS

- Niacin overdose,
- Oculocutaneous albinism and X-linked albinism,
- Chemotherapy (toxic maculopathy),
- Retinitis pigmentosa (Golmann-Favre and other forms),
- Epiretinal membrane and vitreomacular traction syndrome.

DIAGNOSTICS

Clinical examination of macula and retinal periphery is the first step toward diagnosis. Fundoscopic examination can reveal stellate-pattern microcysts in the center or retinal periphery. Fundus photography and optical coherence tomography (OCT) can help in diagnosis of XJR. Fundus photography usually shows transparent anterior ocular media, regular and undamaged optic nerve and circular retinal stretches that accentuate the localization of the macula and foveola. Stellate cystoid cavitations can be seen on both eyes. The optical coherence tomography (OCT) B-scan shows schisis of retina, cystoid changes that are different in size and shape and many consolidated cavitations. They are usually seen in the inner nuclear layer. The outer nuclear layer is thinned and compressed, due to the pressure of large cavities and cysts. Fluorescein angiography (FA) does not aid in the diagnosis of X-linked juvenile retinoschisis. If the doubt in diagnosis still exists, ERG finding with negative-shaped responses helps. DNA sequencing of the *XLRS1* gene can be a useful for a definitive confirmation of XJR.

X-linked juvenile retinoschisis in 15- year old male patient presented by the optical coherence tomography angiography (Figs. 21.1 to 21.4).

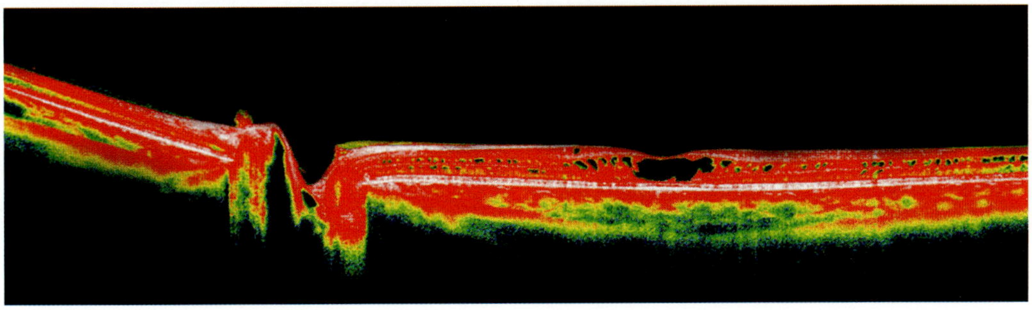

Fig. 21.1: An optical coherence tomography (OCT) B-scan of the macular area and optic nerve. Sagittal cross-section shows multiple microcystic, which are different in size and shape, in the macular center and all along the retinal periphery. They refer to retinoschisis. Cysts are mostly seen in the inner nuclear layer, although they are noticeable also in outer nuclear and plexiform layer. Papilla seems to be regular and PVD can be detected.

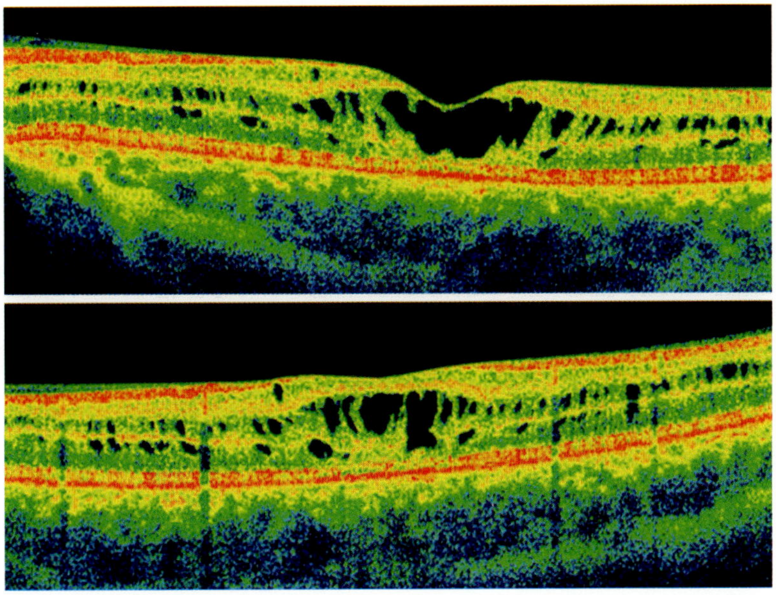

Fig. 21.2: The optical coherence tomography (OCT) B-scan of macular area of the same eye as in previous image, scanned with larger magnification. Sagittal cross-section shows the schisis of retinal tissue and consolidation of cystoid retinal cavities. Most of cysts are found in the inner nuclear layer, although they can also be seen in the outer nuclear layer. There are many fine retinal tissue fibers that are separating cystoid spaces.

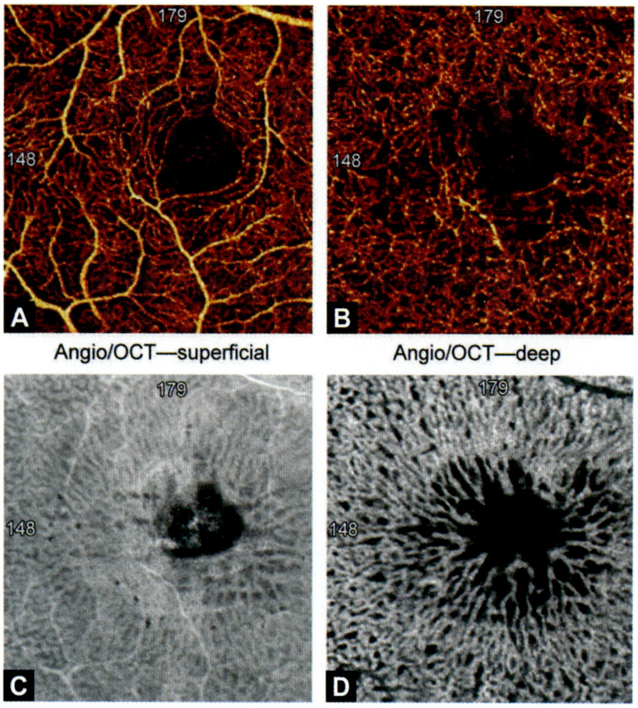

Figs. 21.3A to D: Comparative images of an optical coherence tomography angiography (OCTA) and enface optical coherence tomography (OCT) of superficial and deep vascular plexus, the same eye as in previous Figures (3x3 mm); (A) shows a completely regular superficial capillary network, with a central roundish FAZ and densely arranged capillaries around it; (B) shows the mild irregularities in the deep capillary network. Figure shows many capillary dropouts, along with the enlarged central avascular zone. A mild capillary congestion can also be seen; (C and D) show enface OCT of corresponding retinal layers. Even the superficial part of inner retina shows a mild changes and appearance of the honeycomb. Enface optical coherence tomography (OCT) can very nicely present the X-linked juvenile retinoschisis. It can be noticed that the volume of cysts increases in the deeper part of retina. In the deep layer of inner retina, cavities form a stellate-pattern, due to their symmetric arrangement. This appearance of the enface OCT, which looks like a honeycomb, is a pathognomonic finding for XJR. Angiograms are not specific in diagnosis, due to the fact that superficial plexus may seem regular, while the deep plexus can be mildly altered.

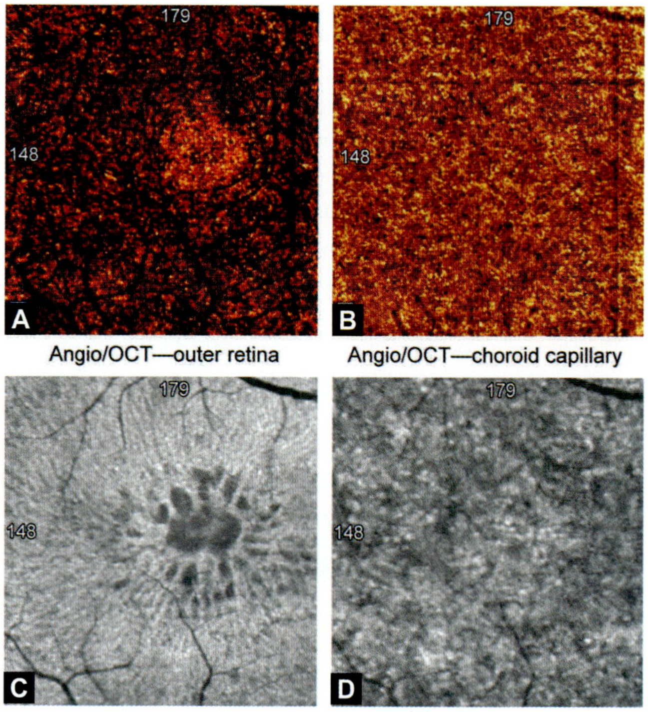

Figs. 21.4A to D: Comparative images of an optical coherence tomography angiography (OCTA) and enface OCT of outer retina and choroid, the same eye as in previous Figures (3x3 mm). (A and B) Angiograms of those two layers show no significant pathological changes. A more visible central vascular projection in the outer retina is an artifact; (C) shows enface OCT of the outer retinal layer, where the specific central stellate-like formation can be seen. (D) shows the enface OCT of choriocapillary layer, which shows no characteristic changes. The finding proves the fact that the schisis occurs mostly in the inner nuclear layer, while the outer retina appears compressed and deformed by the large and consolidated cysts.

TREATMENT

Genetic testing is recommended. Local or oral usage of carboanhydrase inhibitors is recommended for the reduction of the size and number of cystoid changes. However, long-term therapy did not show results. Surgical approach is advised if complications of the disease, such are rhegmatogenous retinal detachment and repetitive vitreous hemorrhages, occur. These conditions represent an indication for vitrectomy. Laser treatment, in the prophylactic purpose, isn't a long-term guarantee that the hemorrhage will not occur. Visual acuity prognosis is poor, due to the progressive maculopathy.

BIBLIOGRAPHY

1. Berenberg TL, Van Tassel SH, Patel SN, et al. Juvenile X-Linked Retinoschisis: A Comparison of Imaging Modalities and Review of Angiographic Findings. Retina. 2016;36(12):e117-9.
2. Chan WM, Choy KW, Wang J, et al. Two cases of X-linked juvenile retinoschisis with different optical coherence tomography findings and RS1 gene mutations. Clin Exp Ophthalmol. 2004;32(4):429-32.
3. Kim JE, Ruttum MS, Koeberl MJ, et al. Genetic and clinical evaluation of juvenile retinoschisis. J AAPOS. 2009;13(2):215-7.

4. Molday RS, Kellner U, Weber BH. X-linked juvenile retinoschisis: clinical diagnosis, genetic analysis, and molecular mechanisms. Prog Retin Eye Res. 2012;31(3):195-212.
5. Renner AB, Kellner U, Fiebig B, et al. ERG variability in X-linked congenital retinoschisis patients with mutations in the RS1 gene and the diagnostic importance of fundus autofluorescence and OCT. Doc Ophthalmol. 2008;116(2):97-109.
6. Salvatore S, Fishman GA, Genead MA. Treatment of cystic macular lesions in hereditary retinal dystrophies. Surv ophthalmol. 2013;58:560-84.
7. Staffieri SE, Rose L, Chang A, et al. Clinical and molecular characterization of females affected by X-linked retinoschisis. Clin Exp Ophthalmol. 2015;43(7):643-7.
8. Stanga PE, Papayannis A, Tsamis E, et al. Swept-Source Optical Coherence Tomography Angiography of Paediatric Macular Diseases. Dev Ophthalmol. 2016;56:166-73.
9. Swept-Source Optical Coherence Tomography Angiography of Pediatric Macular Diseases. Dev Ophthalmol. 2016;56:166-73.
10. Tsang SH, Vaclavik V, Bird AC, et al. Novel phenotypic and genotypic findings in X-linked retinoschisis. Arch Ophthalmol. 2007;125(2):259-67.
11. Yu J, Ni Y, Keane PA, et al. Foveomacular schisis in juvenile X-linked retinoschisis: an optical coherence tomography study. Am J Ophthalmol. 2010;149(6):973-8.

CHAPTER 22

Radiation Retinopathy

INTRODUCTION

Radiation retinopathy is a predictable and often radiation dose-dependent complication following exposure to any type of radiation including external beam and plaque brachytherapy. Specifically, it occurs after external beam radiation as a method of treatment for nasopharyngeal, paranasal sinus, or orbital tumors, where there is limited protection for the eyes, and it can often lead to clinically significant radiation retinopathy. Plaque brachytherapy in the treatment of intraocular tumors can also cause severe damage to the immediate retina and choroid. The time of onset of radiation retinopathy is between 6 months and 3 years. However, it has been known to occur earlier or later.

EPIDEMIOLOGY AND ETIOLOGY

Ocular damage from radiation treatment is a well-established phenomenon. The incidence of the radiation retinopathy is not well known. Many factors are now known to influence the incidence of radiation retinopathy, including total dosage and daily fraction size. Patients who are diabetic, hypertensive, have vascular diseases, are pregnant, or have previously been subject to chemotherapy are more susceptible to radiation retinopathy. It is considered that more than 50% of patients with radiation as the treatment of choice for the eye, orbit, neck, nasopharyngeal, or paranasal sinus develop radiation retinopathy. One study reported 50% of patients developed retinopathy following 60 grays of radiation while another report showed a rise in incidence to 85–95% in those exposed to 70–80 grays. Plaque brachytherapy for the treatment of choroidal melanoma within 5 mm of the macula is a great risk for the development of radiation retinopathy. The risk for radiation retinopathy increases with radiation dosage increasing more than 4,500 rad (45 Gy). The total dose of radiation, along with the fraction size is important in the development of retinopathy. A reported safe dose is 3,000 rads/30 gray, 1,000 rads/10 gray per week in five fractions (200 rads/2 gray per session), although cases have been reported using even lower doses of radiotherapy. Exposure to radiation is thought to cause preferential loss of vascular endothelial cells with a relative sparing of the pericytes. It is hypothesized that differential sensitivity between endothelial cells and pericytes is the result of direct exposure of the endothelial cells to high ambient oxygen and iron found in the blood which generates free radicals and leads to cell membrane damage. The retinal ischemia from areas of retinal nonperfusion ultimately leads to macular edema, neovascularization, vitreous hemorrhage, and tractional retinal detachment.

SYMPTOMS AND SIGNS

Patients with early or mild retinopathy may be asymptomatic. Pathologic changes in the macula cause vision decreasement. Severe radiation retinopathy includes the following pathologic features: retinal microaneurysms, retinal hemorrhages, retinal telangiectatic vessels, retinal hard exudates, macular edema, cotton-wool spots, retinal neovascularization, vitreous hemorrhage, and tractional retinal detachment. Other associated features may include optic disk edema, neovascularization of the iris, neovascularization of the angle, and neovascular glaucoma. Radiation retinopathy may sometimes look like an ischemic optic neuropathy, and occurs usually in younger patients with no history of hypertension.

DIFFERENTIAL DIAGNOSIS

- Diabetic retinopathy
- Central retinal vein occlusion
- Human immunodeficiency virus (HIV) retinopathy
- Leukemia
- Coagulopathy
- Coats' disease
- Ischemic optic neuropathy
- Optic neuritis.

DIAGNOSTICS

Radiation retinopathy is a clinical diagnosis involving symptoms of ischemic retinopathy or papillopathy with anamnestic data of radiotherapy. Clinical examination shows many retinal hemorrhages, microaneurysms, telangiectasia, cotton and hard exudates, macular edema, and optic disk edema. The neovascularization of the optic disk and iridocorneal angle are also possible. The optical coherence tomography (OCT) is useful for the diagnosis and management of the macular edema and also monitoring benefits of the therapy. Fluorescein angiography (FAG) is the diagnostic method which determines retinal ischemia due to nonperfusion, optic disk edema, and the neovascularization. Optical coherence tomography angiography (OCTA) can also provide information of the retinal ischemia, and can also visualize neovascularizations (Figs. 22.1 to 22.3).

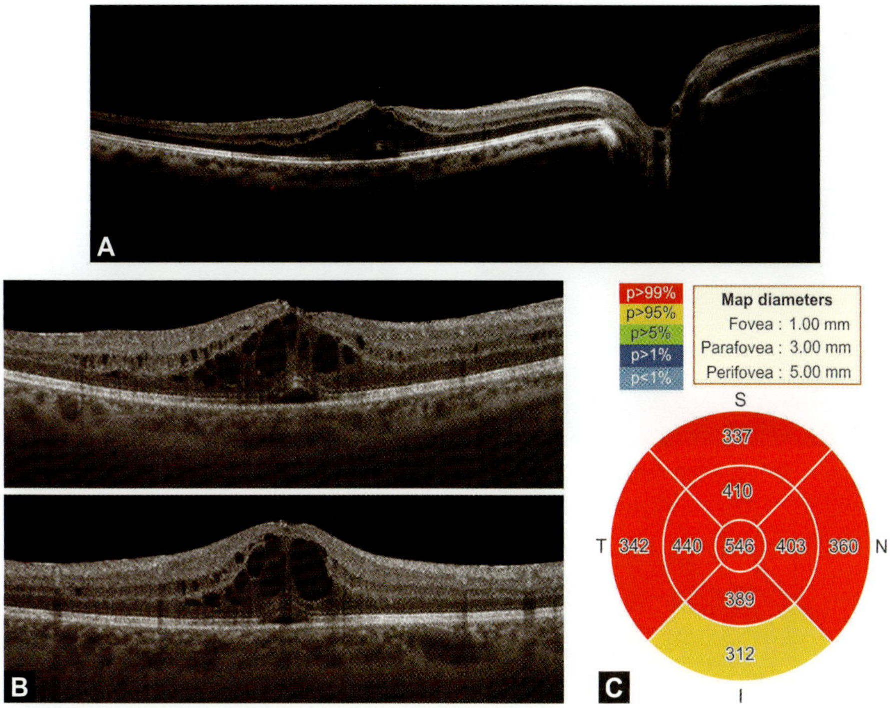

Figs. 22.1A to C: (A and B) An OCT B-scan of the macula and optic disk in a 52-year-old female patient, 4 months after external brachytherapy of a neck neoplasma. The image demonstrates CME and initially, small exudative subretinal detachment with subretinal fluid; and (C) Retinal thickness map shows almost all segments with an increased values of macular thickness (red and yellow colors indicate a significant edema). (CME: cystoid macular edema; OCT: optical coherence tomography)

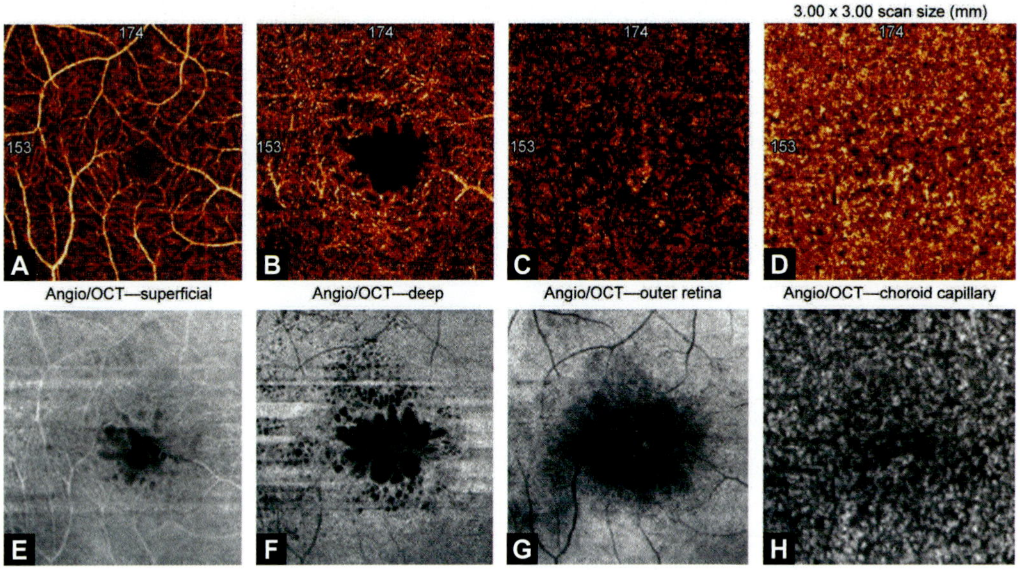

Figs. 22.2A to H: An OCTA SSADA protocol (3 × 3 mm) and en face OCT of the corresponding retinal layers of the same eye as depicted in previous Figure. (A) Angiography of superficial part of retina shows no significant changes. (B) Typical changes are visible in the deep part of the inner retina, both in angiography; (C) Outer part of retina shows no neovascularization; (D) Angiography of the choroid capillary shows normal structure without neovascularization and (F) in en face OCT image. Angiography shows the irregular shape of the FAZ which corresponds to a cystic "dropout" zone without vascularization. A mild congestion and anastomoses are visible in the deep vascular plexus; and (E and G) Additionally, en face OCT also demonstrates cystic, hyporeflective, petal-like changes in central macula, both in superficial part and outer retina. (H) En face OCT of choroid capillary shows no significant changes. (FAZ: foveolar avascular zone; OCTA: optical coherence tomography angiography; SSADA: split-spectrum amplitude-decorrelation angiography)

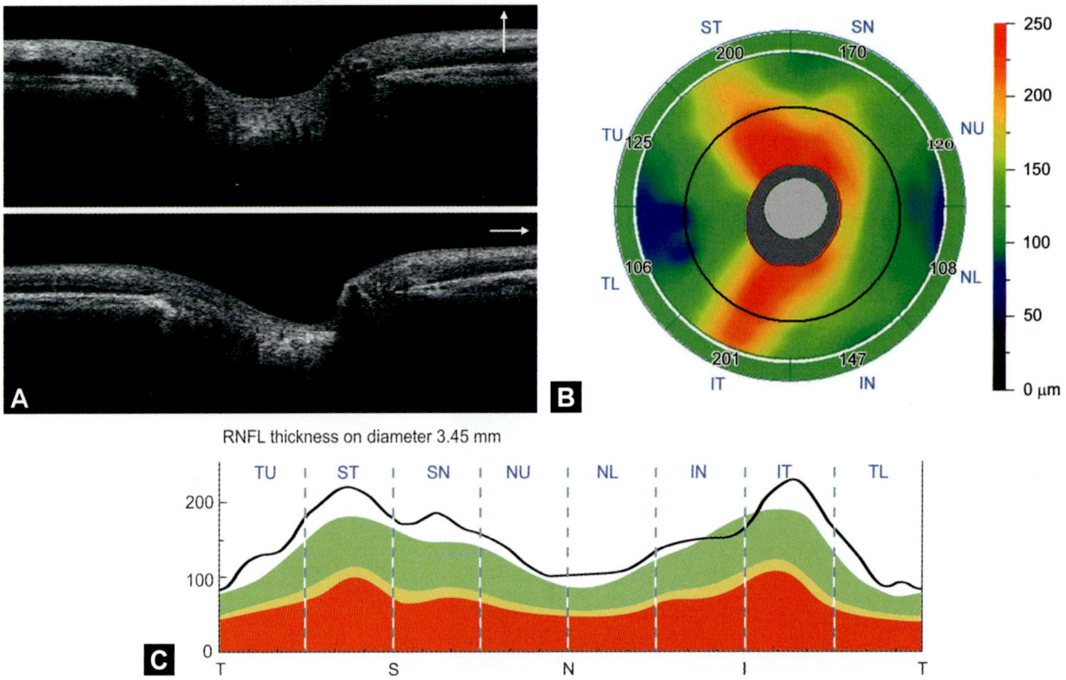

Figs. 22.3A to C: (A) An OCT B-scan of the optic disk with a cross-section of the large blood vessels at the edge of the optic disk; (B) Figure presents an overview of the RNFL thickness, which is shown by a map dividing the papillary circumference into segments. RNFL shows increased values in all of them; and (C) Graphically shows the thickness of RNFL (its thickness is represented by the black sinusoidal line). All the values are above the normal, green zone representing the increasement of RNFL thickness and papillary edema, due to the radiation. (RNFL: retinal nerve fiber layer; OCT: optical coherence tomography)

THERAPY

Therapy is similar to the treatment of diabetic retinopathy and includes laser photocoagulation, an intravitreal injection of corticosteroids or antivascular endothelial growth factor (anti-VEGF), and pars plana vitrectomy. No special treatment is recommended for moderate radiation retinopathy. Progressive and severe radiation retinopathy must be regularly examined. Patients with nonproliferative radiation retinopathy have visual acuity around 20/50 for many years (up to 4 years). If macular edema appears, grid or focal laser treatment is recommended, as well as in diabetic macular edema. Anti-VEGF therapy or intravitreal injection of corticosteroids can be off-label treatment, as it is not confirmed by clinical studies. Follow-up studies reported that anti-VEGF treatment, which is used in patients with ocular melanoma in a year after the radiation, reduces the risk of radiation retinopathy. The retinal ischemia ultimately leads to macular edema, neovascularization, vitreous hemorrhage, and tractional retinal detachment. Neovascularization is a result of the retinal ischemia and can be prevented by panretinal photocoagulation (PRP). Patients with proliferative changes in anterior or posterior part of an eye have much serious, complicated, and poorer prognosis, with the vision acuity less than 20/200 over the period of 6 years.

BIBLIOGRAPHY

1. Finger PT, Chin KJ, Semenova EA. Intravitreal anti-VEGF therapy for macular radiation retinopathy: a 10-year study. Eur J Ophthalmol. 2016;26(1):60-6.
2. Finger PT, Kurli M. Laser photocoagulation for radiation retinopathy after ophthalmic plaque radiation therapy. Br J Ophthalmol. 2005;89(6):730-8.
3. Grange JD. Radiation-induced retinopathy. J Fr Ophthalmol. 2001;24(9):993-1003.
4. Levitz LM. The use of optical coherence tomography to determine the severity of radiation retinopathy. Ophthalmic Surg Lasers Imaging. 2005;36(5):410-1.
5. Li M, Qiu G, Luo W, et al. Clinical investigation of radiation retinopathy fundus and fluorescein angiographic features. Yan Ke Xue Bao. 1999;15(3):183-6.
6. Mendrinos E, Pilly B, Baglivo E, et al. Chorioretinal anastomosis as a rare complication of radiation retinopathy. Acta Ophthalmol. 2009;87(4):473-5.
7. Reichstein D. Current treatments and preventive strategies for radiation retinopathy. Curr Opin Ophthalmol. 2015;26(3):157-66.
8. Spaide RF, Borodoker N, Shah V. Atypical choroidal neovascularization in radiation retinopathy. Am J Ophthalmol. 2002;133(5):709-11.
9. Sánchez-Vicente JL, Muñoz-Morales A, Galván-Carrasco MP, et al. Radiation maculopathy treated with intravitreal bevacizumab. Arch Soc Esp Oftalmol. 2017;92(6):283-6.
10. Zahir F, Tahri H. Radiation retinopathy. Pan Afr Med J. 2015;22:54.

CHAPTER 23

Glaucoma

INTRODUCTION

Glaucoma stands for a group of various eye diseases that have a few things in common—damage of the optic nerve, narrowing and loss of the visual field, increased ocular pressure, and ultimately loss of vision and blindness. The significance and importance of the features offered by optical coherence tomography (OCT) and OCT angiography (OCTA) are unquestionable in all macular and retinal diseases. This gives hope that modern technology could soon be used to estimate vascular peripapillary dropout and optical disk flow in glaucoma patients. This would be a great scientific breakthrough because fluorescence angiography (FAG) has virtually no diagnostic role in glaucoma syndrome, also resulting in better therapeutic results for patients suffering from this disease, as it would ensure early recognition and diagnosing.

The dense capillary network around the disk can be identified and quantified by the RTVue-XR Avanti (Optovue, Fremont, CA USA) software using the software split-spectrum amplitude-decorrelation angiography (SSADA). An ophthalmologist that uses SSADA protocol does not only have access to the angiographic system but also a system that provides a deep penetration and high resolution that clearly identifies previously unreachable elements inside and around the optic nerve head. The AngioVue system allows visualization of an extremely rich and dense vascular net around and in the optic disk that we were not aware even existed until now. Previously, this vascular network was not detectable by FAG.

The capillary vascular network is located just beneath the nerve fiber layer or is mixed with it. It is believed that these blood vessels have a role in nerve nutrition. The correlation between the damage of the capillary net around the disk and glaucoma development has been proven. In cases of glaucoma progression, the peripapillary vascular network can be extremely damaged. In moderate cases of glaucoma, loss of peripapillary flow may occur in one and/or several quadrants around the optic disk.

The discovery of dynamic bloodstream inside the optic disk is also very interesting. The AngioVue system allows the ophthalmologist to observe the rich capillary network inside the disk itself in healthy patients. Earlier, it was thought that the center of the disk contains only nerve fibers. Nowadays, it is known that in a healthy eye, the capillary vessel layer is balanced and uniform both inside and around the disk. In patients with glaucoma, in comparison to healthy eyes, vascularization within the disk itself is also reduced. With the increased resolution of this system, a mesh-like structure called lamina cribrosa can now also be visible. OCTA provides a clear visualization of the structure, arrangement, and size of the pores of lamina cribrosa. Many glaucoma patients have pores with a definite and regular shape; however, the pores can also be enlarged and curved. They are usually thicker and stretched to the side of the papilla excavation.

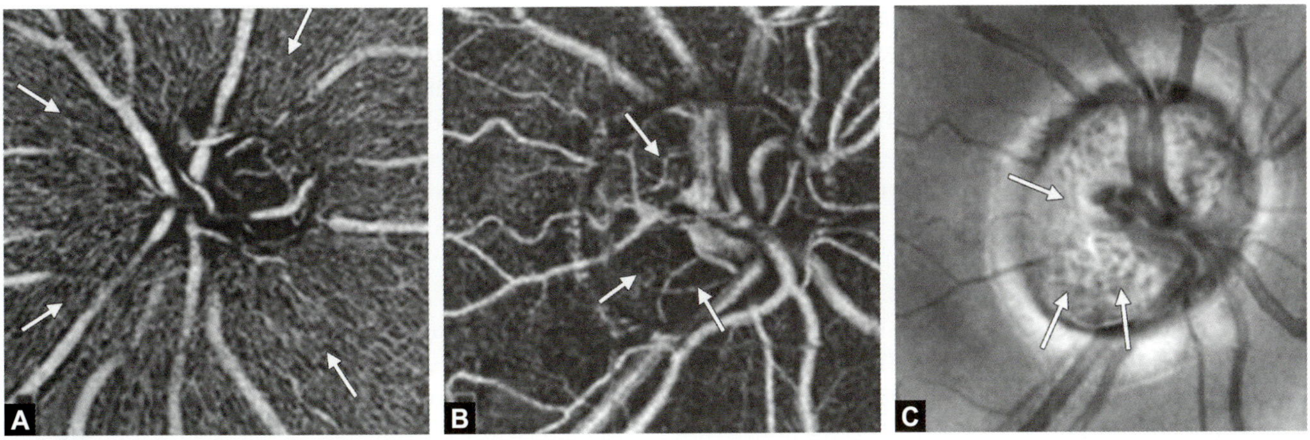

Figs. 23.1A to C: Optical coherence tomography angiography (OCTA) of the optic disk papilla. (A) The arrows indicate a dense superficial peripapillary capillary network around the optic disk head; (B) The arrows indicate a dense capillary network inside the optic disk head. (C) Enface optical coherence tomography (OCT). Large and stretched pores of the lamina cribrosa in a patient with glaucoma are indicated by the arrows. Pores are enlarged and stretched to the side of the papilla excavation.

The AngioVue system offers exceptional possibilities of blood flow analysis inside the optic disk, peripapillary blood flow, and also the size, shape, and number of pores of the lamina cribrosa. OCTA is becoming an important diagnostic tool for the detection and monitoring of glaucoma patients as well as in the very comprehension of the disease pathophysiology.

Comparison of the capillary network density (with OCTA) and other available diagnostic procedures [visual field, estimation of ganglion cell complex, PNO indexes, retinal nerve fiber layer (RNFL) thickness] contributes to easier defining of the stage of glaucoma development.

There are three areas of interest, which are particularly important when analyzing the glaucoma changes shown with OCTA protocol:

1. Peripapillary capillary network analysis
2. Blood flow inside the optic disk
3. Size and shape of lamina cribrosa pores (Figs. 23.1A to C).

ANALYSIS OF PERIPAPILLARY CAPILLARY NETWORK BY OCTA

Optical coherence tomography angiography protocol clearly shows the density, arrangement, and symmetry of the capillary network around the optic disk. Areas with a damaged vascular net or areas without vascular flow are very easily seen as dark regions without capillaries. In some patients with an atrophic optic papilla, no flow in the peripapillary capillary network is visible. In regions with a thinned or damaged RNFL, no flow can be detected. Since vascular reduction is a common and pathognomonic sign for the glaucoma syndrome, it is always necessary to simultaneously analyze the thickness of the RNFL as well as the thickness of ganglia cell complex (GCC) and its atrophy.

Based on these facts, glaucoma patients can be divided into three groups:

1. A group of patients with suspected glaucoma or patients with ocular hypertension with a dense peripapillary vascular network and without any reduction or changes in vascular flow. There are no changes in RNFL thickness, thickness of GCC, and not in the functional visual field test. There is no structural or functional damage to the papilla or peripapillary area.
2. A group of patients with initial or moderate changes due to glaucoma with localized vascular reduction that corresponds to the loss of RNFL in the analogous part of the papilla. The GCC and visual field test show no significant changes or may show incipient to moderate changes.
3. A group of patients with severe glaucoma progression, large areas of flow reduction or the complete loss of capillary blood flow. There is usually a fine vascular peripapillary dropout all around the papilla as well as loss of circulation inside the optic disk head.

It should be emphasized that the changes in capillary blood flow or any deviation in OCTA findings must be compared with the classic fundoscopy findings, map of RNFL thickness, changes in the GCC, and functional visual field test. It is very common for patients with the initial stage of glaucoma not to have a single segment or quadrant of RNFL damaged, to not have any changes in the GCC or any visible scotomas in the visual field test.

Patients with moderate glaucoma usually present with decreased RNFL thickness, initial changes or atrophy of the GCC, and visual field loss that corresponds to defects in the localized peripapillary part.

Patients with severe glaucoma present with serious reduction of peripapillary blood flow with an analogous significant decrease of RNFL thickness in all parts of the optic nerve, fully expressed parapapillary atrophy (PPA), and withdrawal of retinal pigment epithelium (RPE) as well as the atrophy and loss of GCC. The visual field test can show many scotomas or significant arcuate scotomas, hemianopsia, and altitudinal defect.

General experience shows a strong correlation between the blood flow and the quality of the peripapillary capillary network and the rate of glaucoma development. The results suggest a vascular etiology of glaucoma development. It has a particular importance and has given positive results in the diagnostics and monitoring of low-tension glaucoma, normotensive glaucoma, and ischemic ocular neuropathy. Further studies and clinical trials are necessary in order to prove a statistical correlation between flow index values, vascular flow densities, and avascular areas in glaucoma patients. The future development of the AngioAnalytics of the peripapillary capillary network of blood flow within the disk and segmental blood flow is greatly relied upon. This type of analysis is still in the experimental phase and is not available for commercial use in everyday practice.

OPTIC DISK VASCULARIZATION

Optical coherence tomography angiography precisely shows capillary flow inside the optic disk and is able to localize and visualize lamina cribrosa. Changes in the capillary plexus in the optic disk are analyzed in the same way and according to the same criteria as the peripapillary capillary network. Whether it is a healthy eye or one with a mild glaucoma, a regular or reduced capillary flow in the small blood vessels inside the disk is visible. In en face OCTA, the peripapillary blood network and papillary blood flow are not at the same level, as the papilla anatomy and lamina cribrosa itself. According to present findings, the vascular capillary networks around and inside the disk have a significant and leading role in nerve nutrition. In moderate and severe glaucoma, the loss of gentle capillaries inside and around the optic disk is equal and it usually follows one another. However, OCTA merely provides material depicting the flow inside and around the disk subject to assessment by the observer's eye. An objective analysis will be possible after the AngioAnalysis of blood flow inside and around the disk is available for commercial use. Estimating capillary flow density and accurately identifying the location and size of the region without flow will provide new insight into the assessment of damage and the development of disease as well as in monitoring the progression of disease and the success of the treatment.

Optical coherence tomography angiography has fully demonstrated and justified its quality in the clinical practice of macular diseases. In the case of glaucoma, OCTA is a precise diagnostic tool that allows the estimation of blood flow in the optic nerve head and in peripapillary area. The connection between glaucoma disease and the changes in capillary networks inside and around the disk is very clear. These findings and disease are confirmed by changes in the RNFL thickness, thinning and atrophy of GCC, and by changes in the visual field test. The ophthalmologist should be very careful when analyzing angiography because large blood vessels can make it difficult and mask the condition of a gentle surface capillary network. The importance of qualitative and quantitative estimation of the peripapillary capillary network, vascularization inside the optic nerve head and appearance of the lamina cribrosa pores leads OCTA into a daily practice tool useful for early detection and monitoring of changes in glaucoma patients (Figs. 23.2A to F).

GLAUCOMA

The eye with/without various conditions of glaucoma is described below.

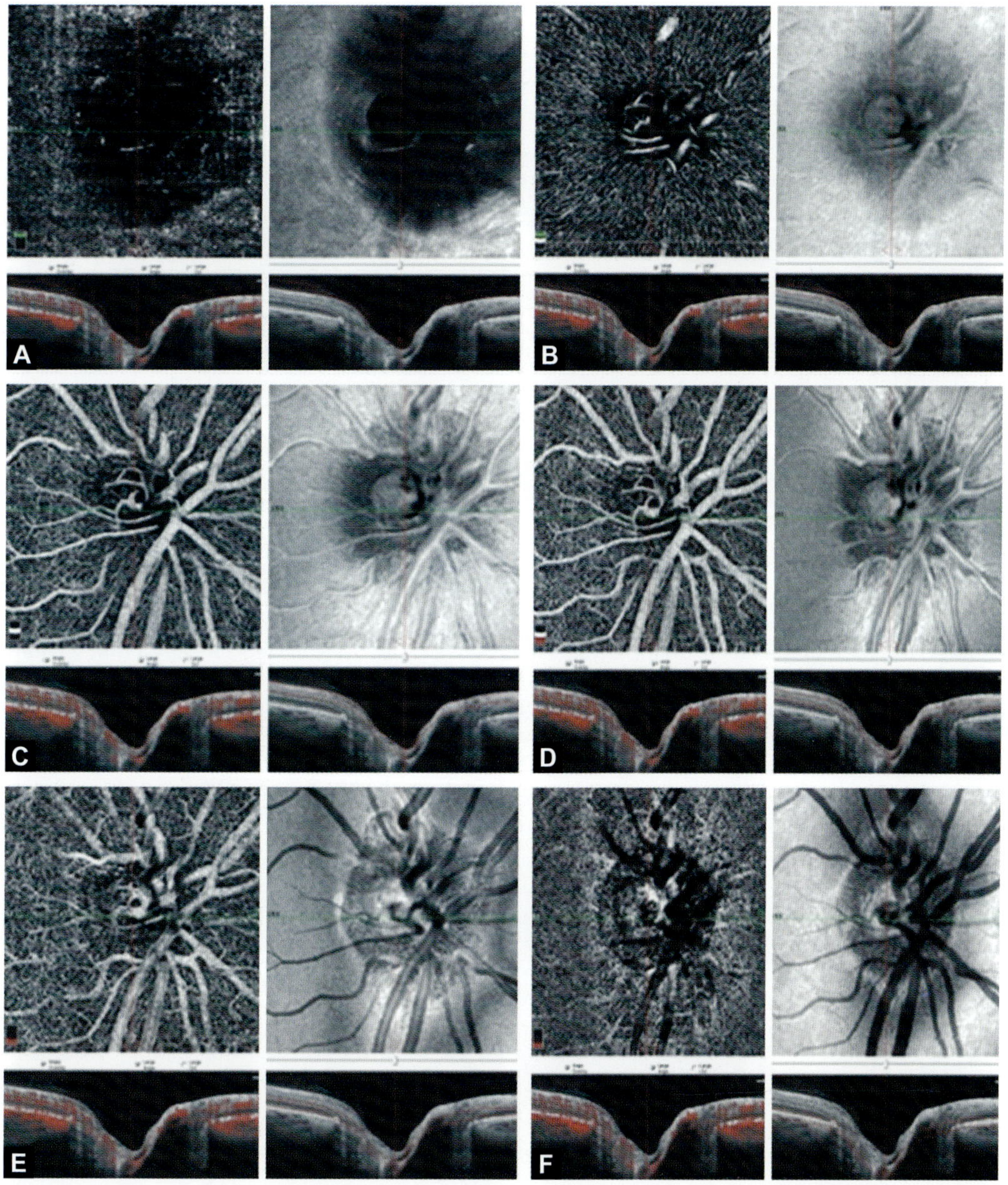

Figs. 23.2A to F: Images of optical coherence tomography angiography (OCTA) and enface optical coherence tomography (OCT) show the importance of selecting the right depth of the observed tissue layer in order to obtain a correct angiographic picture of the parapapillary region in a completely healthy eye. (A) Angiography shows no signs of capillary flow in vitreous, but enface OCT implies the existence of papilla. Details are not visible; (B) OCTA, if observed in level of ILM (inner-limiting membrane), angiographically shows no important results, whereas enface OCT shows a clear contour of the papilla. These two layers (A and B) have no clinical significance except emphasizing the importance of selecting the proper thickness and depth of analyzed tissue; (C) Observation of OCTA finding in the retinal nerve fiber layer (RNFL) demonstrates angiography in which a fine, symmetrical, and gentle capillary network can be seen along with parts of large blood vessels. It is a layer where retinal nerve fibers are mixed with the superficial capillary network. Enface OCT shows papilla and large blood vessels presenting with blurry and unclear edges; (D) The OCTA of the internal vascular layer shows a regular and neat vascular network with numerous thin and delicate capillaries. Large blood vessels are seen throughout this mesh capillary network. Enface OCT shows the optic papilla with fine, sharp edges, central excavation, and properly branched large blood vessels; (E) OCTA of the outer capillary layer demonstrates an almost identical dense, regular, and symmetrical capillary net. Enface OCT shows a papilla with sharp borders, visible excavation, and regular large blood vessels; (F) The image of OCTA shows a deep retinal layer in level of photoreceptors and retinal pigment epithelium (RPE). Large blood vessels and dense meshed capillary network are visible without vascular dropouts. The image is accompanied by an enface OCT with very bold papilla edges and large blood vessels.

Healthy Eye without Glaucoma Presented with OCTA (Figs. 23.3 and 23.4)

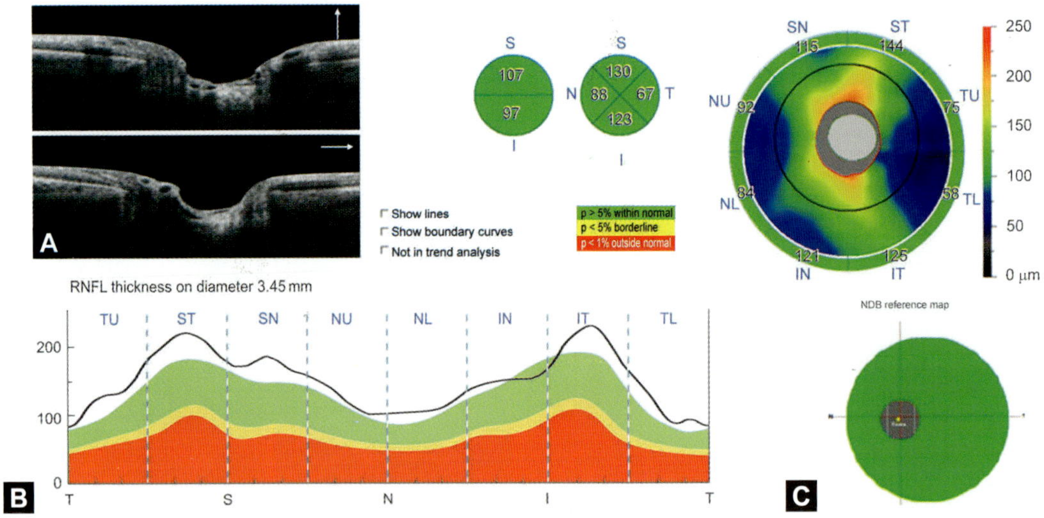

Figs. 23.3A to C: (A) An optical coherence tomography (OCT) B-scan of the optic nerve papilla and the different methods for retinal nerve fiber layer (RNFL) thickness presentation. On the left side of the image is a B-scan of a regular papilla with sections of large blood vessels on the edges of the excavation. In the middle part of the image an overview of the RNFL thickness is shown by a map divided into quadrants and in the right part of the image RNFL thickness is also shown, but by a map dividing the papillary circumference into segments. RNFL shows physiological values. (B) It graphically shows the thickness of RNFL (its thickness is represented by the black line that completely fits the green sinusoidal zone in this patient). (C) Ganglia cell complex (GCC) map—the map is colored green, which means there is no thinning or atrophy of the ganglion cell layer and that the finding is physiological.

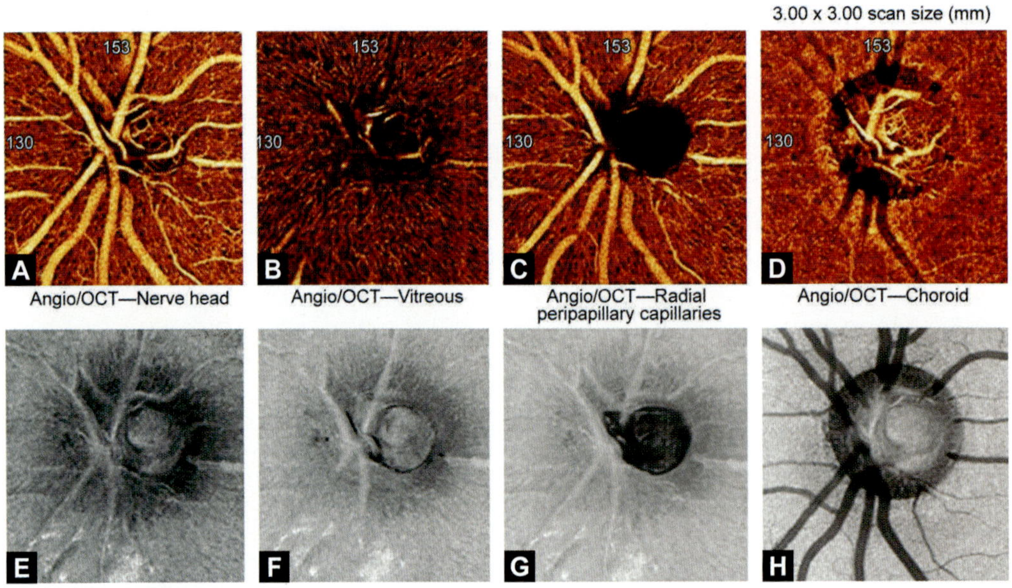

Figs. 23.4A to H: Comparative optical coherence tomography angiography (OCTA) and en face OCT images (3 × 3 mm) of the peripapillary and papillary region by layers. In figures A to D, angiography of these regions is presented. A capillary network at the level of the optic nerve head (A), vitreous (B), the radial peripapillary capillary layer (C), and in the choroidal layer (D) is shown. A neat, densely meshed peripapillary capillary network, with no vascular dropouts, and flow breaks is seen as well as large blood vessels coming out of the papilla. Inside the nerve head smaller meshed tiny capillaries are also visible. Figures E to H show the en face OCT of the papillary and peripapillary regions of the optic nerve. A regular papilla is seen with all its normal anatomical characteristics and large blood vessels. (H) shows the lamina cribrosa with its regular pores and large blood vessels.

Eye with Mild Glaucoma Presented with OCTA (Figs. 23.5 and 23.6)

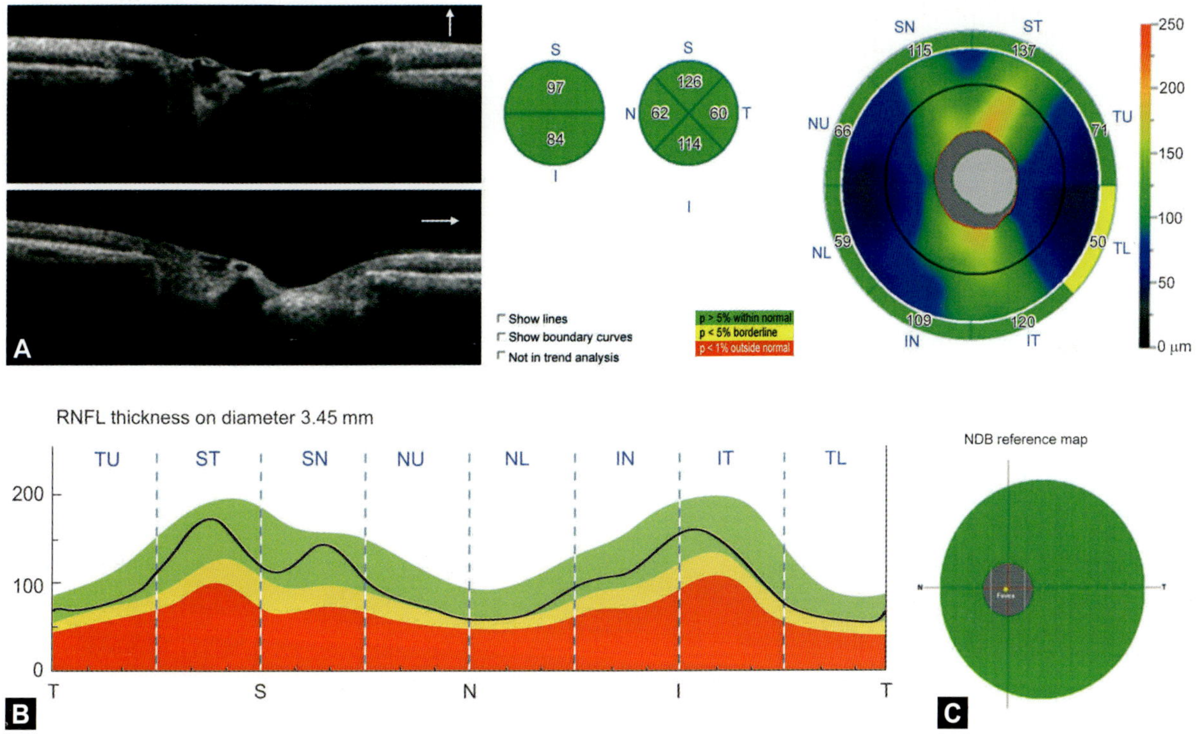

Figs. 23.5A to C: (A) An optical coherence tomography (OCT) B-scan of the optic nerve papilla and retinal nerve fiber layer (RNFL) thickness maps. On the left part of the image, a B-scan of a perfectly normal papilla with large blood vessels at the edges of excavation is shown. In the middle part of the image an overview of the RNFL thickness is shown by a map divided into quadrants, depicting physiological values. However, the right part of the image shows a slight RNFL thinning in the temporal segment of the papillary circumference. (B) Graphically shows the thickness of RNFL with the same localization of thinning. (C) The ganglia cell complex (GCC) map shows no pathological changes but a completely physiologically green color on the eye with incipient glaucoma.

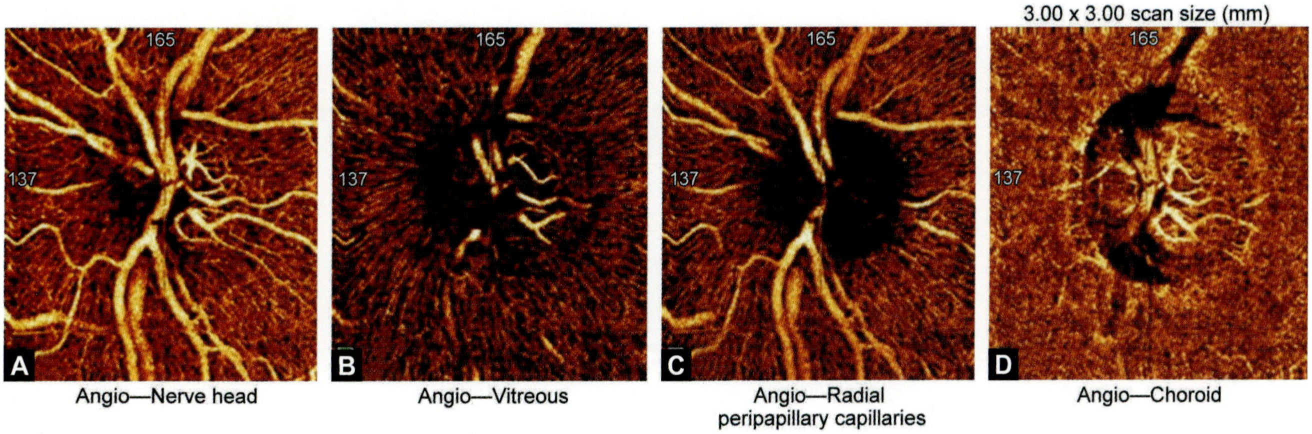

Figs. 23.6A to D: An optical coherence tomography (OCTA) of the optic nerve papilla (3 x 3 mm). Vascularization in the optic nerve head is regular (A). In the vitreous layer the vascularization is normal (B). In the radial peripapillary capillaries layer there are no vascular dropouts (C). Choroid has normal structure (D).

Eye with Moderate Glaucoma Presented with OCTA (Figs. 23.7 and 23.8)

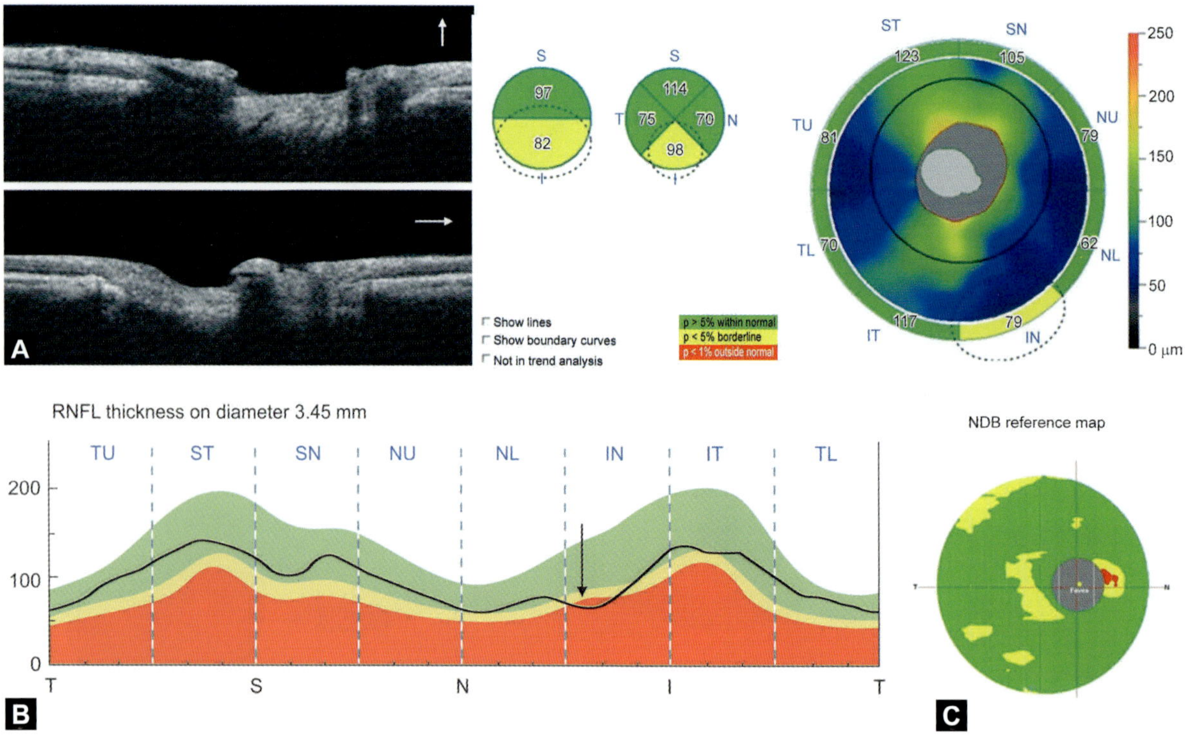

Figs. 23.7A to C: An optical coherence tomography (OCT) B-scan of the optic nerve papilla and retinal nerve fiber layer (RNFL) thickness values (A). On the left side of the image, a small neat papilla with cross-sections of large blood vessels on its edges is visible. In the middle and right part of the image, RNFL thickness maps are presented. In both maps, the inferior parts show slightly decreased RNFL thickness values. Even Figure (B), in which the graph shows the black line moving from the green to the red zone (to the zone of RNFL atrophy), corresponds to the findings explained in Figure A, also pinpointing the zone of thinning in the inferior-nasal part. (C) The ganglia cell complex (GCC) map presents ganglion cell thickness. In this map, small yellow areas seen on the green background can be interpreted as initial signs of the deterioration of the ganglion cell layer in the eye with moderately developed glaucoma.

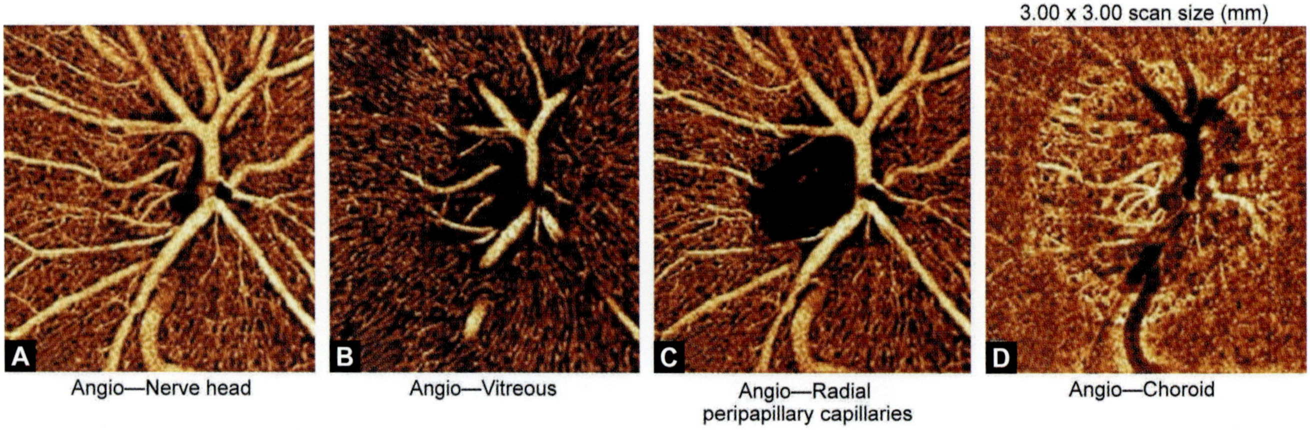

Figs. 23.8A to D: An optical coherence tomography angiography (OCTA) of the optic nerve papilla (3 x 3 mm). There are no major changes in vascularization of optic nerve head (A). Vascularization in layer of vitreous is normal (B), as well as in the layer of radial peripapillary capillaries (C). Choroid has normal structure (D). The angiography finding cannot be declared as pathological in a patient with moderate glaucoma.

Eye with Severe Glaucoma Presented with OCTA (Figs. 23.9 to 23.19)

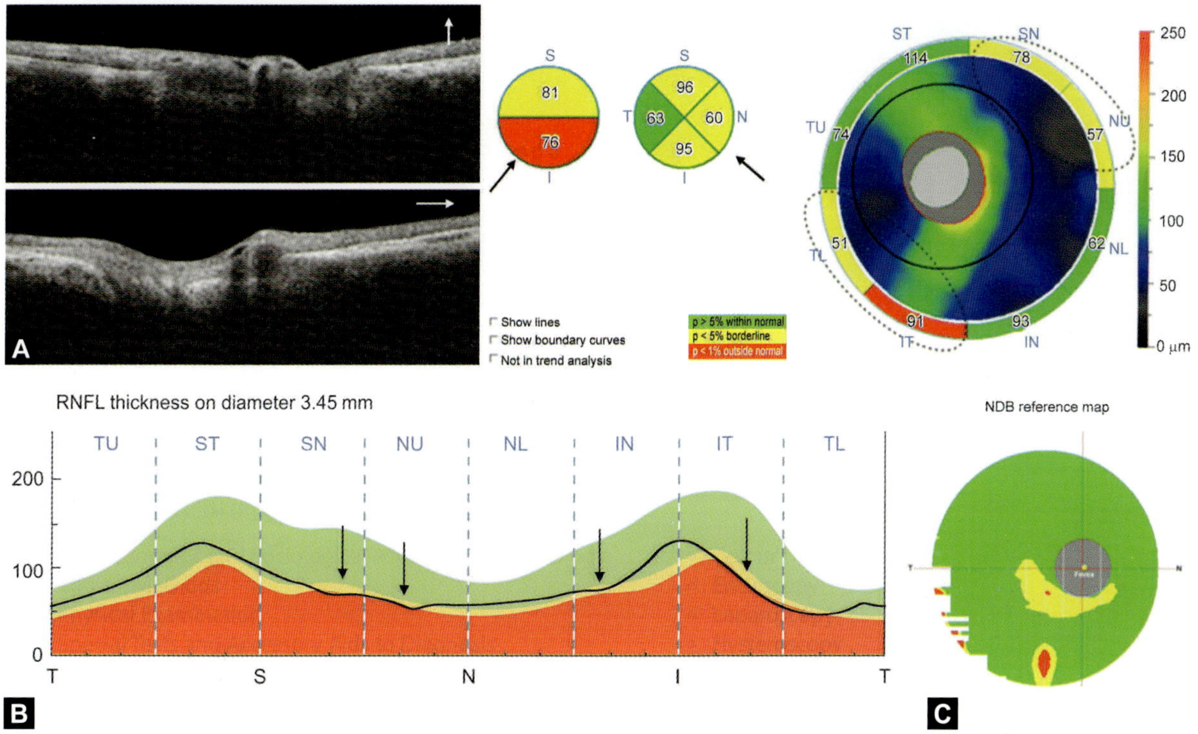

Figs. 23.9A to C: An optical coherence tomography (OCT) B-scan of the optic nerve papilla and retinal nerve fiber layer (RNFL) thickness maps. On the left side of the image, a small excavated papilla with the cross-sections of large blood vessels is visible. In the middle part of the image, a RNFL thickness map divided by quadrants shows decreased thickness values in all parts (A). The RNFL thickness map on the right side of the image shows similar changes, but the values are especially decreased in the nasal and temporal segments. (B) Shows the graph with the black RNFL thickness line, which is located in the yellow–red parts for nearly its entire length, indicating loss and atrophy of RNFL. (C) shows the ganglia cell complex (GCC) map. Inside the yellow areas, there are smaller red areas (atrophy!).

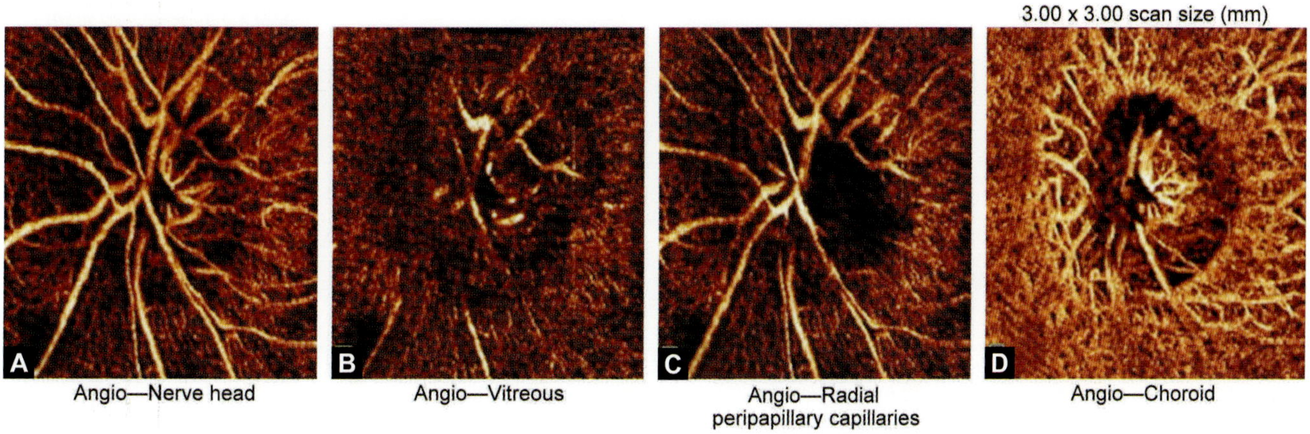

Figs. 23.10A to D: There are vascular drop-outs in all layers of the optic nerve head (A). In the vitreous layer there are drop-outs in inferior and nasal parts (B). In the radial peripapillary capillary layer we see loss of symetry and disappeared capillaries, the localization of ischemic areas corresponds to retinal nerve fiber layer (RNFL), thickness decrease (C). Choroid has normal structure (D).

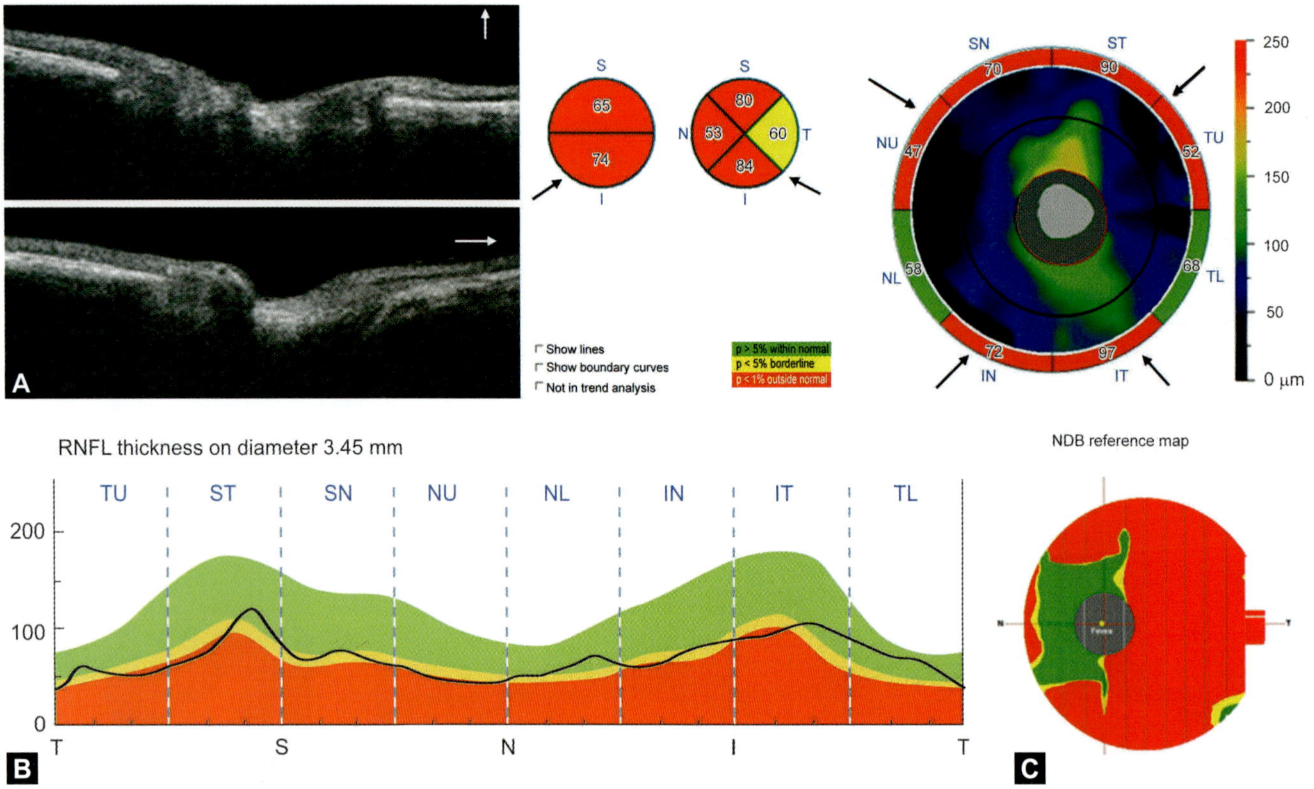

Figs. 23.11A to C: (A) An optical coherence tomography (OCT) B-scan of the optic nerve papilla and retinal nerve fiver layer (RNFL) thickness maps. On the left side of the image, a cross-sectional view of the papilla is shown. The right side of the image shows decreased values of RNFL thickness in all quadrants and in all segments of the papilla circumference. (B) Graphically shows the atrophy of RNFL, where the RNFL thickness line is located in the red and yellow zones all along its course, demonstrating its decreased values. (C) The ganglia cell complex (GCC) map shows clear atrophy of the ganglion cell complex (almost the entire map is colored in red). Only a small nasal area is not affected.

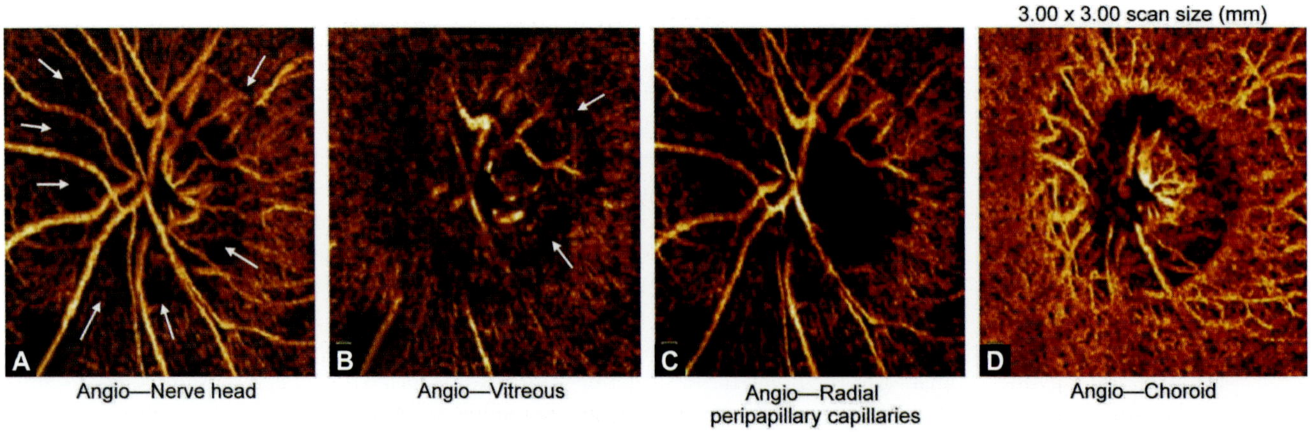

Figs. 23.12A to D: An optical coherence tomography angiography (OCTA) (3 x 3 mm), the same eye as in Figure 23.11. In the optic nerve head angiography we see vascular drop-outs (white arrows) (A). In the vitreous layer we can also see some drop-outs (white arrows) (B). In the peripapillary capillary layer we see drop-outs in nasal and inferior segments (C). Choroid has altered structure (D).

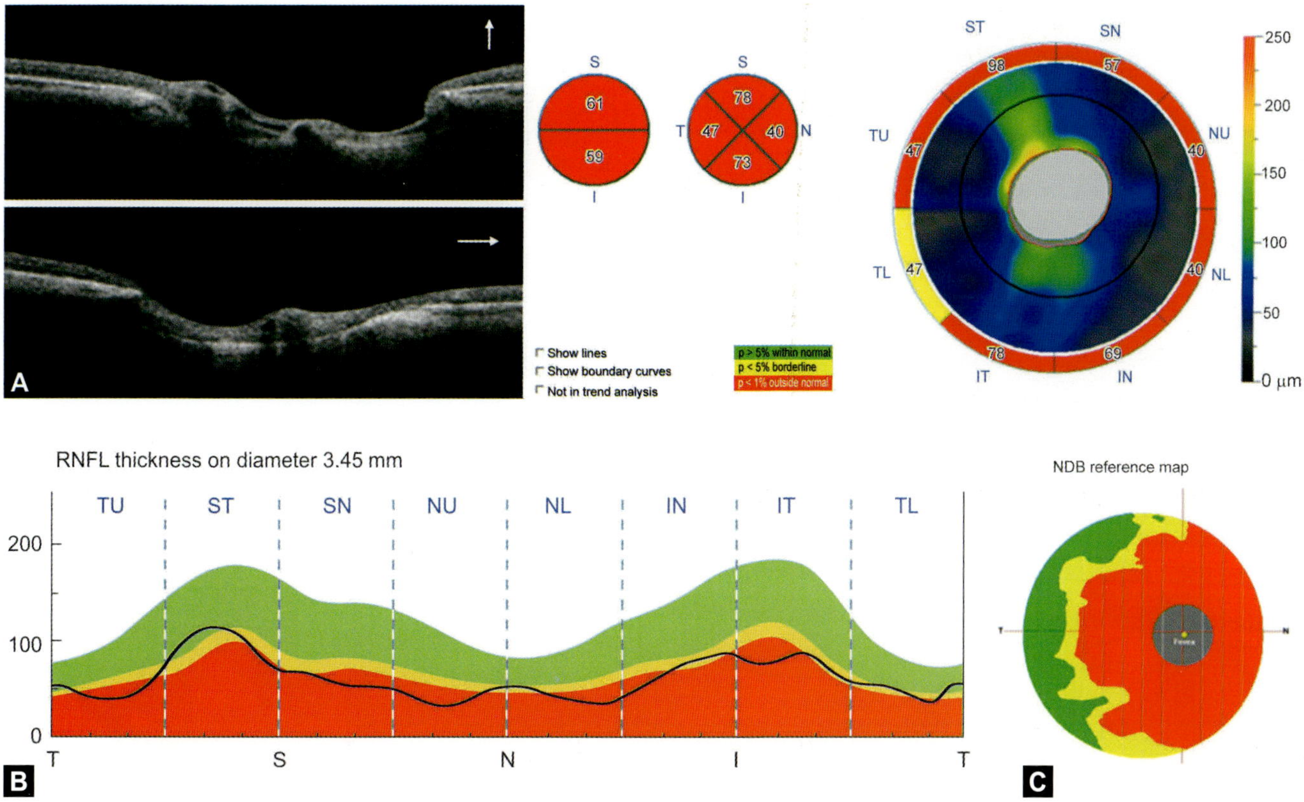

Figs. 23.13A to C: (A) An optical coherence tomography (OCT) B-scan of the optic nerve papilla and retinal nerve fiber layer (RNFL) thickness maps. On the left side, a B-scan of a widely excavated papilla affected by glaucoma is shown. Sections of large-blood vessels are barely visible. In the middle and right parts of the picture, RNFL thickness maps are presented. The red color is prevalent in all quadrants and segments of papilla circumference. This represents decreased values of RNFL thickness. (B) Graphically shows the RNFL thickness represented by a black line. It can be concluded that there is significant RNFL atrophy caused by severe glaucoma. (C) Represents the thinning and atrophy of the ganglia cell complex (GCC) layer (yellow and red colors on the map).

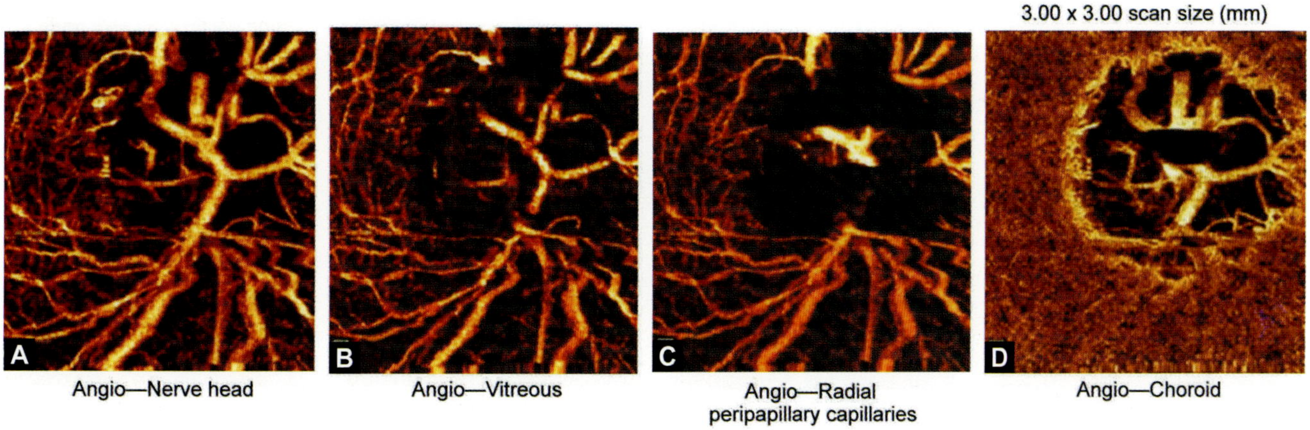

Figs. 23.14A to D: An optical coherence tomography angiography (OCTA) (3 x 3 mm) of the same eye as in Figure 23.13. The apperance of the papilla is altered and the edges have lost their proper shape (A). Vascluar drop-outs are present in the vitreous layer (B). A fine, regular and meshed capillary network is completely lost in all peripapillary segments (C). Choroid has altered structure (D).

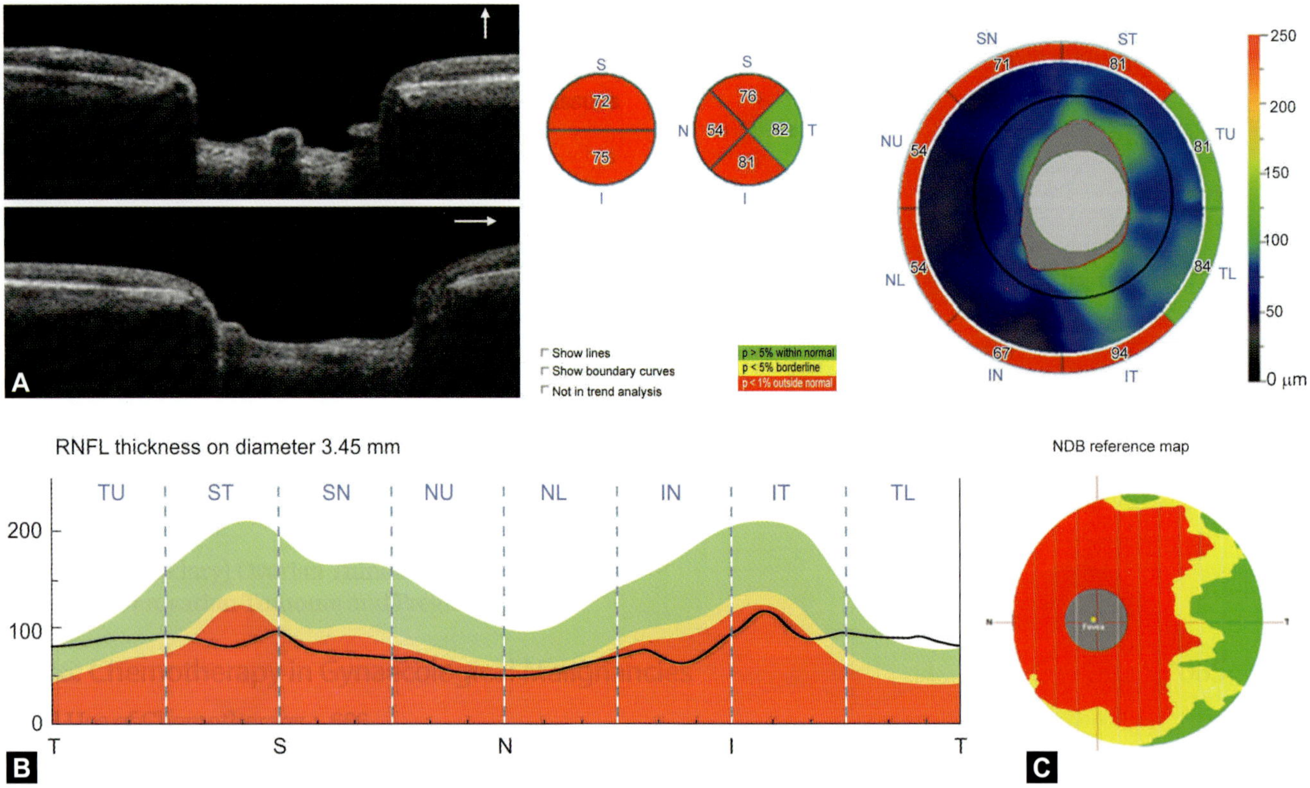

Figs. 23.15A to C: (A) An optical coherence tomography (OCT) B-scan of the optic nerve papilla and retinal nerve fiber layer (RNFL) thickness maps. The left side of the image shows a B-scan of a papilla affected by glaucoma. Glaucomatous excavation is visible and the condition is furthermore affirmed by RNFL thickness maps on the right side of the image. The RNFL maps show thinning and atrophy in all parts of the papilla, except temporally. (B) Graphically shows the thickness of the RNFL, where the atrophy of the superior, nasal, and inferior fiber parts is visible (S, N, I). (C) Ganglia cell complex (GCC) map—thinning and atrophy of the GCC are indicated by the yellow and red color.

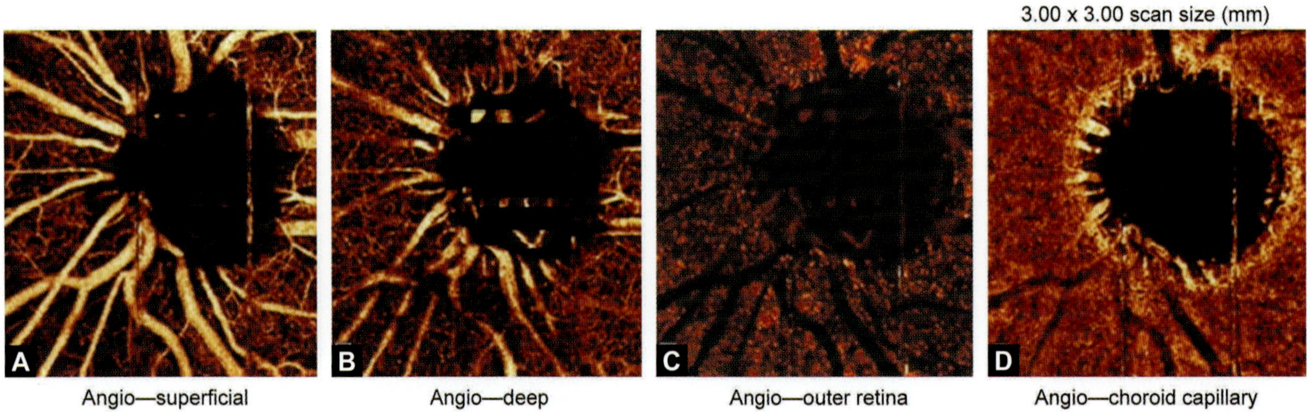

Figs. 23.16A to D: An optical coherence tomography angiography (OCTA) (3 x 3 mm) of the same eye as in Figure 23.15. There are many vascular drop-outs in the optic nerve head (A). In the deep vascular layer drop-outs are shown (B), as well as in outer retina layer (C). Choroid has changed structure (D).

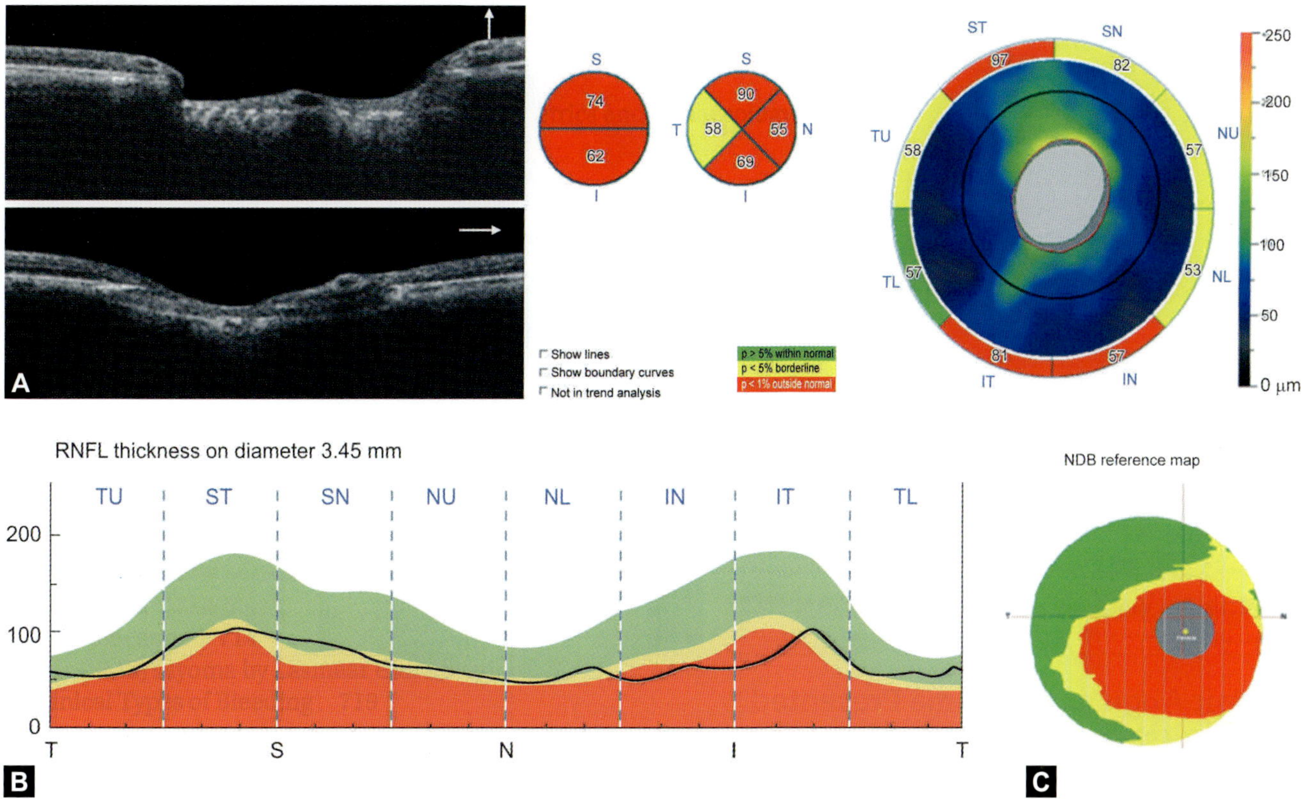

Figs. 23.17A to C: (A) An optical coherence tomography (OCT) B-scan of the optic papilla and retinal nerve fiber layer (RNFL) thickness maps in an eye with severe glaucoma. On the left part of the image, the B-scan of the glaucomatous excavated papilla is presented. The right part of the image shows RNFL thickness values by maps. Decreased values are seen both in the map divided by quadrants and in the map divided by the circumference segments of the papilla. Only the temporal parts of the fibers, although at the lower limit, are still within referential values. (B) Shows the RNFL thickness graph, which completely matches the finding in Figure A. (C) Ganglia cell complex (GCC) map—a big red area surrounded by a yellow ring is shown, representing the thinning and atrophy of the ganglion cell layer.

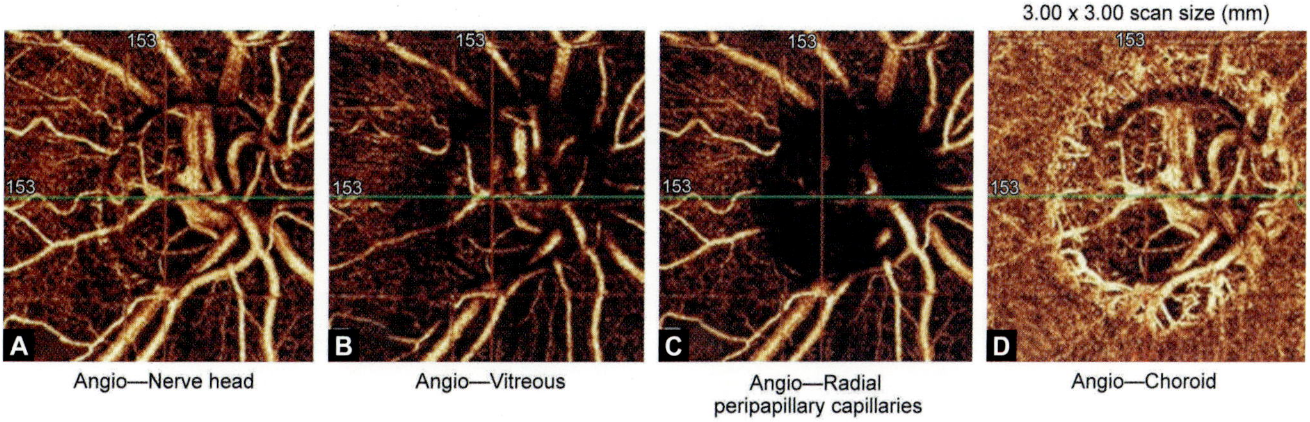

Figs. 23.18A to D: An optical coherence tomography angiography (OCTA) (3 x 3 mm) of the same eye as in Figure 23.17. The blood flow in the optic nerve head is deteriorated (A). There are many drop-outs in the vitreous layer (B). In the radial peripapillary capillary layer we see deterioration in all segments corresponding to the retinal nerve fiber layer (RNFL) atrophy shown in Figure 23.17A (C). In the choroid we see drop-outs (D).

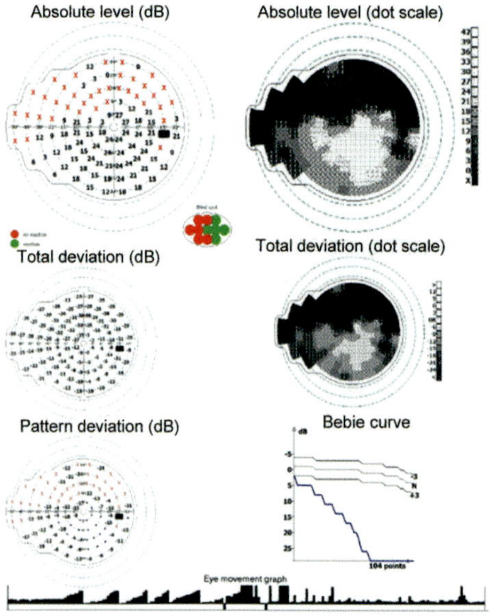

Fig. 23.19: The functional visual field test, the same eye as in previous pictures. The test shows an altitudinal defect in the visual field caused by the severe form of glaucoma.

Chronic Angular Glaucoma Presented by OCTA (Figs. 23.20 to 23.23)

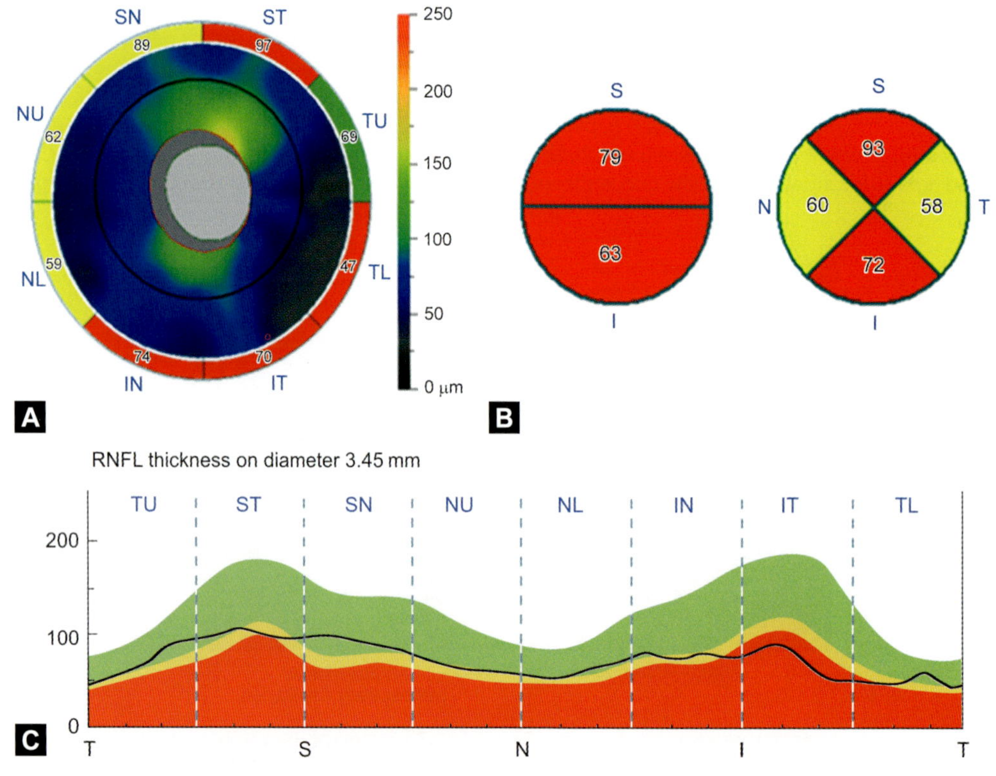

Figs. 23.20A to C: (A and B) Decreased values of retinal nerve fiber layer (RNFL) thickness, presented by the map with quadrants and with the circumference segments of the papilla. (C) The sinusoidal graph also shows decreased values of RNFL thickness; the black sinusoidal RNFL line spreads along the yellow and red zone.

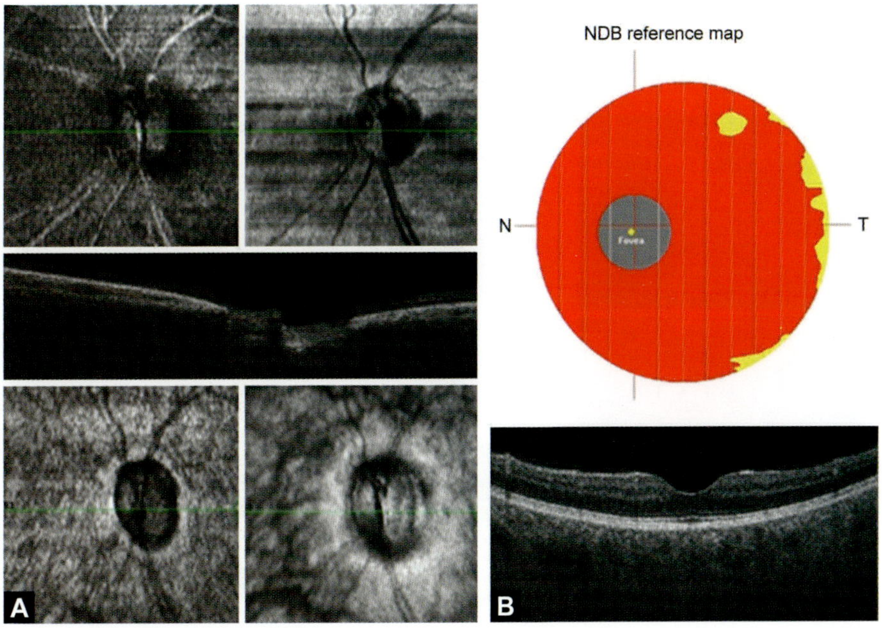

Figs. 23.21A and B: (A) The en face optical coherence tomography (OCT) of the optic disk papilla of the same eye as in the previous image. Large blood vessels and papillary atrophy are presented in all layers. (B) Ganglia cell complex (GCC) map, measured in the fovea, is fully colored in red, representing ganglion cell complex atrophy.

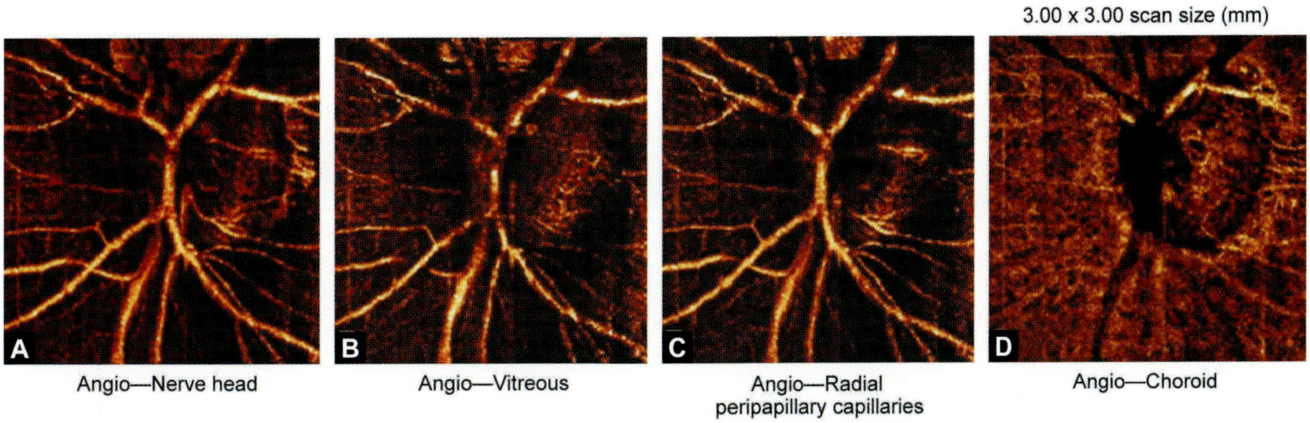

Figs. 23.22A to D: Optical coherence tomography angiography (OCTA) (3 x 3 mm) of patinet with chornic angular glaucoma. Many drop-outs in optic nerve head (A). Circumferential loss of capillaries in the vitreous layer (B). Dark peripapillary areas of dropouts in radial peripapillary capillary layer (C). There are some drop-outs in the choroid (D).

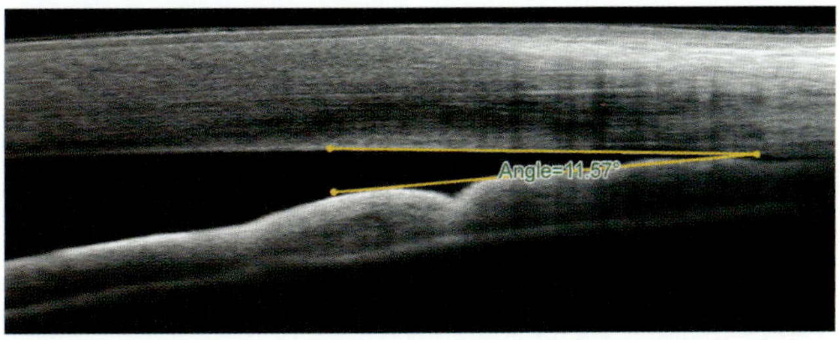

Fig. 23.23: The anterior chamber presented by anterior segment optical coherence tomography (AS-OCT). The narrow, but opened (11.57°) anterior chamber is visible.

Secundar Post-traumatic Glaucoma Presented by OCTA (Figs. 23.24 to 23.26)

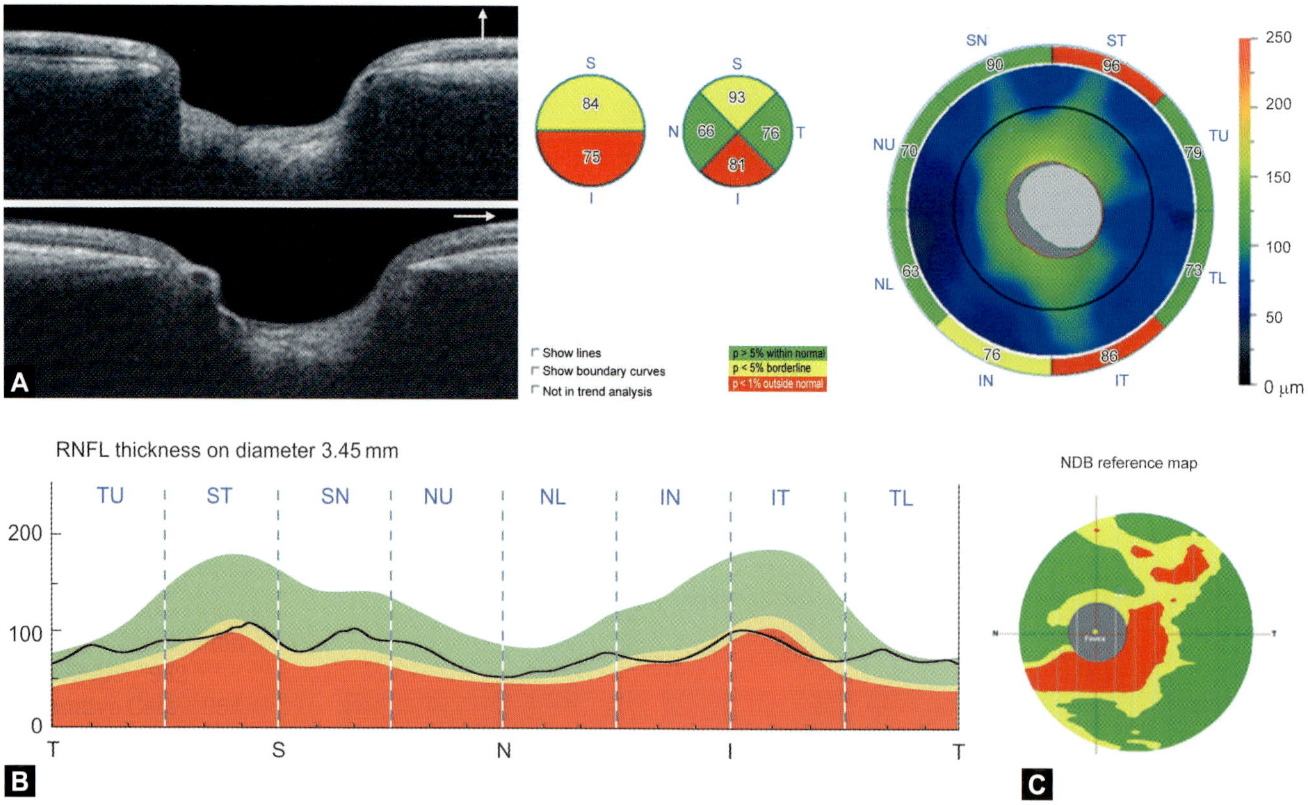

Figs. 23.24A to C: (A) An optical coherence tomography (OCT) B-scan of the papilla along with the retinal nerve fiber layer (RNFL) thickness maps in a patient that experienced a contusion of the bulbus 2 years ago. The image shows a sagittal scan of the papilla and decreased values of RNFL thickness in the inferior and superior parts of the papillary circumference. The sinusoidal RNFL thickness graph on Figure B corresponds to the changes in thickness shown in Figure A. (C) The ganglia cell complex (GCC) thickness map shows a few red areas, which are surrounded with a yellow zone, indicating the atrophy and thinning of the ganglion cell layer.

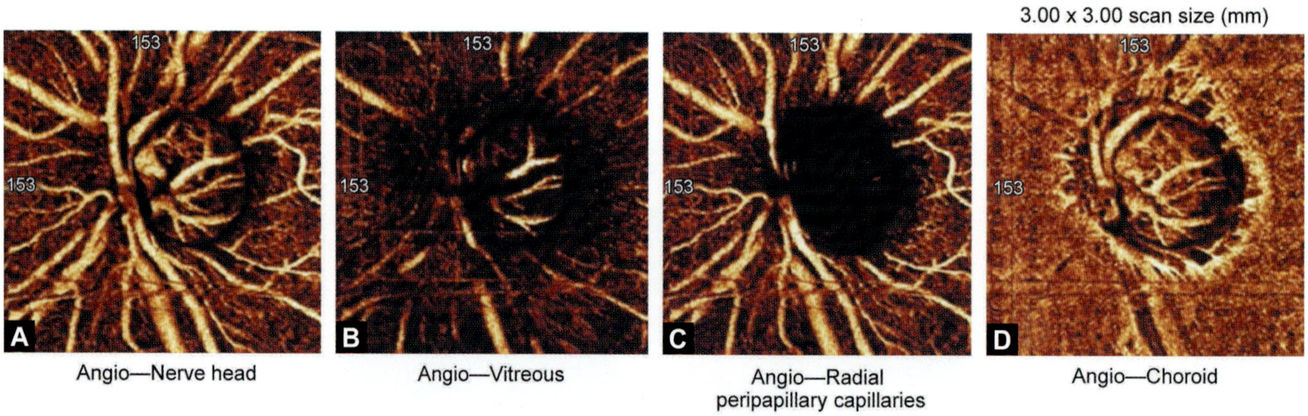

Figs. 23.25A to D: The optical coherence tomography angiography (OCTA) of the papilla in a patient with secondary post-traumatic glaucoma (3 x 3 mm). There are partial drop-outs in the optic nerve head (A). In the vitreous layer there are some drop-outs (B). In the radial peripapillary capillary layer we see drop-outs in the superior and inferior region (C). Choroid has normal structure (D).

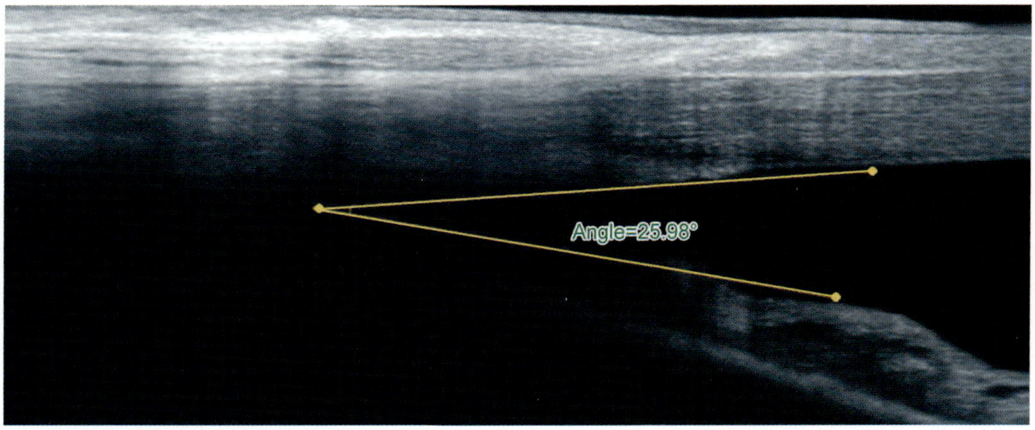

Fig. 23.26: The anterior chamber presented by anterior segment optical coherence tomography (AS-OCT). The patient has an open angle, 25.98° wide.

Congenital Glaucoma Presented by OCTA (Figs. 23.27 and 23.28)

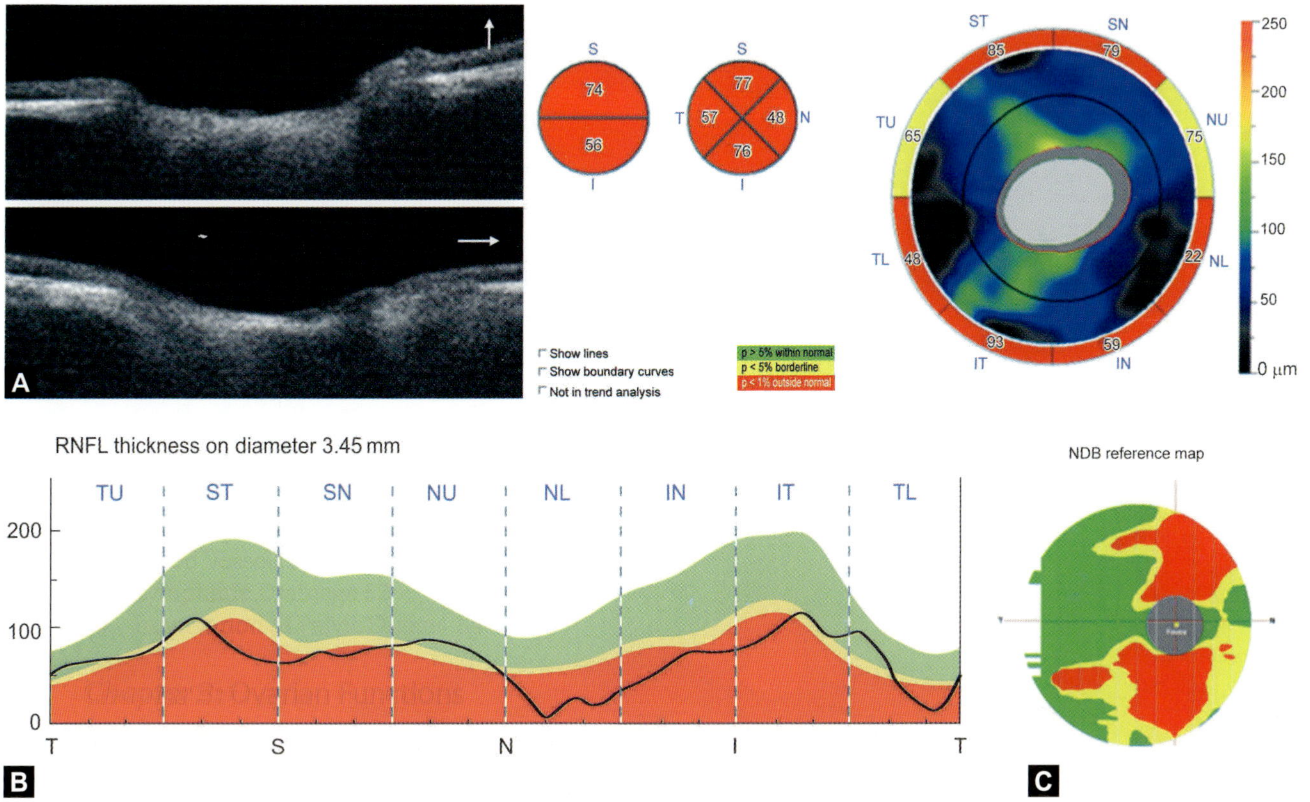

Figs. 23.27A to C: (A) The left part of the image shows an optical coherence tomography (OCT) B-scan of the papilla in a 15-year-old patient. The patient has congenital glaucoma that was operated at the age of 4 months. The visual acuity with –8.0 diopters is 0.6 (20/30). On the right part of the image, maps of retinal nerve fiber layer (RNFL) thickness are presented with a predominate atrophy. Every quadrant and almost every circumference segment is colored in red, pointing the decreased values of the RNFL thickness. (B) The graphic representation of RNFL thickness matches the findings in the Figure A. (C) Shows the ganglia cell complex (GCC) thickness. There are a few areas in GCC map colored in yellow and red, which correspond to the thinning and atrophy of the ganglion cell layer.

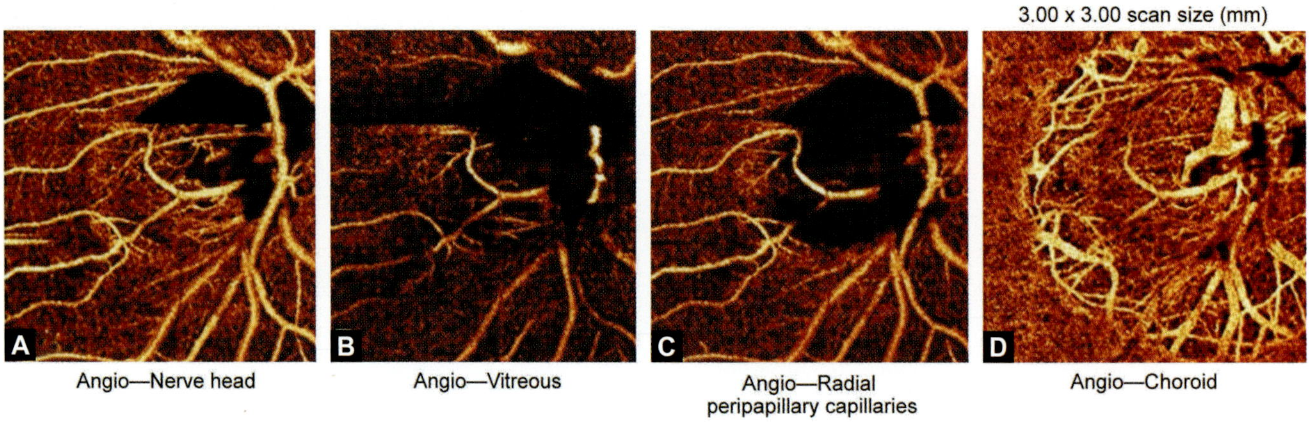

Figs. 23.28A to D: The optical coherence tomography angiography (OCTA) (3 x 3 mm) of patient with congenital glaucoma. A big, bizzare papila with unclear edges (A). The picture of vitreous layer shows altered structure (B). In the radial peripapillary capillary layer there is complete loss of tiny capillary network (C). The choroid layer has altered and bizzare structure (D).

Neovascular Glaucoma Presented by OCTA (Figs. 23.29 to 23.33)

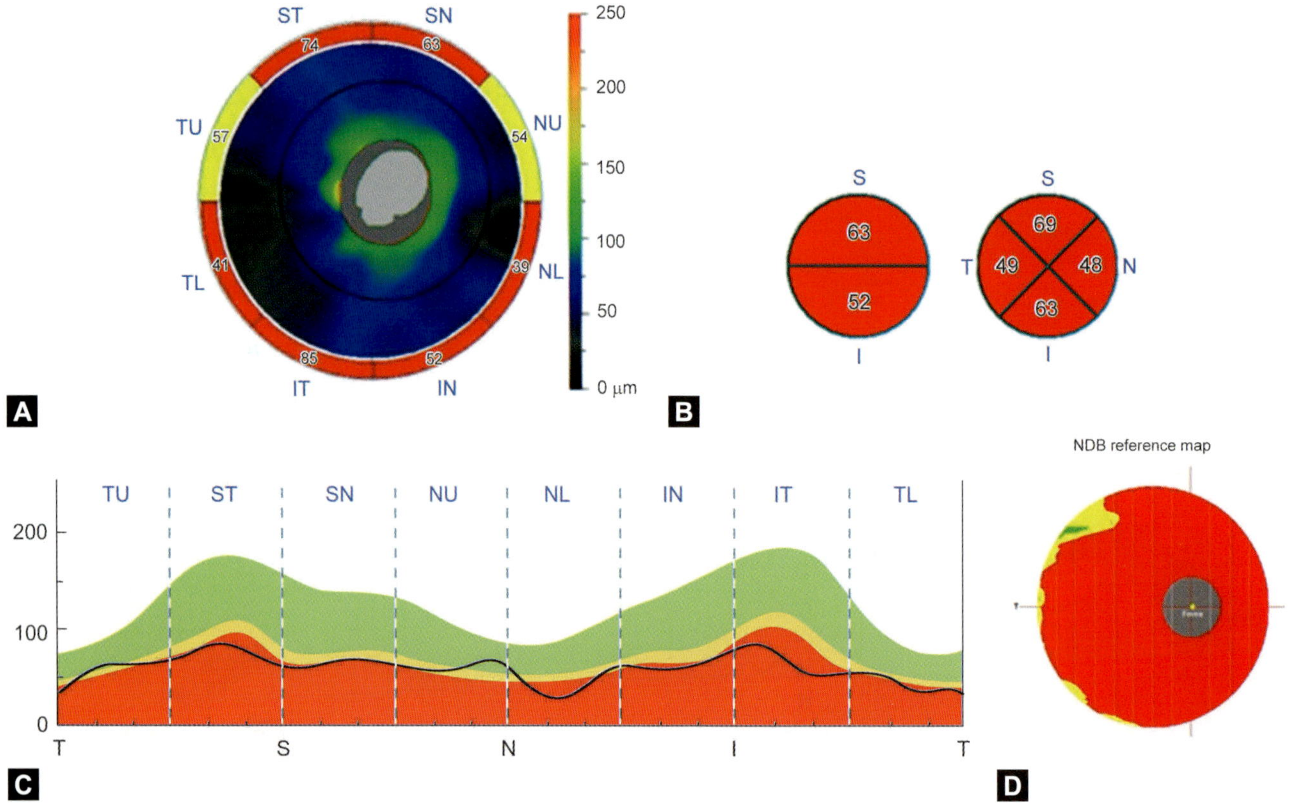

Figs. 23.29A to D: (A to C) The retinal nerve fiber layer (RNFL) thickness maps clearly show RNFL atrophy in all quadrants and circumference segments of the papilla in a patient with neovascular glaucoma. The thickness values are also reduced in the graphical display where the black RNFL line follows the red "atrophy" zone. (D) The ganglia cell complex (GCC) map is completely colored in red, which is a pathognomonic sign of ganglion cell atrophy.

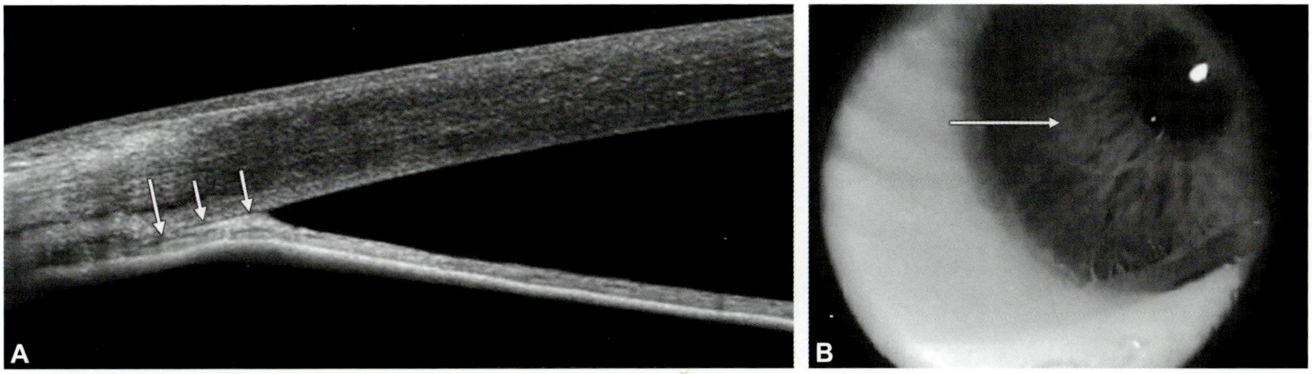

Figs. 23.30A and B: (A) A chamber angle measured with an anterior segment optical coherence tomography (AS-OCT). The fully closed chamber angle is marked with the arrows (*Plateau iris*). (B) The arrow shows the exact spot where the chamber angle is captured.

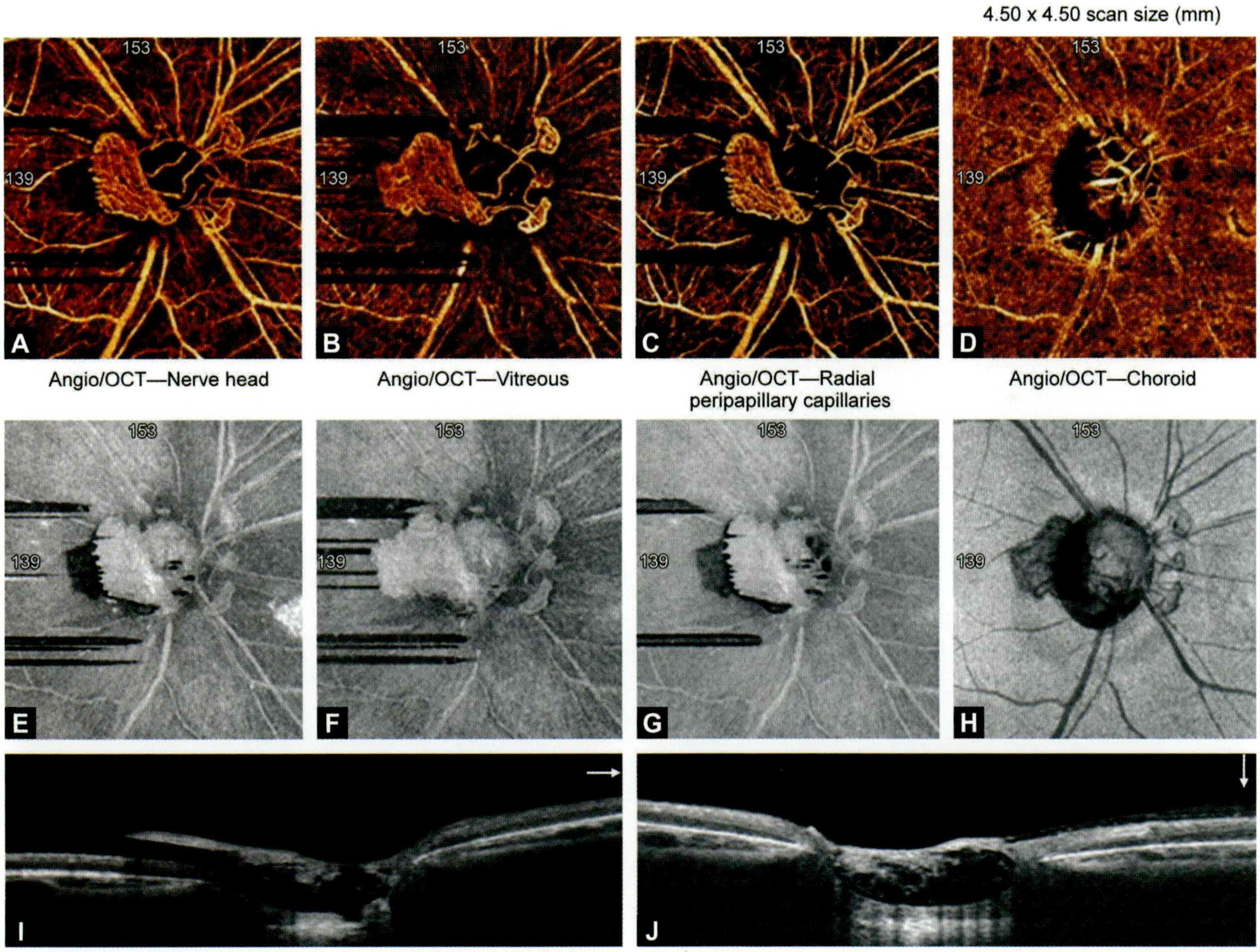

Figs. 23.31A to J: (A to D) The optical coherence tomography angiography (OCTA) of the papillary and peripapillary area (4.5 × 4.5 mm) of the same eye as seen in the previous figures. In all layers, except in the choroid, a clearly bounded ellipsoidal neovascular formation is seen. The horizontal black lines, seen on the angiography images, are artifacts. (E to H) The en face OCT of the corresponding layers (4.5 × 4.5 mm). In all layers, a big white fibrous membrane, which camouflages the edges of papilla, is seen. On the opposite side of the papilla, three smaller and similar membranes are visualized. (I and J) The corresponding OCT B-scans show a "filled" papilla with the hyperreflective neovascular tissue crossing the excavation and making a "bridge-like" formation.

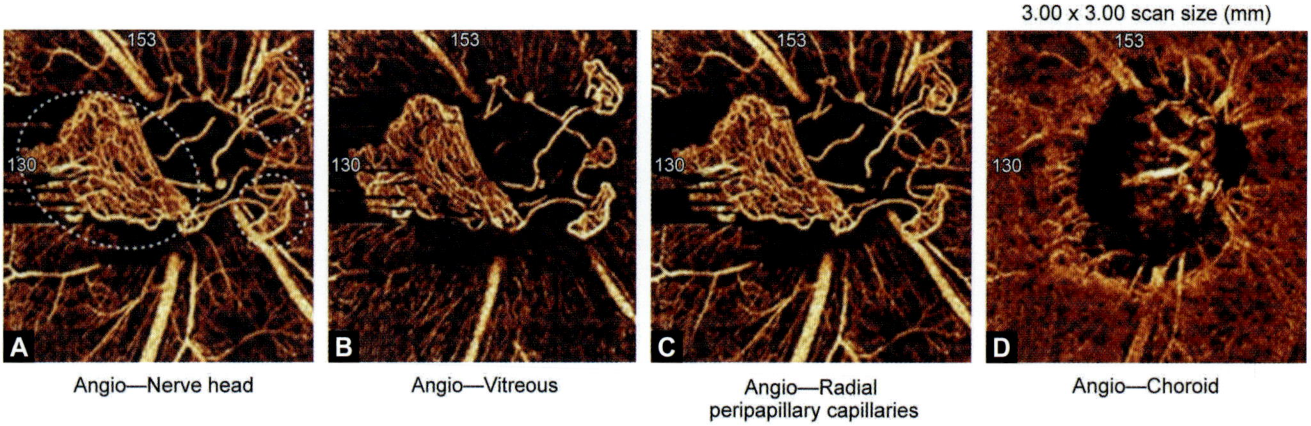

Figs. 23.32A to D: The optical coherence tomography angiography (OCTA) (3 x 3 mm). The neovascularization is accurately shown in the optic nerve head (A). In the vitreous layer we see a large neovascularization (B). In the radial peripapillary capillary layer we see the details of neovascular membrane (C). The neovascularization originates from the choroid (D). Blood vessels are more detailed in higher magnification.

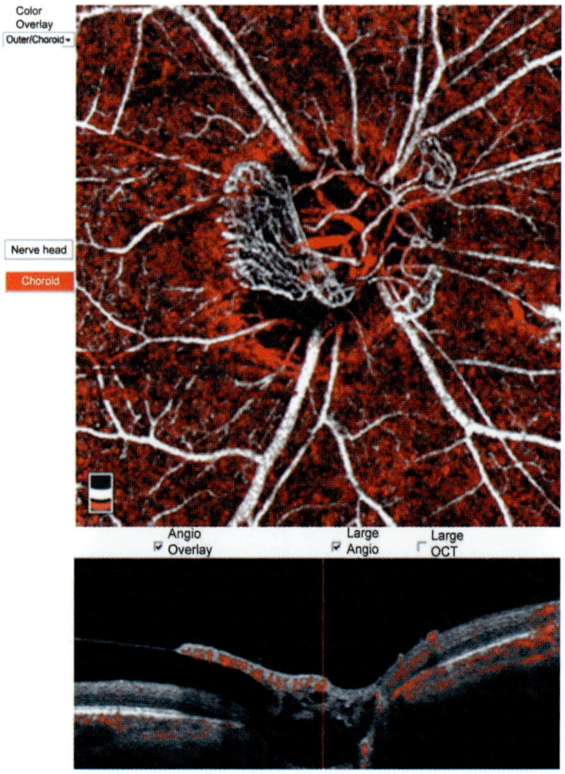

Fig. 23.33: The optical coherence tomography angiography (OCTA) AngioAnalysis of the neovascular membrane. The choroidal neovascularization (CNV) that ascends from the papilla into the vitreous is very clearly visualized. It is obvious that the blood circulation in the flat membrane crossing over the papilla excavation exists (seen on the corresponding B-scan).

BIBLIOGRAPHY

1. Akil H, Huang AS, Francis BA, et al. Retinal vessel density from optical coherence tomography angiography to differentiate early glaucoma, Pre-perimetric glaucoma and normal eyes. PLoS One. 2017;12(2):e0170476.
2. Baumann B, Potsaid B, Kraus MF, et al. Total retinal blood flow measurement with ultrahigh speed swept source/fourier domain OCT. Biomed Opt Express. 2011;2(6):1539-52.
3. Bojikian KD, Chen CL, Wen JC, et al. Optic disc perfusion in primary open angle and normal tension glaucoma eyes using optical coherence tomography-based microangiography. PLoS One. 2016;11(5):e0154691.
4. de Carlo TE, Romano A, Waheed NK, et al. A review of optical coherence tomography angiography (OCTA). Int J Retina Vitreous. 2015;1:5.
5. Holló G. Vessel density calculated from OCT angiography in 3 peripapillary sectors in normal, ocular hypertensive and glaucoma eyes. Eur J Ophthalmol. 2016;26(3):e42-5.
6. Huang D, Chopra V, Lu AT, et al. Does optic nerve head size variation affect circumpapillary retinal nerve fiber layer thickness measurement by optical coherence tomography? Invest Ophthalmol Vis Sci. 2012;53(8):4990-7.
7. Huang D, Puech M, Jia Y, et al. OCT Chapter 28: Angiography and glaucoma, Clinical OCT-angiography Atlas. In: Bruno Lumbroso (Ed). Practical Handbook of OCT Angiography. New Delhi: Jaypee Brothers Medical Publisher (P) Ltd; 2014.
8. Hwang JC, Konduru R, Zhang X, et al. Relationship among visual field, blood flow, and neural structure measurements in glaucoma. Invest Ophthalmol Vis Sci. 2012;53:3020-6.

9. Jia Y, Morrison JC, Tokayer J, et al. Quantitative OCT angiography of optic nerve head blood flow. Biomed Opt Express. 2012;3(12):3127-37.
10. Jia Y, Tan O, Tokayer J, et al. Split-spectrum amplitude-decorrelation angiography with optical coherence tomography. Opt Express. 2012;20(4):4710-25.
11. Jia Y, Wei E, Wang X, et al. Optical coherence tomography angiography of optic disc perfusion in glaucoma. Ophthalmology. 2014;121(7):1322-32.
12. Kumar RS, Anegondi N, Chandapura RS, et al. Discriminant function of optical coherence tomography angiography to determine disease severity in glaucoma. Invest Ophthalmol Vis Sci. 2016;57(14):6079-88.
13. Lee EJ, Lee KM, Lee SH, et al. OCT angiography of the peripapillary retina in primary open-angle glaucoma. Invest Ophthalmol Vis Sci. 2016;57(14):6265-70.
14. Liu L, Jia Y, Takusagawa HL, et al. Optical coherence tomography angiography of the peripapillary retina in glaucoma. JAMA Ophthalmol. 2015;133(9):1045-52.
15. Lumbroso B, Huang D, Jia Y, et al. Optical coherence tomography angiography: New clinical terminology. In: Lumbroso B, Huang D, Jia Y, Fujimoto JG, Rispoli M (Eds). Clinical Guide to Angio-OCT, 1st edition. New Delhi: Jaypee Brothers Medical Publisher (P) Ltd; 2014. pp. 5-7.
16. Mo S, Phillips E, Krawitz BD, et al. Visualization of radial peripapillary capillaries using optical coherence tomography angiography: The effect of image averaging. PLoS One. 2017;12(1):e0169385.
17. Peachauer AD, Jia Y, Liu L, et al. Optical coherence tomography angiography of peripapillary retinal blood flow response to hyperoxia. Invest Ophthalmol Vis Sci. 2015;56(5):3287-91.
18. Sehi M, Goharian I, Konduru R, et al. Retinal blood flow in glaucomatous eyes with single-hemifield damage. Ophthalmology. 2014;121(3):750-8.
19. Suh MH, Zangwill LM, Manalastas PI, et al. Optical coherence tomography angiography vessel density in glaucomatous eyes with focal lamina cribrosa defects. Ophthalmology. 2016;123(11):2309-17.
20. Tokayer J, Jia Y, Dhalla AH, et al. Blood flow velocity quantification using split-spectrum amplitude-decorrelation angiography with optical coherence tomography. Biomed Opt Express. 2013;4(10):1909-24.
21. Wang X, Jiang C, Ko T, et al. Correlation between optic disc perfusion and glaucomatous severity in patients with open-angle glaucoma: An optical coherence tomography angiography study. Graefes Arch Clin Exp Ophthalmol. 2015;253(9):1557-64.
22. Wang X, Jia Y, Spain R, et al. Optical tomography of optic nerve head and parafovea in multiple sclerosis. Br J Ophthalmol. 2014;98(10):1368-73.

CHAPTER 24

Optic Neuritis and Papilledema

INTRODUCTION

Optic neuritis (ON) is an acute, inflammatory demyelinating disorder of the optic nerve that occurs most often in young adults.

Papilledema is swelling of the optic nerve due to increased intracranial pressure (ICP).

EPIDEMIOLOGY AND ETIOLOGY

Optic neuritis is the most common cause of optic neuropathy in the population of younger people, especially female. It can be an idiopathic, inflammatory, or autoimmune disease isolated to the optic nerve or can be associated with a more widespread demyelinating disorder of the central nervous system (CNS) such as multiple sclerosis (MS) or neuromyelitis optica.

Papilledema refers to swelling of the optic disk from increased ICP. It must be distinguished from optic disk swelling with different origins, which is simply termed as *optic disk edema*. Since the root cause of papilledema is increased ICP this is an alarming sign which may precede conditions such as brain tumors, CNS inflammation, or idiopathic intracranial hypertension (IIH). It is assumed that there is reduced axoplasmic transport through the retinal nerve fiber layer (RNFL), due to the chemical and structural causes, which lead to the leaking of fluid, proteins, and other cellular components into the extracellular space of the optic disk. Papilledema is usually bilateral and may occur within hours or weeks. The unilateral appearance of papilledema is rare.

SYMPTOMS AND SIGNS

The most common symptoms of ON are sudden vision loss, dyschromatopsia, and defects in the visual field. The typical clinical profile consists of sudden loss of vision, which can vary in severity from a slight deficit in the field of vision to complete loss of light perception, followed by spontaneous improvement over several months. Most patients have lasting symptoms of visual impairment, and even when visual acuity returns to normal, abnormalities are common in other aspects of visual function, such as the visual field, color vision, and contrast sensitivity. Early papilledema may be asymptomatic, but it can also be presented as a simple headache, which is followed with vomiting and/or nausea. Loss of color vision, central visual acuity, and peripheral visual field, especially inferonasally, also occur. Optic disk swelling is observed by the fundus examination. A detailed fundus examination shows bilaterally swollen hyperemic disks with blurry edges, dilated, tortuosus retinal veins, papillary or peripapillary retinal hemorrhages (usually flame shaped), and loss of venous pulsations. In early papilledema disk swelling may be asymmetric. As chronic papilledema progresses to the optic atrophy, the hemorrhages and cotton-wool spots

Table 24.1: Differential diagnosis of optic neuritis and papilledema.

Optic neuritis	*Papilledema*
▪ Optic neuromyelitis ▪ Hereditary or nutritional optic neuropathy ▪ Wegener's granulomatosis ▪ Branch retinal artery occlusion ▪ Central retinal artery occlusion ▪ Necrotizing herpetic retinopathy in immune compromised individuals and patients coinfected with Herpes simplex.	▪ Intraocular inflammation with optic disk swelling ▪ Central retinal vein occlusion ▪ Optic neuritis ▪ Diabetic papillopathy ▪ Hypertension papilledema ▪ Nonarteritic ischemic optic neuropathy (NAION) ▪ Infiltrative optic neuropathy and tumors (lymphoma, leukemia) ▪ Scleritis.

resolve, peripapillary gliosis and narrowing of the peripapillary retinal vessels occur, and optociliary shunt vessels may develop on the disk.

DIFFERENTIAL DIAGNOSIS

The differential diagnosis of optic neuritis and papilledema is given in Table 24.1.

DIAGNOSTICS

During the clinical examination and visualization of the optic disk in patients with ON, there are often no abnormalities of the optic disk (retrobulbar neuritis), while in some patients disk swelling may be detected (papillitis anterior or enlarged ON). Most commonly is only one eye affected and therefore patients are often unaware of the decreasement in vision. Optical coherence tomography (OCT) is an imaging tool for diagnosing and long-term monitoring of ON. OCT B-scan, in patients with acute ON, shows edema and swelling of the optic disk. Analysis of the optic disk and thickness of the RNFL reflects changes due to optic disk swelling, as well as progressive changes associated with long-term loss of axons and optic disk atrophy. OCT angiograms confirm the diagnosis and depict a clear picture of the papillary swelling, where the blood vessels cross over the blurred disk margins, giving the impression of overflow. The loss of optic disk excavation is shown, the optic papilla is extremely large (over 6 mm^2), and its normal configuration is lost.

Considering papilledema, fundoscopy is the first step in diagnostics, where one or more signs of the optic disk swelling can be found. The OCT can show an increased thickness of the entire retina, along with the thickening of the RNFL. An increase in retinal thickness is much more significant than the thickness of RNFL in the initial, early stages of papilledema, as well as in cases of severe papilledema. In the early stages, increasement of RNFL thickness may be absent, while in the late severe stages, software disruptions occur where the values of RNFL cannot be certain. OCT is the most useful in the detection and monitoring (follow-up) the moderately developed papilledema. Some studies have shown that the increasement of parapapillary RNFL is associated with an increased ICP in newly diagnosed patients with papilledema. In severe long-lasting papilledema, spectral domain optical coherence tomography (SD-OCT) has a limiting value in the prediction of increased intraocular pressure. A visual field, as a functional test, can be normal or show different sizes and shapes of scotomas, especially in peripheral parts. An optical coherence tomography angiography (OCTA) shows the phenomenon of "overflow", where blood vessels inside the optic disk seem to be falling over the optic disk margin. The central excavation is lost and the parapapillary nerve layer thickness is extremely high (over 200 μm). The patient is recommended to undergo one of the medical imaging techniques for the CNS evaluation [magnetic resonance imaging (MRI) or computed tomography (CT)].

An eye with acute papillitis shown by the OCTA is described in Figures 24.1 and 24.2.

Images of the same eye, 2 months after a steroid therapy is described in Figures 24.3 and 24.4.

An eye with papilledema shown by the OCTA is described in Figures 24.5 to 24.9.

The papilledema after plaque radiation therapy of the choroidal melanoma is described in Figures 24.10 to 24.13.

THERAPY

Optic neuritis is most commonly treated with steroid therapy, with the aim to decrease the optic disk inflammation.

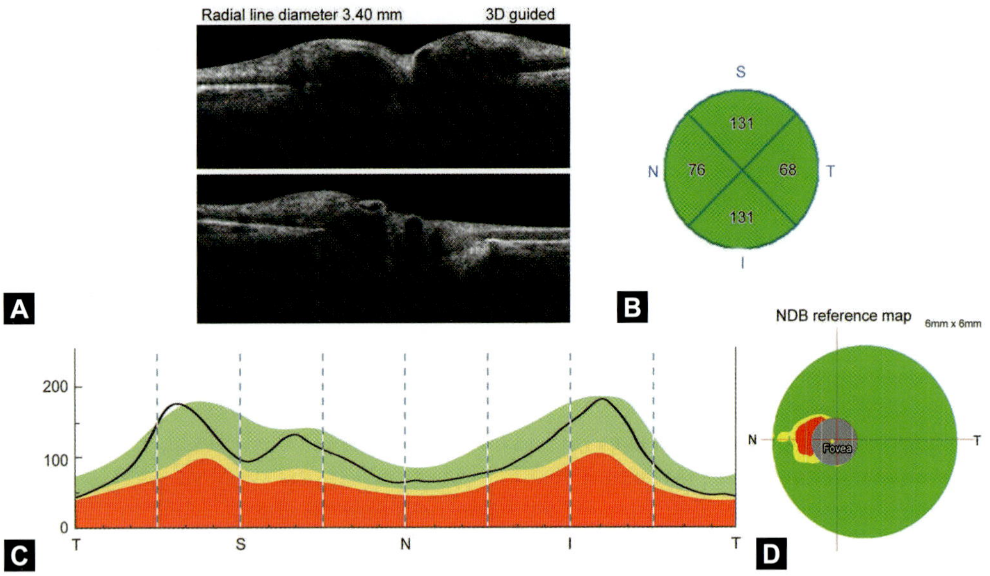

Figs. 24.1A to D: (A) An OCT B-scan in a patient with acute papillitis. The loss of the central excavation is visible, as are the extremely elevated disk margins with the loss of large blood vessels cross-sections; (B) Figure shows an overview of the RNFL thickness by a map divided into quadrants. RNFL thickening can be numerically observed in the superior and inferior part parapapillary, along with regular values of the nerve fiber thickness nasally and temporally; (C) Graphically shows the RNFL thickness which is within the physiological range. However, increasement of RNFL can be noted in the same parts as in Figure B; and (D) Figure shows a map of the ganglion cell complex thickness. The nasal part shows a red area with a yellow surrounding zone indicating thinning of that region, due to the extracellular fluid pressure on the ganglion layer. (RNFL: Retinal nerve fiber layer; OCT: Optical coherence tomography)

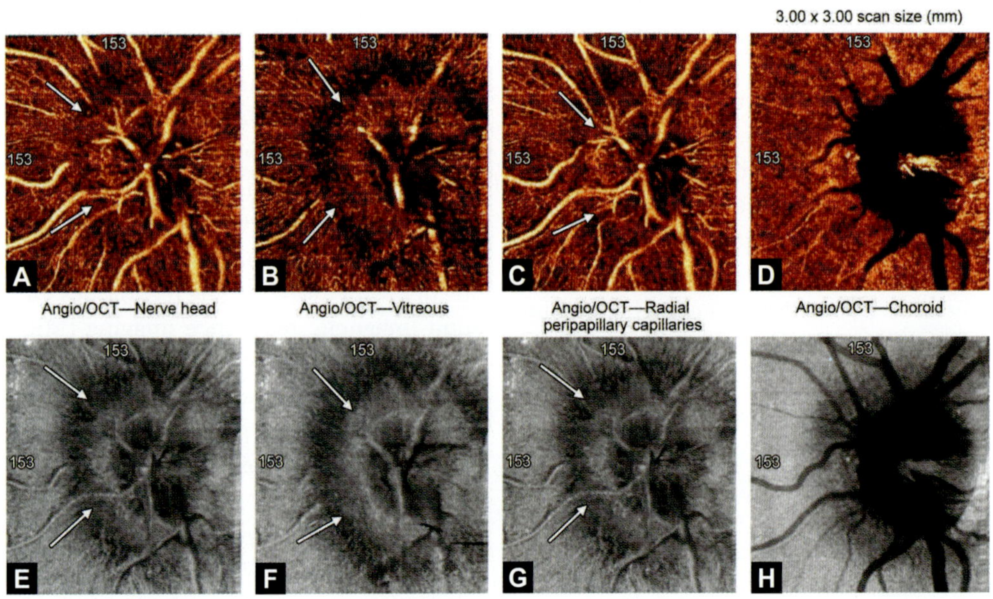

Figs. 24.2A to H: An OCTA SSADA protocol (3 × 3 mm) and en face OCT images of the corresponding layers; the same eye as depicted in previous figures. (A to D) Figures show blood vessels and capillaries of the swollen optic disk. Arrows mark the zone with the phenomenon of "vessels overflow", where blood vessels inside the optic disk seem to be falling over the optic disk margins. Vessels seem to be disrupted and they cannot be followed all along their length, due to the extremely fast blood flow in some parts, which cannot be detected by a software; and (E to H) Figures show en face OCT images with a hyporeflective margin of the unclear and enlarged optic papilla. Large blood vessels are interrupted and have segmented flow. (OCTA: Optical coherence tomography angiography; SSADA: Split-spectrum amplitude-decorrelation angiography)

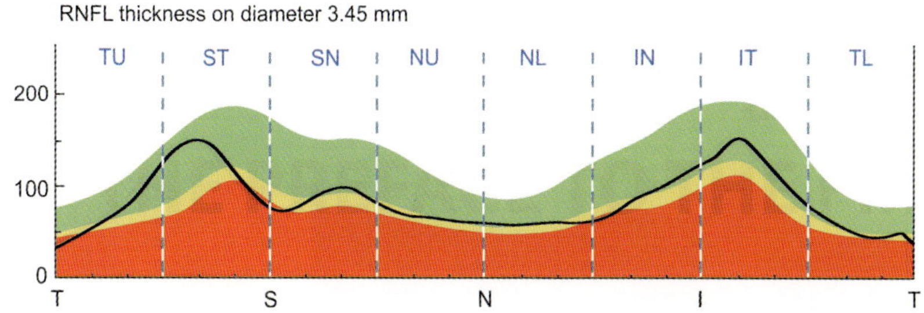

Fig. 24.3: Map which graphically represents the retinal nerve fiber layer (RNFL) thickness shows significantly decreased RNFL values in all segments parapapillary.

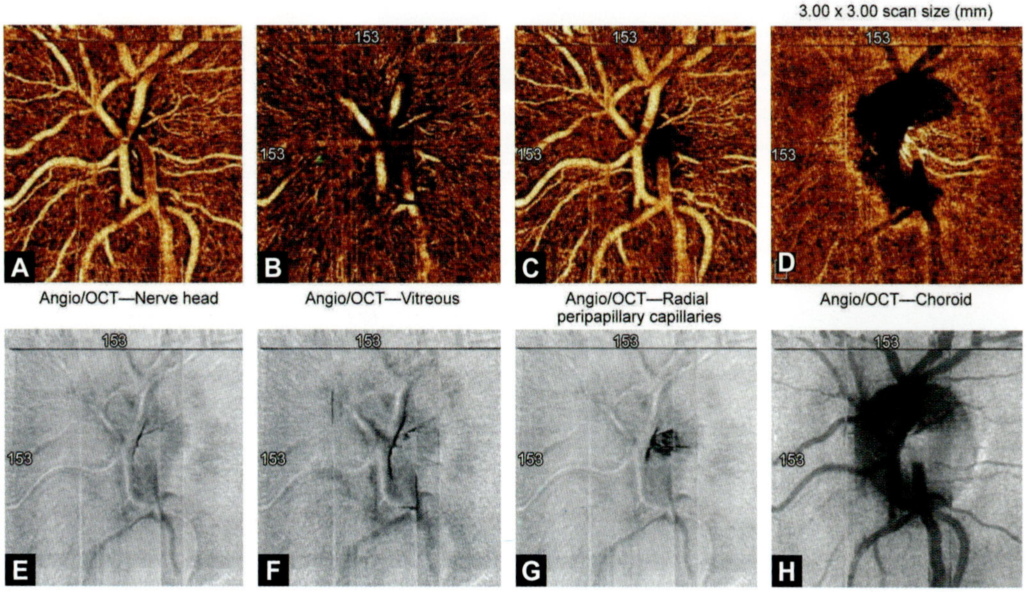

Figs. 24.4A to H: The OCTA SSADA protocol (3 × 3 mm) and en face OCT images of corresponding layers of the optic disk and parapapillary region. (A to D) Figures show a regular vascularization in all layers down to the choroid, with a symmetrical, dense capillaries parapapillary. The phenomenon of "overflow" cannot be seen; and (E to H) Figures show en face OCT images with a clearly visible papilla and its margin, large blood vessels, and a flow that is seen all along the vessels. (OCTA: Optical coherence tomography angiography; SSADA: Split-spectrum amplitude-decorrelation angiography)

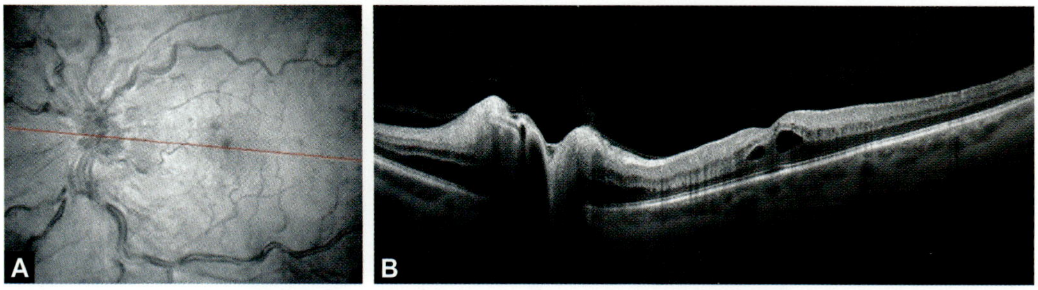

Figs. 24.5A and B: (A) Fundus photography of the left eye in a 40-year-old male patient. The photograph shows blurry, unclear margins of the optic disk, dilated, tortuous, "sausage-like" retinal veins, and segmented flow. Retinal arteries are rigid, almost invisible. The flame-shaped retinal hemorrhages are seen all along retinal vessels; and (B) Figure is an optical coherence tomography (OCT) B-scan, which shows a sagittal cross-section of the optic disk and macula. The optic disk is swollen, it shows elevated disk margins, and faded central excavation. Peripapillary, serous retinal detachment, which almost reaches the macula, can be seen. Also, a macular area shows pathological changes. On the scan, two cysts of intraretinal fluid can be seen.

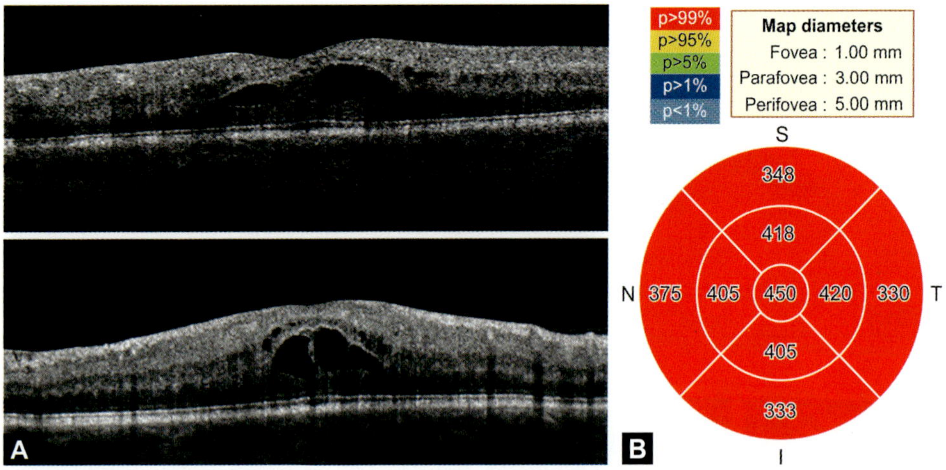

Figs. 24.6A and B: (A) An OCT B-scan of the macula in larger magnification, which more clearly shows cystoid macular edema and many intraretinal cysts. RPE and the Bruch's membrane are preserved; and (B) Figure presents the retinal thickness map, which is completely colored in red, indicating macular thickening (macular edema). (RPE: Retinal pigment epithelium; OCT: Optical coherence tomography)

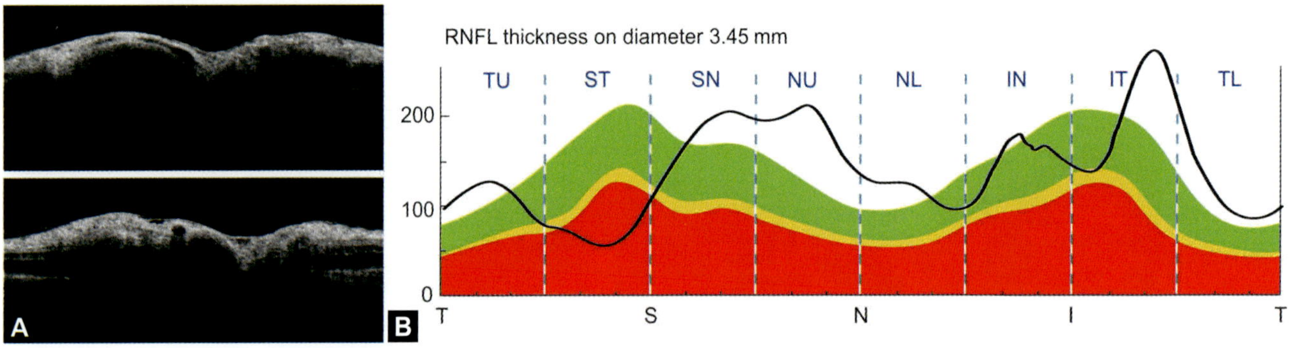

Figs. 24.7A and B: (A) An OCT B-scan of the optic disk shows papillary edema and elevated disk margins. Central disk excavation is completely lost; and (B) Figure shows a RNFL thickness graph, with irregular and increased RNFL thickness values in all segments. (RNFL: Retinal nerve fiber layer; OCT: Optical coherence tomography)

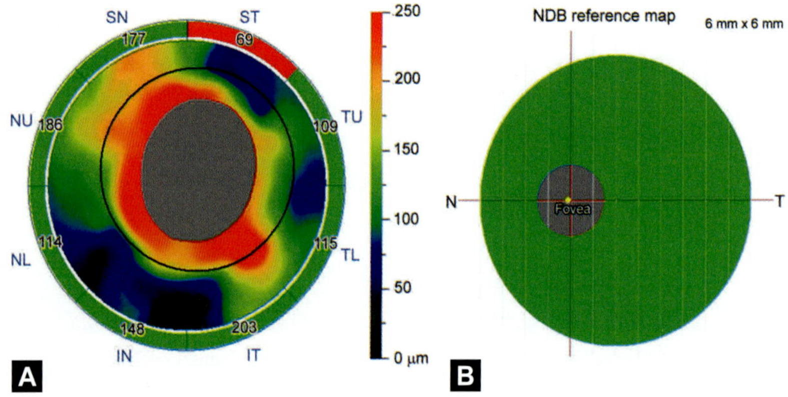

Figs. 24.8A and B: (A) Another presentation of retinal nerve fiber layer (RNFL) thickness, but by a map dividing the papillary circumference into segments. RNFL thickness is increased in almost all segments of the papillary circumference. The thickness ranges from 114 µm to 203 µm, except in the superior-temporal segment (69 µm); and (B) Figure shows a GCC layer thickness map which is completely colored in green, indicating that it is in physiological range.

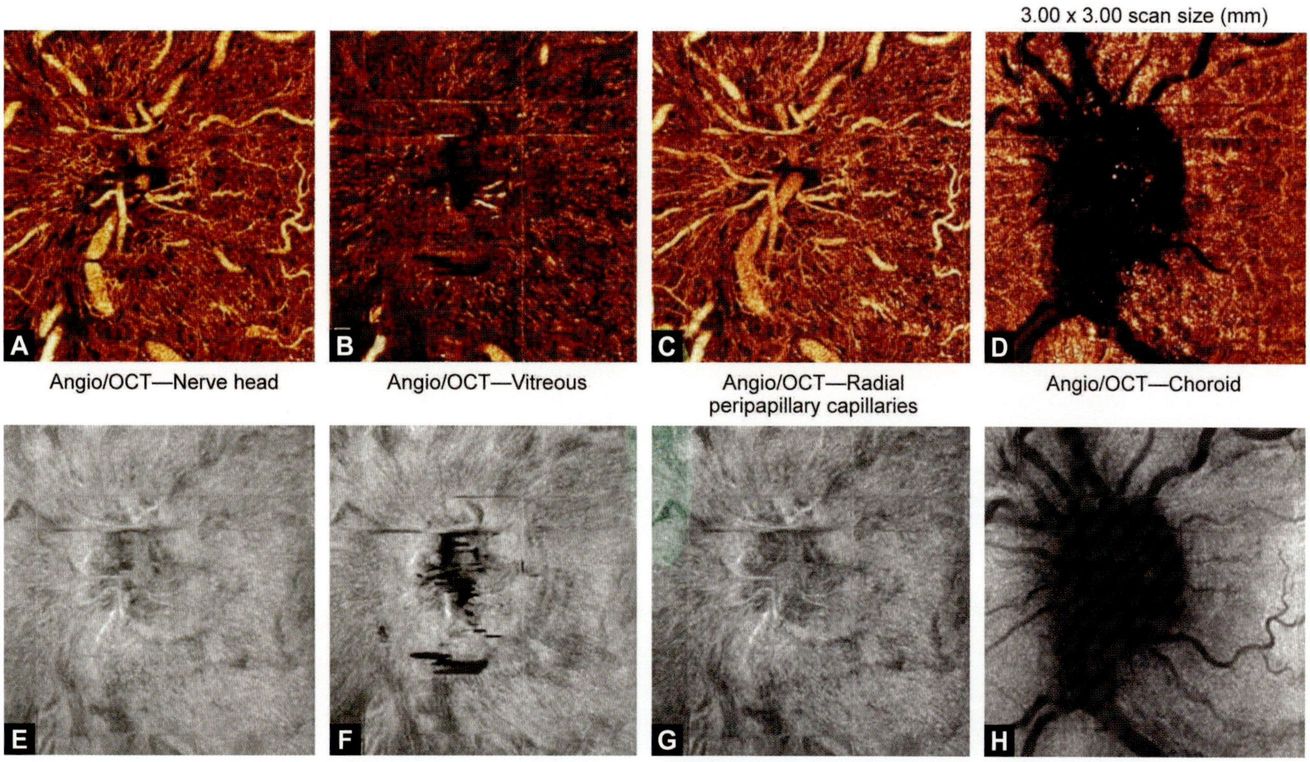

Figs. 24.9A to H: An OCTA SSADA protocol (4.5 × 4.5 mm) and en face OCT images of corresponding layers of the optic disk and parapapillary region. (A to D) Figures show the changes in peripapillary vascularization as well as in the vascularization of the optic disk. A regular meshwork is interrupted, capillaries and larger blood vessels are tortuous and irregular, all the way from ILM to the choroid layer. Also, they show a segmented flow, since it is extremely fast and software cannot detect it; and (E to H) Figures show en face OCT scans with an optic disk, its blurry and faded margins, and large blood vessels that are almost invisible. (ILM: Internal limiting membrane; OCTA: Optical coherence tomography angiography; SSADA: Split-spectrum amplitude-decorrelation angiography)

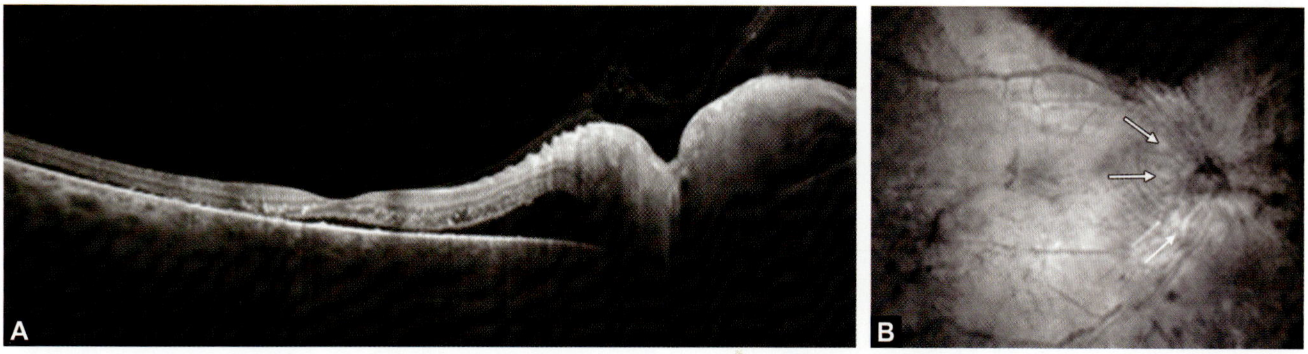

Figs. 24.10A and B: (A) An OCT B-scan of the optic disk and macula of the right eye, in a 42-year-old patient. Sagittal cross-section shows an extremely large optic disk with elevated disk margins and a significantly changed central excavation, along with the peripapillary serous retinal detachment. RPE and the Bruch's membrane are preserved. Shallow detachment of sensory retina extends from the optic disk to macula; and (B) Figure shows a fundus photography, where the optic disk is presented with blurry, faded edges, and circular wrinkles of the ILM. In the upper part of the fundus photograph, a large dark hyporeflective region is seen. This region was exposed to the radiotherapy. (ILM: Internal limiting membrane; OCT: Optical coherence tomography; RPE: Retinal pigment epithelium)

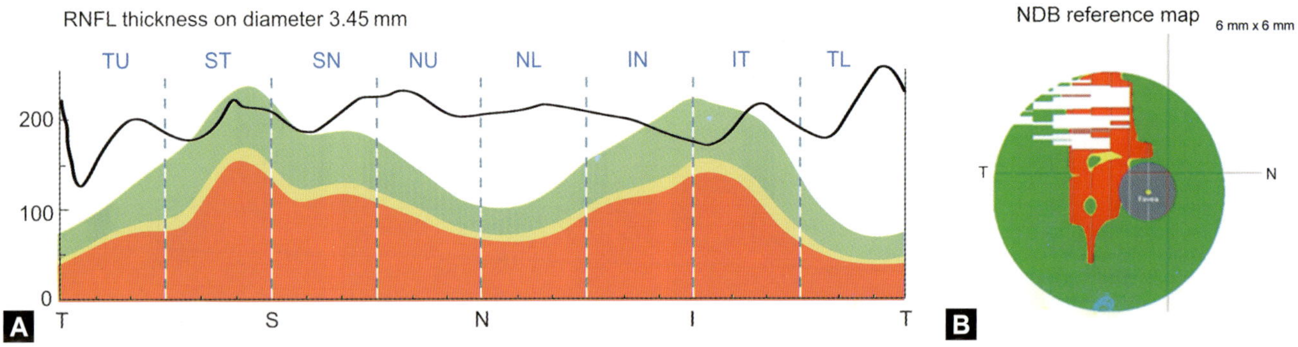

Figs. 24.11A and B: (A) The retinal nerve fiber layer (RNFL) thickness graph shows an increased RNFL values in all segments; and (B) figure with a GCC map and ganglion layer thickness shows signs of the ganglion cell atrophy.

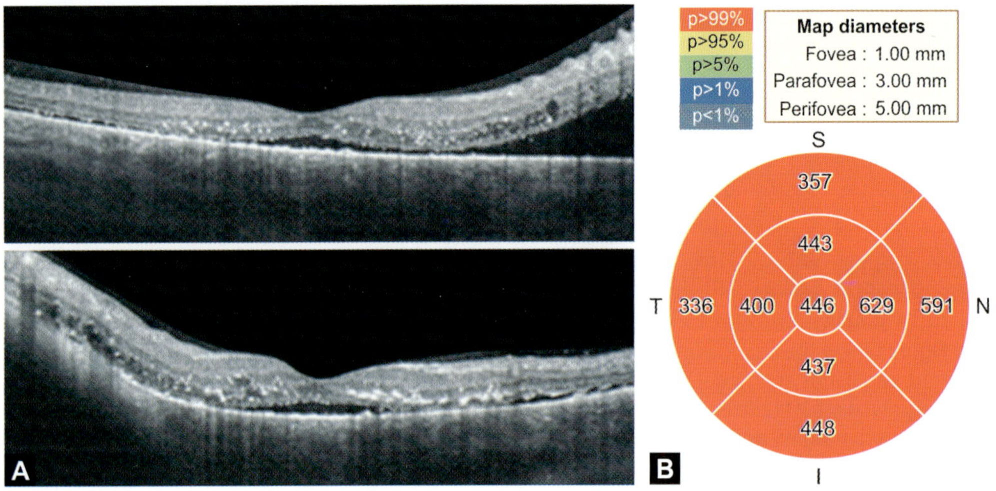

Figs. 24.12A and B: (A) An OCT B-scan of the macular area shows a shallow detachment of retinal layers, which extends and completely elevates toward the optic papilla. RPE is preserved, but appears granular and irregular; and (B) Figure shows the retinal thickness map with increased values of all macular segments, due to the subretinal detachment. (OCT: optical coherence tomography; RPE: Retinal pigment epithelium)

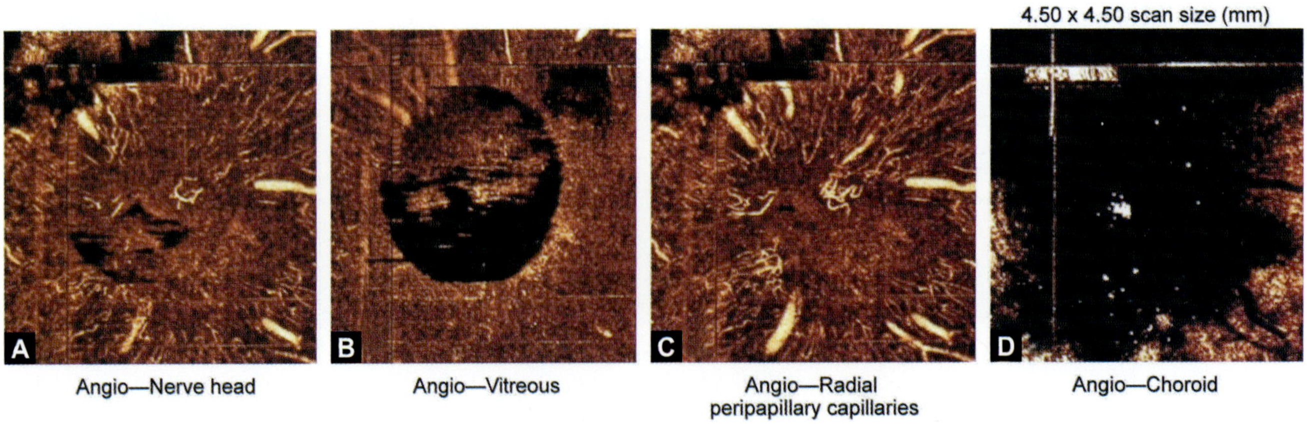

Figs. 24.13A to D: An optical coherence tomography angiography (OCTA) of the optic papilla and peripapillary area (4.5 × 4.5 mm). Edges of the optic disk are unclear and faded, and no flow can be seen, although the extremely high velocity of the flow inside the optic papilla and around it is present, but the software cannot detect such a fast flow. The flow of large blood vessels seems to be interrupted.

Most commonly, steroids are given intravenously, and this way of application accelerates vision recovery (pulse therapy). The recovery of visual acuity depends on the primary cause. Most patients regain almost normal visual acuity within 12 months after the ON episode.

The treatment of papilledema depends on the primary cause. Since papillary edema occurs due to the increased ICP, it may be an indicative sign of a cranial tumor or other intracranial process, such as CNS inflammation. If confirmed to be a tumor, the treatment is based on an operation and/or radiation, with the aim to eradicate or reduce the tumor. In order to reduce ICP, medications that increase the absorption of cerebrospinal fluid or those that reduce its production can be given. Some of these drugs are diuretics such as acetazolamide and furosemide. If inflammation contributes to the ICP elevation, steroids may be prescribed for reducing the inflammation and preventing vision loss. Other types of treatment include repetitive lumbar puncture to remove excess fluid that increases ICP.

BIBLIOGRAPHY

1. Fleischman D, Perry JT, Rand Allingham R, et al. Retrospective analysis of translaminar, demographic, and physiologic parameters in relation to papilledema severity. Can J Ophthalmol. 2017;52(1):26-9.
2. Higashiyama T, Nishida Y, Ohji M. Optical coherence tomography angiography in eyes with good visual acuity recovery after treatment for optic neuritis. PLoS One. 2017; 12(2):e0172168.
3. Kardon R. Optical coherence tomography in papilledema: what am I missing? J Neuroophthalmol. 2014;34 Suppl:S10-7.
4. Kling F, Cochener B, Colin J. Bilateral papilledema in young women: Two case reports of benign intracranial hypertension? J Fr Ophthalmol. 2002;25(8):835-9.
5. Lamirel C, Newman NJ, Biousse V. Optical coherence tomography (OCT) in optic neuritis and multiple sclerosis. Rev Neurol. 2010;166(12):978-86.
6. Petzold A. Neuroprotection and visual function after optic neuritis. Curr Opin Neurol. 2017;30(1):67-73.
7. Rebolleda G, Diez-Alvarez L, Casado A, et al. OCT: new perspectives in neuroophthalmology. Saudi J Ophthalmol. 2015;29(1):9-25.
8. Rebolleda G, Muñoz-Negrete FJ. The role of OCT in the differential diagnosis between buried optic nerve drusen and papilloedema. Arch Soc Esp Oftalmol. 2016;91(9):431-8.
9. Steffen H. Optic nerve neuritis: From an ophthalmological perspective. Nervenarzt. 2013;84(12):1525-34.
10. Toosy AT, DF Mason DF, Miller DH. Optic neuritis. Lancet Neurol. 2014;13(1):83-99.
11. Wang X, Jia Y, Spain R, et al. Optical coherence tomography angiography of optic nerve head and parafovea in multiple sclerosis. Br J Ophthalmol. 2014;98(10):1368-73.
12. Zhang J, Foroozan R. Optic disc edema from papilledema. Int Ophthalmol Clin. 2014;54(1):13-26.

Index

Page numbers followed by *f* refer to figure.

D

E

F

G

H

O

P

R

S

T

V

W

X

Z